The Impact of Religiosity on Fertility

Sandra Hubert

The Impact of Religiosity on Fertility

A Comparative Analysis of France, Hungary, Norway, and Germany

Springer VS

Sandra Hubert
Bochum, Germany

Dissertation at Ruhr-University Bochum, 2014

ISBN 978-3-658-07007-6 ISBN 978-3-658-07008-3 (eBook)
DOI 10.1007/978-3-658-07008-3

The Deutsche Nationalbibliothek lists this publication in the Deutsche Nationalbibliografie; detailed bibliographic data are available in the Internet at http://dnb.d-nb.de.

Library of Congress Control Number: 2014948496

Springer VS

Printed on acid-free paper

Springer VS is a brand of Springer DE.
Springer DE is part of Springer Science+Business Media.
www.springer-vs.de

Danksagung

Mein erstes Dankeschön richte ich an meinen Doktorvater und Erstgutachter Prof. Dr. Jörg Althammer, denn er hat meine Arbeit betreut und fachlich beraten. Herrn Prof. Dr. Klaus Peter Strohmeier spreche ich meinen Dank für die Übernahme des zweiten Gutachtens aus.

Das Zentralinstitut für Ehe und Familie in der Familie (ZFG) an der Katholischen Universität Eichstätt-Ingolstadt hat mich finanziell unterstützt. Vielen Dank!

Im Deutschen Jugendinstitut e.V. München blieb neben den eigentlichen Aufgaben oft Zeit übrig, um die Dissertation nicht vollständig auf die Freizeit verlegen zu müssen. Das hat vor allem Dr. Christian Alt ermöglicht. Herzlichen Dank Christian! Dr. Ulrich Pötter danke ich für den statistischen Support. Dank dir, Uli! Ich möchte auch allen weiteren Kolleginnen und Kollegen am Deutschen Jugendinstitut danken, die mich unterstützt haben.

Maximilian Sommer war immer für mich da, hat zugehört, ermutigt, auch mal angetrieben und kritisiert sowie R- und LaTeXProbleme gelöst. Liebsten Dank Max!

Meine Familie hat mir Kraft gegeben, mir einen Rückzugsort geboten, jederzeit an mich geglaubt und sich um mich gekümmert, wenn ich mal erschöpft war. Danke, dass es Euch gibt!

Danken möchte ich auch meinen früheren Lehrern in Beverstedt, Frau Pfeiffer und Herrn Knerr, der im letzten Jahr viel zu früh verstarb. Sie waren hervorragende Pädagogen, wie man sie sich als Schülerin nur wünschen konnte und haben vier Jahre lang den Weg in die Zukunft geebnet.

Contents

List of Figures

List of Tables

1 Introduction

1.1 Subject focus and the principle research questions

Academic interest in religion has re-escalated during recent years. The topic has again taken a front seat on the European agenda. On the one hand this is associated with immigration processes creating multi-religious societies. Immigrants are not longer willing to hide their religiosity and request their own places of prayer where they can express their religiosity. On the other hand, it is due to events and conflicts for which religion is held responsible. A third explanation are religious minorities whose higher fertility and – from a secular perspective – partly deviant behavior make them highly visible.

For some decades research on religion and religiosity almost ceased, which was also due to the "belief" in the victory of secularization over religion and religiosity. This premature conclusion had to be revised, also with respect to demographic behavior. Religiosity is a major cultural trait that shapes values. In the past however, fertility research in Europe generally focused on economic factors. Much less attention was paid to values-based variables. It seems worthwhile to neither neglect the first nor the latter but to combine economic and cultural factors to explain fertility. Furthermore, surrounding events, developments, and factors have to be taken into account.

This dissertation investigates the impact of religiosity of both women and men on completed fertility in comparative perspective. It is assumed that religious individuals do not only desire more children and have more positive attitudes towards family and children, but also that they realize a higher fertility. Furthermore, it is supposed that the effect can be demonstrated independently of the institutional context and policy-making, social norms, state-church-relations, and the national degree of religious vitality which is associated with the denominational cultural tradition. These factors, that vary across countries, build the frame for fertility decisions but also react to changes in individual behavior. Furthermore, a variety of individual characteristics and resources are associated with fertility decisions and fertility behavior. The most important traits are labor supply and educational achievement as well as their related domains.

Fertility and religiosity levels not only vary across individuals within a country but also between countries. The national degree of religiosity sheds light on the size of the religiosity effect on aggregated fertility, which makes cross-country analyses promising. Second, while the common focus is mostly on women's fertility, it could be more interesting to compare demographic behavior of women and men by religiosity. Do they differ and if so, how? A third point is the time perspective. Has the influence of religiosity changed over the course of time? A fourth and final issue is to distinguish the micro (individual) and macro (national) level. Secularization can also be differentiated at these levels and so should the effect of religious institutions and religiosity on demographic behavior. Until now, there has been no detailed study with such a multi-dimensional approach.

The theoretical approach argues that individual religiosity promotes fertility both directly and indirectly. The direct effect makes recourse to denomination-specific norms and rules with respect to family behavior. The indirect effect is derived from the religious composition of a couple. Confidence in marital stability should have a positive impact on fertility while the anticipation of divorce discourages investments in the marriage. It is assumed that the religious composition of a couple and union stability are clearly linked to each other. Furthermore, the approach considers that fertility has decreased, also among the religiously affiliated. It therefore associates behavioral changes with changing environmental conditions. Indirect effects also arise from interactions of religiosity with other factors that affect fertility.

The following study compares five countries with different demographic and denominational patterns: France, Norway, West Germany, Hungary, and East Germany. (1) France has high fertility and strongly supportive policies. In addition, it can be referred to as a laicist state, i.e. state and church are strictly separated, with Catholic roots. (2) Norway is a universalistic welfare state geared to gender equality (in recent decades). Fertility is also high. The country has a Lutheran state church and hence a Protestant imprint. Family-related policies have been influenced by Protestant ideals. (3) West Germany (Federal Republic of Germany (FRG) before 1990) has had a persistently low level of fertility for almost 40 years. In terms of denominations, it is mixed with balanced shares of Protestants (rather in the North) and Roman Catholics (rather in the South). The number of desired children was and is well below the replacement level. Christian churches and the state cooperate, and are hence not strictly separated. (4) Hungary experienced state socialism which included the promotion of fertility and the discrimination of religion. Fertility during that time period was stable and relatively high, but dramatically sank after the system transformation. The country has a pluralist religious structure with Roman and Greek Catholics, Reformed and Lutheran Protestants, and further Christian as well as non-Christian minorities. (5) East Germany was also a socialist state in the form of the German Democratic Republic (GDR). After the fall of the wall, the fertility level declined. Even if demographic developments around 1990 were similar, East Germany and Hungary differ in a variety of factors and characteristics. For example, the Protestant imprint in East Germany was already fading due to the religion-hostile ideology of the regime of the Socialist Unity Party (SED), while Hungary remained Christian though not highly religious. East and West Germany will – with one exception – be treated separately from each other due these far-reaching differences. Moreover, the selected countries have different historical and institutional contexts, cultures, social norms, and church-state-relations.

Empirically, assumptions will be tested by estimating regression models on the basis of wave I of the *Generations and Gender Survey* (GGS). The advantage of the GGS is the opportunity to internationally compare completed fertility and fertility differences between several religious groups within diverging settings due to the availability of relevant indicators. In Germany, a supplemental survey was carried out to collect data from Turkish migrants. Information on migrant groups are generally scarce. Therefore, the additional survey offers a good opportunity to involve Muslims and their demographic behavior in this study. The respondents considered were born between 1930 and 1962. The youngest respondents were 45 years old at the time of data collection, the oldest were 74 years old.

In addition to the empirical analyses, a literature-based analysis is conducted to determine intermediate macrolevel effects of religious institutions on fertility. Taken together, the following study contributes to religion-related research by working multi-dimensionally. Firstly, the comparative perspective is the cross-country dimension. Secondly, considering both women and men gives information on gender-specific differences with respect to demographic behavior by religiosity. Thirdly, micro-macro associations are considered. And fourthly, by regarding a broad time period (1950–2007), changes in the influence of religiosity over time can be taken account of.

1.2 Structure

The study proceeds as follows: chapter 2 outlines and compares demographic patterns – based on alternative fertility as well as divorce indicators – of France, Hungary, Norway, and Germany. Chapter 3 defines religion and religiosity and introduces the multi-dimensional concept of religiosity. Thereafter, it deals with historical-cultural patterns that explain diverging levels of religious vitality between the selected countries. Religious vitality is reflected by the degree of secularization, whose three-dimensional character will be clarified. The historical-cultural pattern will be described by modernization, state-church relations, and the denominational cultural tradition. The latter refers to denomination-specific characteristics that encourage or discourage religious activity. The chapter concludes with a review of some existing findings concerning the association between religiosity and fertility. Usually, they document a positive impact at the individual level.

Chapter 4 theorizes the impact of religious affiliation and religiosity on fertility. Some of the common explanations for the religiosity-fertility connection beyond a higher affinity for children are depicted. Additionally, denomination-specific norms, rules, and principles guiding family behavior of adherents are summarized for Catholics, Protestants, and Muslims. Most studies researching the effects of religiosity on fertility restrict themselves to these explanations and denomination-specific norms. However, indirect effects of religiosity on fertility, such as considering religious traits of both spouses, may play a decisive role and are therefore also included in the chapter. Since not only religiosity (of both partners) influences divorce probabilities and hence the union stability, the chapter discusses important characteristics that stabilize or de-stabilize unions.

In the first part of chapter 5 the frame for fertility decisions is described and compared both cross-nationally as well as inter-temporally. Prominent factors, mainly policies – including state-church-relations – are discussed. The second section considers some individual traits and factors associated with fertility. They are gender, education as well as closely related characteristics such as qualifications and labor force participation.

Chapter 6 presents and interprets the results of the empirical analyses and examines the hypotheses formulated in chapter 4 on the basis of the GGS data. The data and variables employed are introduced and the statistical method is explained. A descriptive overview of the relevant data is given and the correlations between religiosity and marital stability, predicted in chapter 4, are tested against reality. Furthermore, the results of several regression estimations are discussed. In this context, direct religiosity effects are tested and then a variety of controls are introduced – among them union stability – and their interactions with religiosity investigated. An additional section analyzes the effects of religiosity on fertility among Muslims based on the supplemental sample to explore whether Muslims' higher fertility can be attributed more to religiosity or to lower educational level due to their origin from a country with a lower level of modernization. A conclusion summarizes the dissertation.

2 Demographic Patterns in Comparative Perspective

This chapter outlines the demographic patterns in France, Hungary, Norway, and Germany by means of several indicators that reflect the demographic situation and its development. Section 2.1 defines some fertility measures, discusses the country values and concludes with a cross-country comparison. Section 2.2 deals in the same way with marriage and divorce indicators. There is a large variety of indicators. Suitability and availability do not always accord with each other. Consequently, diverging measures for different countries have to be used. Only the least suitable indicator – the crude (divorce and marriage) rate – is available for all countries.

2.1 Fertility

2.1.1 Average number of children: definitions

Fertility is described by the average number of children per woman. Two indicators are available: the total fertility rate (TFR) and the cohort fertility rate (completed fertility). While the former is a theoretical concept, the latter is an empirical term. Official data are only provided for the total fertility rate. Data on completed fertility are only available from survey data. The more accurate indicator is the cohort fertility rate. However, the cohort fertility rate cannot be calculated unless a cohort's fertile period has ended. The last birth cohort completed fertility can be ascertained for is 1968. These women celebrated their 45th birthday in 2013 and no definitive statements can be made for younger cohorts. This is why the TFR, which is related to a period of one year, is most often used instead. It states

> [t]he mean number of children that would be born to a woman during her lifetime if she were to pass through her childbearing years conforming to the age-specific fertility rates of a given year (European Union 2010: 176).

This rate is the completed fertility of a hypothetical generation, under the presumption that the fertility pattern of the period lasts, and that deaths do not occur. It is computed by adding the fertility rates by age for women in a given year (Statistics Norway 2012i). The TFR assumes that age at childbearing does not change, which is an assumption that did not hold during recent decades.[1] Family formation is put off and (partly) caught up at a later point in time, a fact the TFR only accounts of with delay. Therefore, the cohort fertility rate usually exceeds the total fertility rate. Variance in the TFR is generally much higher than in the cohort fertility time series. The final number of children that cohorts of women have changes slowly due to inertia, while the total fertility rate can react fiercely to events and changes in regulations and laws. However, these are mostly timing effects. Nevertheless, the two rates are also closely linked to each other.

2.1.2 Total fertility rate

In 2009, the total fertility rate in France was exactly 2.0 children per woman (see the figures 2.1 and 2.2). In 1998, the TFR was 1.78 and since then it has continuously been between these two values with a generally upward trend (Eurostat 2010d). While fertility at ages younger than 28 years stopped to decline in the middle of the 1990s, it has been continuing to rise at ages above. This fact contributed to the increase in the TFR since 1994, when it was only 1.66 for a very short period of two years (Toulemon/Pailhé/Rossier 2008: 510). Roughly speaking, the TFR has been stable since 1975 – compared to the variations before – with a long-term stationary average of 1.8 children per woman. A drop below the value of 1.9 is not expected for the future (Prioux 2005: 376). After World War II, France experienced baby boom periods starting in 1946 with a TFR of three children. This first period cooled down to 2.67 in 1953. Afterward, the level rose again in the first half of the 1960s. The TFR reached a level of 2.8 to 2.9 in those years. From the middle of the 1960s until the middle of the 1970s the fertility level strongly declined by more than one third to 1.85 children per woman.

[1] This has led to a deficit in annual fertility, whose magnitude is proportional to the childbearing delay.

Fig. 2.1. Total fertility rates of France, Hungary, Norway, and Germany (separated)

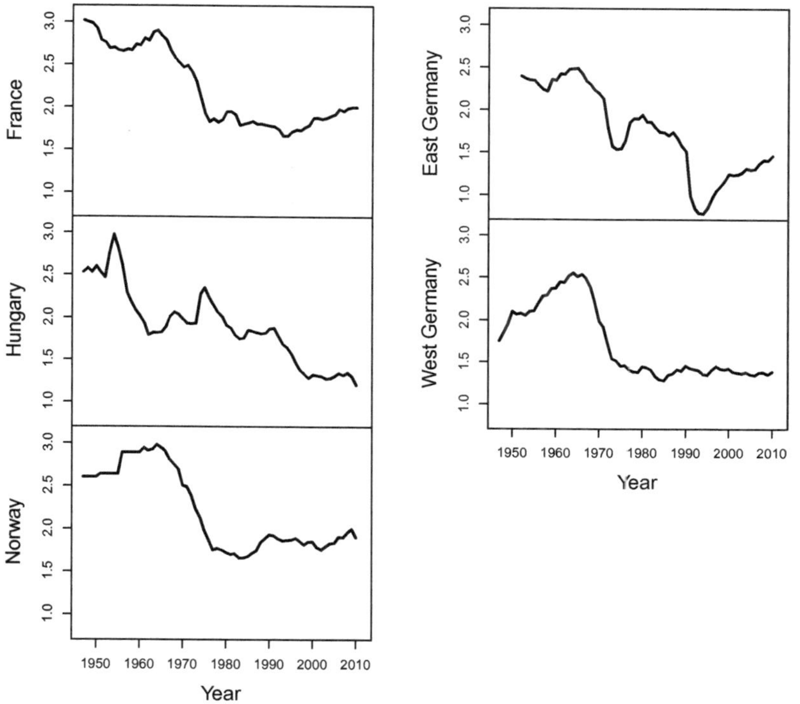

Source: Eurostat 2012d.

Norwegian fertility was (also) 2.0 in 2009. Statements for France could almost be repeated for Norway. The rates ran a synchronous course at identical levels from 1963 to 1979 including the deep fall of the rate usually called the second demographic transition, while it was similar afterwards: in some years the French rate was higher (1980–1986, 2002), and in some years it was the other way round (1990–1997). Since 1963, the largest difference between the rates was 0.25 in 1981. The drop in the Norwegian rate started from a slightly higher fertility level and lasted longer: in France the fall stopped in 1978 while in Norway the rate continued to sink until

1984. In those years, the Norwegian rate was only higher than the West German rate. Before 1963 larger differences were observable at generally much higher fertility levels of between 2.6 and 3.0 children. Between 1947 and 1951 the Norwegian rate was greatly exceeded by the French one. While for some years (1953–1955), women in Norway and France gave birth to the same number of children, the position of the both changed between 1956 and 1962.

Germany had a TFR of 1.36 children in 2009 (Eurostat 2010d). In West Germany, the extremely low fertility level has persisted since the mid-1970s with little variation (see figure 2.1).[2] After the recovery at the end of the 1940s back to pre-war levels, the rate rose to 2.54 in 1966 followed by a pronounced downward movement in the subsequent decade. The drop amounted to more than one child per woman which is equal to 40%. Insofar, the fertility rate can be subdivided in three phases with two trend changes: an upward trend between 1947 and 1966 with values from 1.8 to 2.5, a downward trend between 1966 and 1977 with values from 2.5 to 1.4, and a stable phase at an extremely low level between 1.28 and 1.45 afterward which has lasted until the present.

The East German rate partly underwent another development: initially (between 1952 and 1958) the rate decreased from 2.4 to 2.2, and increased a bit again until 2.5 in 1965. The time afterward can be characterized by a two-phase downward movement: the first one lasted until 1971 and was flatter than the second phase which was very steep and merely two years (1972 and 1973). The whole decline also amounted to one child per woman (to 1.5). It stopped and after a short period was replaced by an upward movement which reached the value of 1.95 in 1980. The following decrease in the rate started and attained the level of 1.5 in 1990. Afterward, the TFR plunged to dramatically low levels and reached a trough in 1994 (0.77). In this respect, the drop was again a two-phase downward movement. Since then, the rate has been steadily and slightly rising again. The two German rates started to converge, or, more accurately: the East German rate has approached the West German one. In 2008, it was even slightly higher for the first time since unification (East: 1.40, West: 1.37). Earlier, between 1957 and 1975 the fertility rates in both parts developed almost synchronously. However, whereas the rate of the FRG experienced a longer decrease and stabilized afterward, the GDR rate already started to rise again so that fertility in the German Democratic Republic from the middle of the 1970s until 1989 was

[2] The country has one of the 20 lowest fertility rates worldwide (Population Reference Bureau 2008).

Fig. 2.2. Total fertility rates of France, Hungary, Norway, and Germany (integrated)

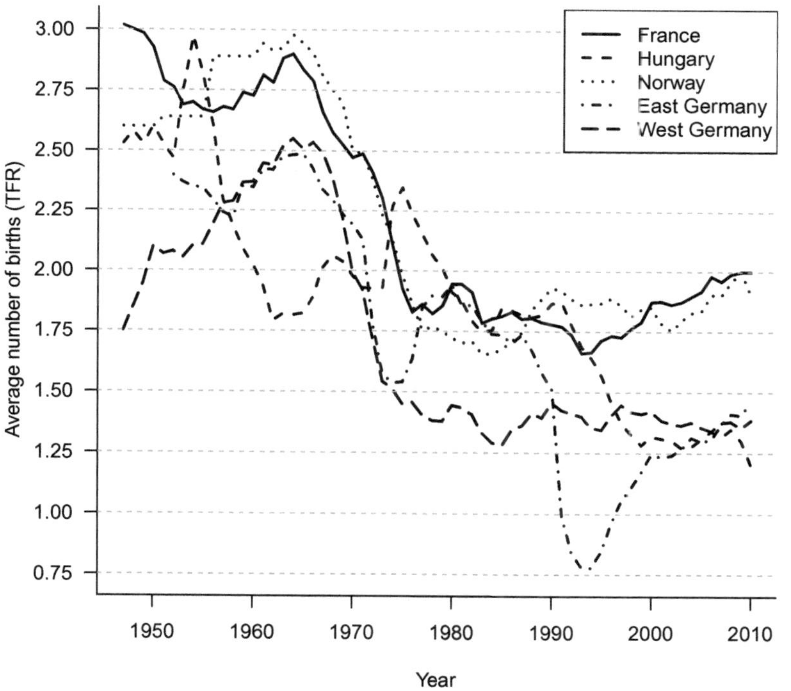

Source: Eurostat 2012d.

noticeably higher than in the Federal Republic of Germany. In 1990 the rates crossed and afterward the situation reversed due to the severe collapse of the East German rate.

As was typical for most of the ex-socialist countries of Central and Eastern Europe (CEE), profound changes in the demographic behavior of the Hungarian population started in the late 1980s and hence, compared to Western European countries, with a delay. In the CEE countries the demographic pattern can in general be summarized as follows: Until the late 1980s marriage and divorce rates were high, most families had two children and age at marriage and childbearing was very low. Since then, behavior developed differently. In 2009, Hungary had – together with Latvia and Portugal – the lowest fertility level of all member states of the European Union. The value was 1.32 children (Eurostat 2010d). In some of the previous years Hungary's TFR was even (marginally) lower – the lowest value was 1.27 in 2003 – and during the last 12 years the TFR has never exceeded 1.35. The Hungarian TFR exhibits a development that is different to the other countries considered here. It already had a post-war peak in 1954 with a value of almost 3.0 children and crashed steeply afterward to the value of 1.8 in 1962. In those years, West European countries experienced their "baby boom" era. Hungary was the first European country that underwent below-replacement fertility after World War II and moreover the nation with one of the lowest rates in the world (Spéder/Kamarás 2008: 603). Between 1967 and 1980 the total fertility rate again displayed values between 1.9 and 2.35. The last decline occurred in the 1990s when the TFR dropped from almost 1.9 to the current low value. Altogether, the total fertility rate of Hungary followed a completely different course and in contrast to the other time series, the TFR of Hungary exhibits – apart from some upward fluctuations (mainly 1953–1956 and 1974–1977) – a long-term downward trend during the last 50 years.

Between 1958 and 1970 Hungary had – with values between 1.8 and 2.24 – the lowest total fertility rate of all five countries, also a much lower rate than the second socialist country GDR whose rate followed the typical Western European course at that time. The Hungarian rate increased again as all other rates took a downward movement. In those years (1974–1980), Hungary had the highest rate of all countries while especially the curve of the GDR dropped down to the low level of the sister state FRG for a short period. Between 1973 and 1990, the rate of the Federal Republic of Germany was by far the lowest until the East German rate fell below this low level until 2003. Between 2000 and 2006 the East German and the Hungarian rates were the lowest at a very low average of 1.3. Compared to the former GDR, the Hungarian rate also dropped from 1990 onwards, but while the rate of East Germany collapsed for four years until 1994, the decline in Hungary lasted longer (until 1999) and the drop was more moderate (from 1.85 to 1.3). Since then, the Hungarian rate has been stable, while the East German rate has been steadily increasing. Since 2007, the East German rate has even marginally outpaced the Hungarian rate. Finally, it is apparent that the curves of France, Norway, and West Germany developed almost parallel with the latter at a much lower level. The difference amounts to about 0.5 units. Only in the last few years have the French and Norwegian rates taken an upward trend while the West German rate has remained stable. The parallel course has ended.

To conclude this subsection, table 2.1 shows the size of the populations of the relevant countries. Differences are considerable.

Table 2.1. Size of population in France, Hungary, Norway, and Germany

	Size in millions	date
France métropolitaine	62.8	2010
Hungary	10.0	2010
Norway	5.0	2012
Germany	81.8	2010

Sources: Institut national de la statistique et des études économiques 2010b, Statistics Norway 2012c, Statistisches Bundesamt 2010b: 28; *France métropolitaine* is the part of France situated in Europe. The population of Hungary already started to decrease in 1980 due to high mortality and morbidity levels as well as the lack of immigration (Speder/Kamaras (2008): 600). 82% of all inhabitants of Germany live in the Western part of Germany, 18% live in the Eastern part.

2.1.3 Cohort fertility rate (completed fertility)

Women in Norway born in 1965 have a cohort fertility of 2.04 children equaling women born in France who have 2.03 children on average (see figures 2.3 and 2.4).[3] Women had 2.5 to 2.65 children until the 1937 birth cohort. The number of children started to decrease with birth cohort 1936 and did not stop falling until cohort 1949 in France and 1955 in Norway. In subsequent birth cohorts, fertility leveled off. Several French birth cohorts (1949–1962) are slightly more fertile than their Norwegian peers while cohorts born between 1935 and 1948 do hardly differ. In contrast, older French women (born before 1935) gave birth to observably more children than older Norwegian women.

The last birth cohort of women in Germany that managed to replace its mother's birth cohort was the 1885 one: the average number of children was 3.36, the replacement level 3.44 at that time (Dorbritz 2008: 565). Since then, even the fertility of

[3] Within Europe, only Irish women have given birth to more children.

Fig. 2.3. Cohort fertility rates of France, Hungary, Norway, and Germany (1930–1965; separated)

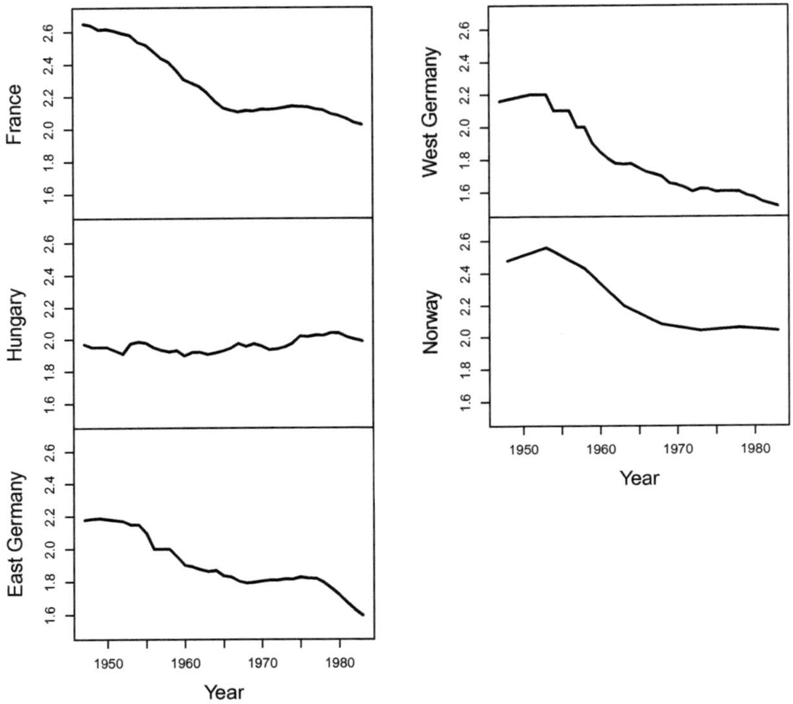

Sources: Max Planck Institute for Demographic Research/Vienna Institute of Demography 2012 based on national data (France: National Institute of Statistics and Economic Studies (INSEE); Norway: Statistics Norway; Hungary: Central Statistical Office; Germany: Statistisches Bundesamt and Federal Institute of Population Research (since 2001 West Germany without West Berlin and East Germany without East Berlin)).

cohorts that had their childbearing period during the so-called golden age of family has marginally fallen below the – at that time current – replacement level of 2.3. Now it has sunk to 2.1 in highly developed countries and cohort fertility even further. East German women born in 1958 have 1.8 children on average, their West German peers 1.6 (Statistisches Bundesamt 2009b). While between 1930 and 1941 cohort fertility was almost equal, completed fertility in the GDR was higher than in the FRG in subsequent birth cohorts. Birth cohorts that recently concluded their fertile phase are closing the gap more and more. On average, the numbers of children of cohort 1967 are almost identical, with 1.44 in West Germany and 1.47 in East Germany (Dorbritz 2008: 566). This cohort has not yet completed its fertility but it is expected to be lower than that of preceding cohorts (Statistisches Bundesamt 2009b).

The cohort fertility rate time series from Hungary show hardly any variance. Cohorts born between 1930 and 1965 completed fertility continuously with between 1.9 and 2.0 children on average. Younger cohorts have fewer children, but this may partly be ascribed to the not yet concluded fertile period: while women born in 1962 have 2 children, those born eight years later are assumed to have only 1.7 children at the end of their childbearing age. Because of the low values of the total fertility rate since 1998, further decrease can be expected.

The large fertility gap between the French and the Norwegians on the one hand and Germans on the other is remarkable and a consequence of the former's consistently much higher annual fertility level. The parallelism of the total fertility rates mentioned above is also observable in the cohort fertility rates. The Hungarian rate was the lowest in the birth cohorts 1929 through 1940. After this point this position changed because the German rates dropped. Due to the fall of the French and Norwegian rates, the Hungarian birth rate approached them. In the cohorts born in the 1960s no significant difference can be measured any more. Therefore, two developments are responsible for the changed position of the Hungarian rate: its inertia and the other rates' decline.

Fig. 2.4. Cohort fertility rates of France, Hungary, Norway, and Germany (1930–1965; integrated)

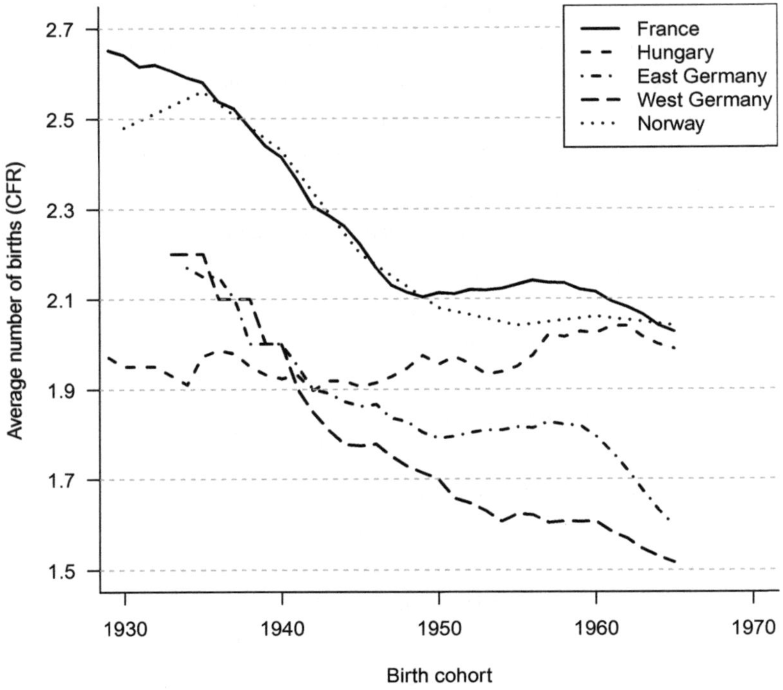

Sources: Max Planck Institute for Demographic Research/Vienna Institute of Demography 2012 based on national data (France: National Institute of Statistics and Economic Studies (INSEE); Norway: Statistics Norway; Hungary: Central Statistical Office; Germany: Statistisches Bundesamt and Federal Institute of Population Research (since 2001 West Germany without West Berlin and East Germany without East Berlin)).

2.1.4 Further fertility indicators

In the following, further fertility indicators are addressed: parity progression ratios and parity distributions, mean age at birth, proportions of children born outside marriage, and the desired number of children. With respect to parity distribution, proportions of childlessness as well as of families with many children in France, Hungary, Norway, and Germany will receive special attention. “Families with many children” are those who have at least three children.

In France, the parity progression ratios to a first child have been almost stable for 50 years.[4] 11% of women born in 1960 are childless (Toulemon/Mazuy 2001: 634). The same proportion is expected for cohort 1970, while 12% of the 1980 cohort will probably close the fertile phase without having children (Toulemon/Pailhé/Rossier 2008: 516, 518). Hence, France is – along with Norway and other Northern European countries – one of the nations that has experienced hardly any increase in the proportion of childless women. The progression ratios to a second, third, and fourth child have not changed since 1975. When comparing the birth cohorts 1950 and 1940 with each other, no differences can be observed with regard to progression ratios to a first and a second child (Toulemon/Pailhé/Rossier 2008: 515). The distribution of the number of children French women have, is presented for cohort 1950 as an example: 10% do not have any children, every fifth woman has one child, a relative majority of 40% has two children, and almost one third has many children with 20% having three and 10% having more than three children (Toulemon/Pailhé/Rossier 2008: 518). Significant changes did not occur until cohort 1960 (Toulemon/Mazuy 2001).

Just like many of the Central and Eastern European countries, Hungary had progression rates to a first child well above 90% – until recently (Frejka/Sardon 2007: 320). Childlessness was a rare event. The birth cohort of 1969 will be the first one (after 1935) that exceeds the rate of 10%. It is however a cohort whose fertile phase has not yet ended, even though the probability of a women having her first child after her 40th birthday is generally still low. The progression rate to a second child has slightly decreased.[5] Almost two thirds of the birth cohort 1968 will have at least two

[4] Civil registration data by birth order are not accurate in France and Germany. Couples are asked about the number of children born in that marriage or relationship and not about the actual birth order of the newborn child of the same mother. A specific 1% sample is thus drawn within each census and delivers precise information about fertility history (Toulemon/Pailhé/Rossier 2008: 514).

[5] Progression rates to a second child differ greatly across the countries of Central and Eastern Europe (Frejka/Sardon 2007: 325).

children (1965: 69%; 1960: 72.5%; 1940: 65%). Progression rates to higher order births are available until birth cohort 1965. No decline in rates of families with many children have been reported – rather the contrary. Almost one fourth of all families have more than two children while only 20% of birth cohort 1940 have three or more children. The percentage has continuously grown since then. Compared to other European countries this third order birth trend cannot be characterized as typical. The incidence of large families with more than three children has strongly declined. 30% of the birth cohort 1928 had four or more children but only 10% of the 1955 birth cohort. Since then, the proportion is slightly on the rise again (Frejka/Sardon 2007: 328).

The share of childless women rose by just 3% within 30 years in Norway: while 9.6% in the birth cohort 1935 remained childless, it was 12.5% in the 1965 cohort. The increase only occurred after birth cohort 1950 (Statistics Norway 2012d, Statistics Norway 2012g). The share of women with an only child also increased. While 10.4% of women born in 1935 have one child, the proportion was 14.2% among women born 30 years later. The proportion of two-child families did not develop linearly: it strongly grew by 50% from the female birth cohort 1935 (30.4%) to the one of 1950 (45.4%) and decreased somewhat afterward (1965: 40.2%). In contrast, the proportion of women with many children strongly declined from almost 50% (birth cohort 1935) to one third (birth cohort 1965). While the proportion of women with three children registered merely a small drop, the majority of the decrease is owing to the reduction of families with four and more children: it declined from 22.2% (1935) to 8.4% until birth cohort 1950 and became stable afterward.

In Germany, 21% of women born between 1964 and 1968 remained childless (Statistisches Bundesamt 2009b: 9).[6] In contrast, the percentage of childless women born between 1933 and 1948 is low with proportions between 11% and 12%. This indicates a sharp rise. Rates of childlessness among men are higher: one fourth of the 1950–1960 birth cohorts have no children (Schmitt/Winkelmann 2005: 6). Compared to other OECD member states, these rates are among the highest (Sleebos 2003). However, it is important to differentiate between East and West Germany when it comes to parity distributions, although on average fertility rates accord. To have no children is – in all age-groups – more widespread in the West (Statistisches Bundes-

[6] The proportion is based on the 2008 Microcensus. Before the Microcensus 2008 the exact extent of childlessness was not known. All data were based on estimates. 22% of the cohorts 1955–1963 remained childless (Höhn/Ette/Ruckdeschel 2006: 18, 65).

amt 2009b: 16). Less than 8% of the East German women born before 1960 remain childless. Among younger cohorts the proportion is increasing: 11% of the 1966 birth cohort have not had a child – whereas one-child families are a common phenomenon. Additionally, the share of one-child families grows.

No precise data on the parity distribution for women who have already completed their fertility seem to be available except for those aged between 35 and 39 years, corresponding to the birth cohorts 1952–1957. The following information is known: 8% of the East and 25% of the West German women were childless, 28% in both parts had one child, 50% respectively 35% were mothers of two children, and 14% in the East and 12% in the West had large families with three or more children (Kreyenfeld 2004: 289). Furthermore, the information available for mothers is: 82% of the women born between 1931 and 1971 (age at data collection: 35–75 years) have children (90% in East and 81% in West Germany). An additional cohort effect exists. This means that a higher percentage of women aged between 50 and 75 years (birth cohorts 1931–1956) have their own family compared to younger women (Statistisches Bundesamt 2007: 26–27). Of these older mothers, 47% in East and 45% in West Germany have two children. 27% respectively 30% have only one child, and one quarter (26%) in both regions have many children. The distributional similarity has changed in younger cohorts. In the East, the proportion of mothers with only one child has risen by 10% to 37%, while in the West it has stagnated. The share of mothers with large families has declined. This development is more pronounced in the Eastern part of the Republic (East: 16%, West: 21%). Finally, the proportion of mothers with two children is more stable respectively increased slightly (East: 48%, West: 49%).

In addition to the number of children, the mean age at (first) birth has changed during recent decades. As young Europeans in (almost) all countries have started to delay family formation, their age at first birth has risen: In 2009, the age was lowest in Hungary (27.2 years), followed by Norway (27.6 years) and France (28.7 years). Germany has the oldest first-time mothers (OECD Family database 2011) aged 30 years on average. East German women are still a bit younger than West German women. This seems to be a consequence of the very early childbearing age in the GDR even if the adjustment has almost been completed. However, the difference can only be stated for age at birth in general, not for age at first birth. It totals one year (Eurostat 2010c).

The postponement in births since 1970 can be subdivided into two periods: the change before and after 1995. In Hungary, the delay amounts to 4.4 years whereas the largest part of the delay (3.4 years) happened after 1995. In Norway the delay was just 1.8 years and the majority also took place after 1995. In France, women enter 4.2 years later into parenthood than in 1970. In contrast to Hungary and Norway, the delay largely occurred before 1995 (3.7 years). Finally, in Germany women postpone family formation by 6 years compared to 1970, which is again and by far the highest value among all OECD countries (3.4 years before 1995 and 2.6 years after). Summarized, this means that in 1970 Hungarian women experienced the transition to motherhood first (before their 23rd birthday) while Norwegian women experienced it last. They were almost 26 years on average when they became mothers. Higher-order births are less strongly postponed. For example, in Hungary, fourth- and higher order births are not postponed at all (Spéder 2006: 258–259). This may provide evidence that individuals who plan to have large families still start early and are not too much affected by environmental – institutional, political, and societal – issues.

In most European countries more and more children are born out of wedlock. This development is accompanied by a rise in cohabitation. Extra-marital childbearing is different from childbearing within a cohabitation because the latter ignores other partnership statuses. In the early 1960s, its incidence was rare with far less than 10% of all births. Today, the rate of children born outside marriage in Norway is one of the highest in European comparison: it was 55% in 2009 following Iceland and Estonia and followed by Sweden – all countries with higher birth rates overall (Eurostat 2010b). Norway was the first country that experienced an increase in childbearing within cohabitations. However, traditional behavior did not change before the late 1970s. The share especially rose in the 1980s and did so more strongly than elsewhere (followed by France; Perelli-Harris et al. 2009).

In Germany, the proportion of children born to unmarried women is much lower: in 2006 it amounted to 30% of all newborn children, and to 32.7% in 2009 (Eurostat 2010b). A decade earlier (in 1998) the rate was only 20%, and 10.5% in 1990. The differences between East and West Germany are substantial: 60% of all children are born to unmarried women in the Eastern part but only 24% in the Western part (Dorbritz 2008: 560). The East German percentage is the second highest following Iceland. This means that it is also higher than the Norwegian one. In the GDR, the proportion of extra-marital births already started to increase in the 1970s (Dorbritz 2008:

574) which was not the case in the FRG. In Hungary, almost 41% of all children were born outside marriage in 2009 (Eurostat 2010b). Eleven years previously (in 1998), the proportion was 26.6% so that the percent rise (14.4%) was little higher than in Germany (12%), that had a lower initial share, as well as in France (11%), that had a higher initial share. The process began before the system transformation (Perelli-Harris et al. 2009: 12). In 1990, the percentage amounted to more than 13%.

In France, the proportion has been increasing since the late 1960s and is today – with 53.7% in 2009 – (also) one of the highest in Europe following East Germany, Norway, and Sweden. The extra-marital proportion started to rise slightly earlier than in Norway. With regard to first-born children, the share is perceptibly higher: 63% are born outside marriage (Institut national d'études démographiques 2010c). This observable difference between first and higher-order births exists in all four countries but it is most pronounced in France and Norway (Perelli-Harris et al. 2009, Perelli-Harris et al. 2012).[7] Also in Norway and France, a significant proportion of cohabitations still lead to marriage before the birth of a second or third child – if this happens at all.[8] Hence, marriage remains the dominant kind of relationship between parents to raise children.

The desired number of children in France is high and exceeds the number of realized births. While almost half of the French (between 15 and 45 years of age) consider two children and 40% regard three children to be the ideal family size according to *Eurobarometer* data, they desire 2.34 children on average (Testa/Grilli 2006: 118). The French mean ranks second behind Ireland. Not even one out of twenty of the French can imagine to live without children. Here a slight North-South divide exists as people from the Southern part of France almost completely reject childlessness (Testa/Grilli 2006: 123). According to the *Population Policy Acceptance Study*[9] (PPAS), Hungarian women desire more than two children (2.19) while the value for men already falls below two, amounting to 1.9 (European Commission 2007: 46–47).

[7] The analyses are based on the Generations and Gender Survey and include the time period 1970–2004 in France and Norway, and until 2001 in Hungary. A comparison with vital statistics suggests that the German GGS understates fertility in the older cohorts and under-reports partnerships. For that reason, the authors of the study restricted their analyses for West Germany to the time period 1980–2004 (Perelli-Harris et al. 2009, Perelli-Harris et al. 2012).

[8] However, it is also possible to assume that marital fertility is higher than fertility in cohabitations. In that case the validity of the statement would indeed be questionable (Perelli-Harris et al. 2009: 20).

[9] 14 countries participated in this study – among others Germany and Hungary took part, but not France and Norway.

Less than 5% of Hungarian women do not want any children. Marginally more men desire childlessness.

The desired number of children in Germany is the lowest in European comparison (Köppen/Mazuy/Toulemon 2007: 89). On average, in 2003 women aged 20–39 years in Germany would have liked to have 1.75 children (East: 1.78, West: 1.73). The corresponding value among men is far lower: they desired only 1.54 children (East: 1.46, West: 1.59; Höhn/Ette/Ruckdeschel 2006: 16, Dorbritz 2008: 583–584). 23% of men did not want to have any children. Some regional differences exist: 27% of West German men and to 21% of the East German men did not want children. The regional differences are larger with regard to women. While 17% of West German women do not want to have any children, only 6% of East German women do (Dorbritz/Lengerer/Ruckdeschel 2005: 36). This extent of desired childlessness is historically new whereas high levels of actual childlessness are not. To have many children is less desired than not to have any (except for East German women): 15% of all women, almost 20% of West German men as well as 10% of East German men desire a large family (Dorbritz 2008: 583). According to actual behavior, more East Germans consider one child to be the ideal family size: 24.2% of female and 28.7% of male East Germans prefer a rather small family size (West Germans: women: 14.5%, men: 13.0%). Finally, a majority of women (East: 50.6%, West: 53.7%) and a relative majority of men (East: 45.0%, West: 40.0%) regard two children as ideal.

To conclude, the countries will be compared with each other concerning the fertility indicators just dealt with. Childlessness is by far more widespread in West Germany. East Germany, Norway, and France hardly differ in this respect. The percentage of people with large families is more than twice as high in France and Norway as in Germany. The French desire by far more children than Germans. Childlessness is almost universally unwanted while many Germans consider this to be a real alternative. The proportion of extra-marital children born in West Germany is not half as high as in France and Norway. The share is highest in East Germany. Status changes of cohabiting, pregnant women occur significantly more often in West Germany than in France until the first birthday of the child. Age at first birth was highest in Germany in 2009 and in Norway in 1970.

Childlessness rarely occurred in East Germany and Hungary and has not risen in both regions until recently in younger cohorts. In Hungary, the two-child-family still dominates while in East Germany the one-child-family is gaining more and more importance. Many Hungarians have three children, the proportion is even increasing again, whereas in East Germany it is strongly decreasing. Families with more than three children are rare. The mean age at first birth is almost equal in the two regions and still a little lower than in the countries of Western and Northern Europe. The proportion of children born out of wedlock in Hungary is far below the corresponding number in East Germany, France, and Norway but much higher than in West Germany. While the values of the TFR are almost equal in Hungary and East Germany, the numbers of desired children greatly differ. One fourth of East Germans prefer to have a small family with only one child. Most Hungarians prefer two children and also two on average. The percentage of women who do not want any children is almost equally low in both regions, while the percentage of men strongly diverges. In East Germany, it is much higher.

2.2 Nuptiality

Recent decades have witnessed a strong growth in the number of divorces, remarriages, and non-marital cohabitations while the number of first marriages has decreased. The age at marriage has increased. The first subsection deals with marriage-related rates and the second one treats divorce-related rates.

2.2.1 Marriage-related rates

The crude marriage rate refers the number of marriages per year to 1,000 inhabitants.[10] The total (first) marriage rate is

> the sum of age-specific (first) marriage rates. It may be quite different from the final proportion of persons who marry at least once in a birth cohort (cohort marriage rate; Institut national d'études démographiques 2009b).

In France, marriage affinity began to decline after having peaked in 1972 (see the figures 2.5 and 2.6). The number of marriages dropped by more than 25% in the course of 14 years. In the late 1980s, less than three-quarters of all marriages were first marriages. In 2005, the total first marriage rate was 0.52 while it was still 0.6

[10] The crude marriage rate ignores the share of the population being at risk of marriage and moreover the marriage order. This means, it does not differentiate between first and higher-order marriages. However, it is the only rate for which continuous values are available for all countries.

Fig. 2.5. Crude marriage rates of France, Hungary, Norway, and Germany (separated)

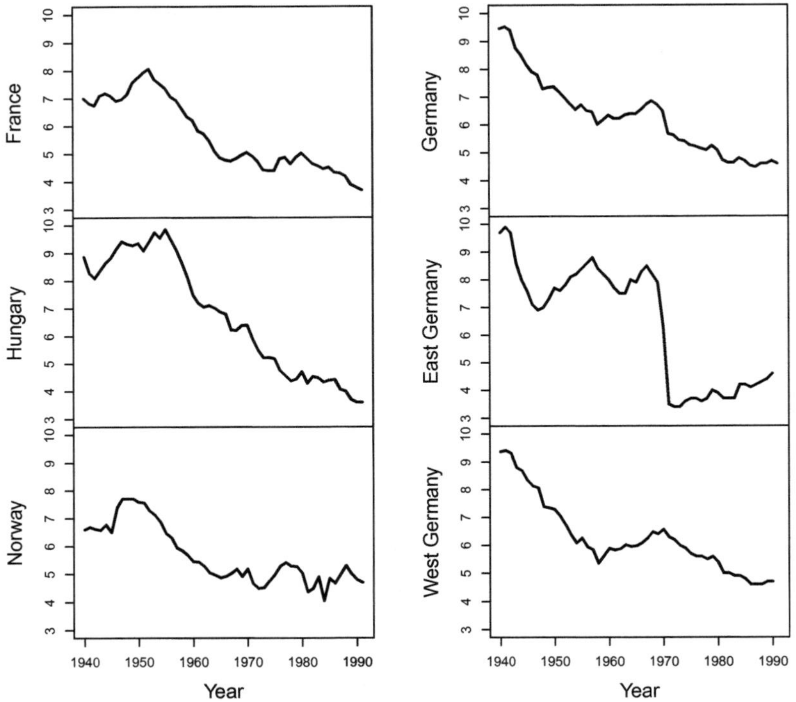

Sources: Eurostat 2012b, Federal Institute for Population Research 2012c, Federal Institute for Population Research 2012b.

in 2000 (Toulemon/Pailhé/Rossier 2008: 524; Prioux 2005: 388). More informative than the total marriage rate is cohort nuptiality, i.e. the share of a cohort that marries at least once in a lifetime (here: at least once before the 50th birthday). In the male birth cohort 1963 this proportion was 72% indicating a steep decline from the birth cohort 1958 where the rate still amounted to 79% and it was 85% in birth cohort 1953. Men born in 1963 first married on average at age 28.2, which is an increase compared to older birth cohorts (e.g. 26.4 years in birth cohort 1958 and 25.0 years in birth cohort 1953). Women were younger than men at first marriage. Their age has also risen over the course of time: those born in 1971 married on average at age 28.1 years, the female birth cohort 1960 married at the age of 24.3 years while women born in 1955 were only 22.9 years old (Institut national d'études démographiques 2012). The percentage of women who marry before reaching the age of 50 years was around 92.5% in the birth cohorts 1930–1946 and experienced a strong decrease to 82% for women born in 1960 and to 73% in birth cohort 1967 (Institut national de la statistique et des études économiques 2012). When concentrating on the age at marriage, the duration of relationships before marriage is disregarded. The premarital period has expanded, however. Evidence is provided by the fact that more and more unions start with a cohabitation: during recent years the share amounted to 90% (Toulemon/Pailhé/Rossier 2008: 525).

At the end of 1999 a law was enacted that permitted a new form of union beside marriage.[11] The *Pacte civil de solidarité* (PACS) is

> a contract concluded between two physical persons (...) of different or the same gender, for the purposes of organizing their life in common. It establishes rights and duties between the co-signatories in terms of material support, housing, inheritance, taxation and social welfare (Institut national d'études démographiques 2010a).

The new union is considered to be a great success and the number of contracts signed has disproportionately risen in recent years (Prioux 2006: 338). The decline of conventional marriages must be partly ascribed to this success (Prioux 2008: 387). The ratio of marriages to PACS was 1:0.7 in 2009. The proportion of heterosexual couples committing to such a contract was 17 times higher than the proportion of homosexual couples (Institut national d'études démographiques 2010b). The contract can be dissolved by joint declaration of both signatories at the district court – the place where it was signed. PACS seem to be more fragile than marriages (Prioux 2008: 387).[12]

Between 1966 and 1975, the average age at marriage was 22.8 years for women and 25.3 years for men in Norway (1961–1965: 23.4 and 26.4 years, respectively). After that date it started to increase by more than 8 years for both women and men. In 2008, the average age at first marriage was 31.1 years for women and 34 years

[11] It can also be entered into by homosexual couples.

[12] Same-sex PACS are the most fragile form of institutionalized relationships.

for men (Statistics Norway 2012b). The increase in mean age coincides with the decline of marriage rates starting in the early 1970s (see also figures 2.5 and 2.6). Additionally, the share of first marriages related to all marriages decreased. While it amounted to 87–89% between 1961 and 1975, the share fell to 70.4% after the turn of the millennium (Statistics Norway 2012e). The estimated share of unmarried persons at age 50 has been steadily on the rise. While it was negligibly low in the 1960s at well under 10% for both sexes, it has increased to 40% in 2011 (Statistics Norway 2012b).

In West Germany, the probability to marry has also decreased. In 1971 the total first marriage rate was 0.93 for women and 0.87 for men. This changed until 2004: the rate fell to three fourths (0.76) for women and two thirds for men (Dorbritz 2008: 576). In the GDR, the rate was (even) higher in 1971: about 0.96 for both women and men. Marriage was a universal phenomenon. Until the end of the 1980s it sank, but was still much higher than in the FRG. From 1989 the rate in East Germany fell rapidly for two years and was far lower than that in the Western part (and all the other countries considered here). In 2004, it was 0.69 for women and 0.57 for men. The East German rate is the only one that has risen slightly in recent years. Concentrating on younger women until age 40, further East-West differences become discernible that may certainly be associated with the lower marriage rates mentioned above. A larger share of women in the Eastern part of Germany in the age-group 16–29 years (East: 91%, West: 84%) is unmarried. The same applies to women aged between 30 and 39 years (East: 42%, West: 30%) (Dorbritz 2008).

The share of unmarried German women and men has risen. It was an utmost of 10% in the birth cohorts 1930, 1940, 1945, and 1950 (Grünheid 2011: 14)[13] and has increased since then. About 30% of the male cohort 1965 was unmarried at age 45 and 20% of the female cohort. This reflects both higher mean ages at marriage as well as lower marriage probabilities in total. The share of first marriages was 63–64% during recent years in Germany (Statistisches Bundesamt 2012a).

The age at first marriage shifted upwards strongly by about eight years for both men and women within a period of 40 years: from 22.7 years in 1971 to 30.5 years in 2011 for women and from 25.1 years to 33.3 years for men (Statistisches Bundesamt 2012b, Federal Institute for Population Research 2012a). The age at first marriage was lower for both sexes in the Eastern part of Germany (Grünheid 2011).

[13] Only the male birth cohort 1950 exceeded this share totaling 13% unmarried men.

Fig. 2.6. Crude marriage rates of France, Hungary, Norway, and Germany (integrated)

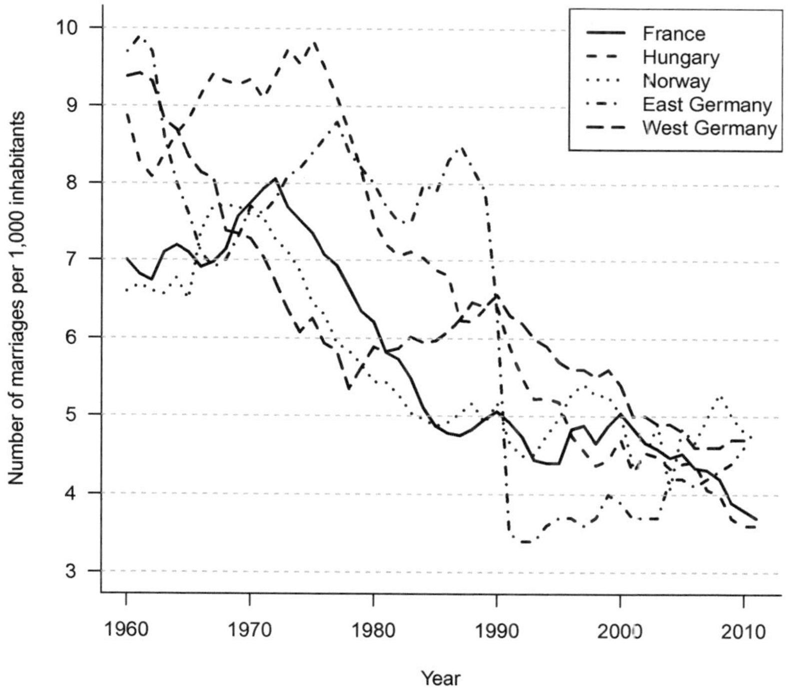

Sources: Eurostat 2012b, Federal Institute for Population Research 2012c, Federal Institute for Population Research 2012b.

This changed after the turn of the millennium when the mean age of women and men in East Germany exceeded the mean age in West Germany. While in the GDR in 1960 mean age was 22.5 years (women) and 23.9 years (men), it amounted to 23.7 years and 25.9 years respectively in the FRG. In some years the difference was higher (e.g. in 1985 when it totaled three years for men: 24.3 (GDR) versus 27.2 years (FRG)).

Until the 1980s, Hungary was characterized by the general practice of early marriage and high marriage rates. The values for the total first marriage rate were around 0.9–1.0 in the 1960s and 1970s. The age at marriage of women exhibited even more stability and was between 21 and 22 years until 1990. The mean age of men was 24 to 25 years (Spéder/Kamarás 2008: 619–621). The behavior pattern for marriage started to change in the 1980s and it has been fundamentally transformed within 15 years – the rate almost halved until 1997 and has remained stuck at around 0.45 in recent years. Age at marriage has meanwhile risen to 27.5 (women) and 30 years (men) in 2007.

The probability to marry (at a very young age) was very high in Hungary and East Germany. This was the typical marriage pattern in the socialist countries of Central and Eastern Europe (Besemeres 1980: 13–14). After 1989, the probability decreased in both countries by about 50% and is a trifle lower in Hungary today. Between 1965 and the middle of the 1980s, marriage rates in Hungary and East Germany were far higher than in the countries of Western and Northern Europe. After the mid-1980s the rates in Hungary and East Germany approached the others. The time series of Norway and France developed somewhat more similarly towards each other compared to the West German one, which was higher, for example, in the 1960s.

2.2.2 Divorce-related rates

Separation and divorce have become widespread in most European countries. Different indicators document this fact. (i) The crude divorce rate relates the number of divorces per year to 1,000 inhabitants, and is therefore a rather problematic indicator as marriage affinity decreases. It measures two effects which cannot be kept apart and neglects the population that is at risk of divorce. However, it is the only indicator available simultaneously and as continuous time series for all countries considered here. (ii) The total divorce rate – which is available for Hungary – indicates "the number of divorces in a fictitious cohort of marriages whose divorce rates for each duration of marriage are the same as those observed in given year. It may differ from the final proportion of divorced couples in a marriage cohort" (Institut national d'études démographiques 2009a). (iii) Divorce rates of marriage cohorts express the proportion of divorced marriages in a marriage cohort. (iv) A fourth indicator is defined as a ratio and relates the number of annual divorces to 1,000 married women (available for France and Norway) or marriages (available for East and West Germany).

Divorce rates solely capture the legal termination of marriages and not actual marital breakdowns (Smith 2002: 213). But not all separations end in divorce. The proportion and hence the extent of distortion depends on law reforms and the costs of divorce. The costs comprise the legal, i.e. economic, as well as the social costs of divorce which may also act as divorce barriers. Social pressure or stigmatization can be barriers (Bodenmann et al. 2006: 2). Furthermore, divorce rates do not account for dissolutions of cohabitations and other forms of non-institutionalized relationships although these have gained much importance. Reality has shown that cohabitations are the more fragile form of relationship compared to marriages.[14] This means that divorce rates become less informative the lower the marriage rates are and the more children are born out of wedlock. As marriage rates started to decline at a later point in time than most of the periods considered here, presenting divorce rates should be acceptable.

In France, the number of divorces per 1,000 married women was 2.85 in 1960, rose only moderately to 3.3 in 1970, then much more strongly to 6.3 in 1980, was 8.4 in 1990, 9.3 in 2000 and 10.7 in 2008 after having reached its peak in 2005 with a figure of 12.4 (see figure 2.7). The greatest relative increase occurred between 1976 and 1977, when the number rose by more than 17% in the course of one year. In that year fundamental legal changes were implemented that considerably lowered the barriers to divorce (Smith 2002: 214): the unilateral divorce law came into force and replaced the mutual-consent (bilateral) divorce law. Unilateral law allows one spouse to obtain a dissolution of the marriage without the consent of the other: divorce became much easier (Alesina/Giuliano 2006).

The Norwegian divorce rate exhibits a very similar gradient to the French one (see figure 2.7) – merely the level has been somewhat higher, in contrast to fertility. The volatile upward movements can be ascribed to the necessity of using five-year-means. The course diverged after 1985 as the increase in Norway developed more steeply. Both time series peaked in 2005 whereas the French peak had the characteristic of an outlier. In Norway *de facto* unilateral divorce law has already existed since 1929, and *de jure* since 1993 as opposed to France and Germany (Kneip/Bauer 2007).

[14] See e.g. Prioux 2005: 389 for France, Spéder/Kamarás 2008: 630-631 for Hungary, generally: Sobotka/Toulemon 2008: 97–103, Perelli-Harris et al. 2009, Perelli-Harris et al. 2012. As many cohabitations are transformed into marriages after a while, they are a prelude to a stage in the marriage process (Sobotka/Toulemon 2008: 99–102). Only in France is cohabitation (including PACS) regarded as an alternative to marriage.

Fig. 2.7. Divorces per 1,000 married women in France and Norway

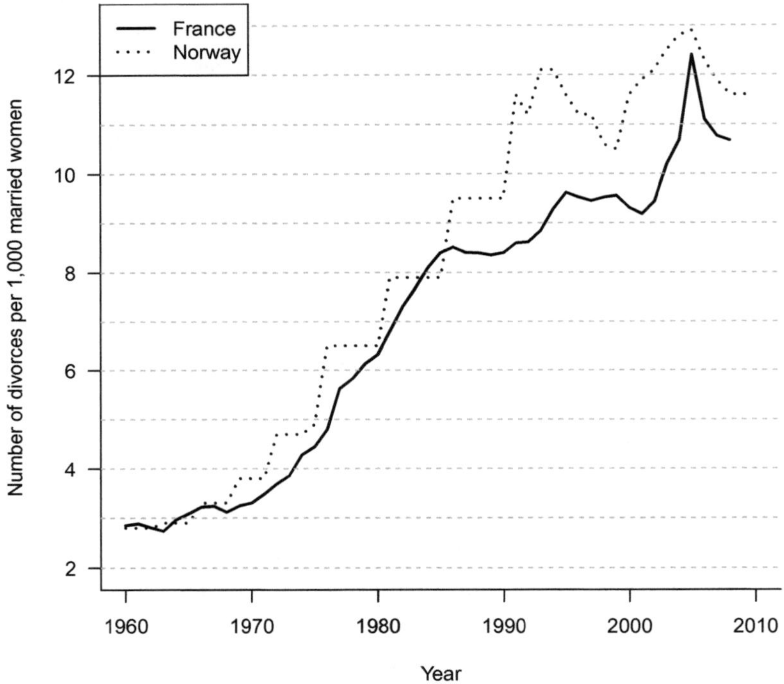

Sources: France: Institut national de la statistique et des études économiques 2009; Norway: Statistics Norway 2012f.

The divorce rate in the GDR was higher than in the FRG at (almost) steadily increasing values. After unification, the rate in East Germany plummeted – exactly the same that happened with the fertility rate – and has been exhibiting lower values until today (see figure 2.8). In 2008, the ratio was 8.3 in the East and 11.0 in the West (overall: 10.6). In 1977 and subsequent years, the number of divorces in the FRG declined dramatically. Divorce laws were amended as was the case in France in 1976. However, in West Germany a year-long judicial separation became a precondition

Fig. 2.8. Divorces per 1,000 existing marriages in Germany

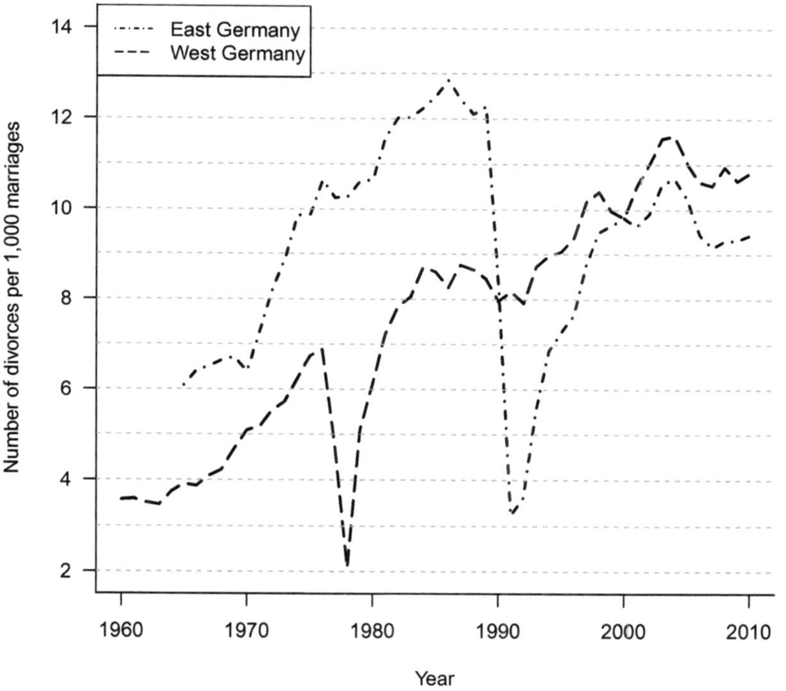

Source: Federal Institute for Population Research 2012e.

to file for divorce. Such a year of separation has never existed in France (Boele-Woelki et al. 2004). This may explain contrary reactions towards divorce law reforms. When comparing different marriage cohorts with each other, the rising divorce risk in West Germany also becomes obvious. Moreover, the risk of divorce increases with the duration of the marriage (Statistisches Bundesamt 2009a). For example, the share of divorces after 25 years of marriage was 20% for the marriage cohort 1964 and has risen to 35% in the 1983 cohort.

The rise in the total divorce rate in Hungary follows a continuous upward trend in the long run – interrupted only by a period of some years around 1990 (see figure 2.9). In 1960 the total divorce rate was 15.3, in 2006 it was 44. Within one year, between 1987 and 1988 the value slid from 30.3 to 24.7, remained at this lower value until 1993 to take up the original trend in the next year (starting again with the value of 30.4). The subsequent gradient was slightly steeper than the preceding one (between 1960 and 1988).

Fig. 2.9. Total divorce rate of Hungary and East Germany

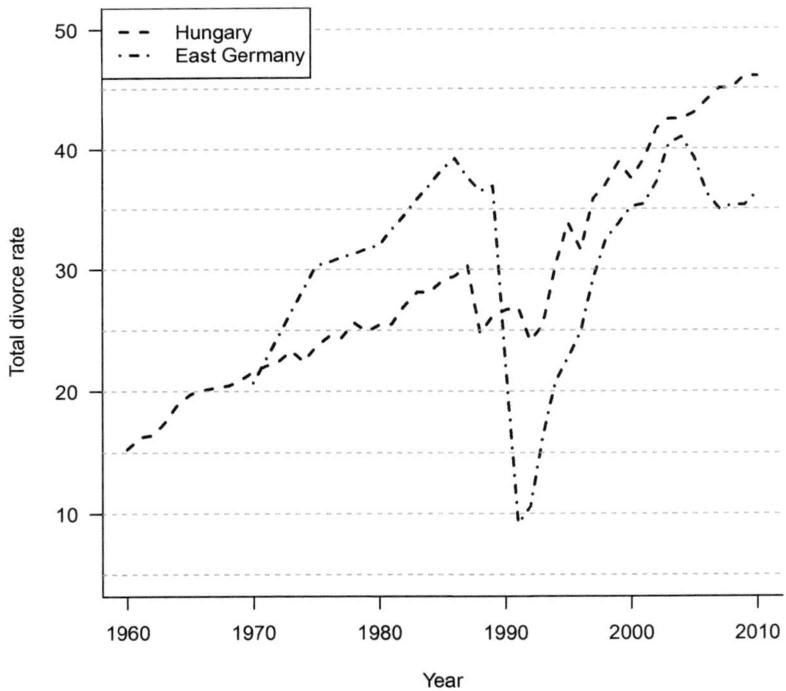

Sources: Hungary: Council of Europe 2003, Spéder/Kamarás 2008, Földházi 2010; East Germany: Federal Institute for Population Research 2012f.

To be able to compare the divorce levels of the two ex-socialist countries with each other, figure 2.9 illustrates both time series. Around 1970, the divorce probabilities exhibited similar values. The following upward trend was, however, much steeper in the GDR. There the rate rose up to 39.2 in 1986 whereas in Hungary it only increased, as mentioned above, up to 30.3 in 1987. After the regime change the rate in East Germany dropped to the lowest value of 9.2 (1991) within two years and started to climb again afterward. In Hungary, the decrease in the rate was much more moderate. This is associated with lower values before the transformation as well as with higher values afterward. The Hungarian rate started to rise again in 1993. Since 1990, the Hungarian divorce rate has been higher than the East German one. Owing to German unification, ongoing processes and legal adjustments around 1990 were more radical in East Germany than in Hungary. This is reflected in the divorce rate's time series. In recent years, the difference has re-grown with changed positions compared to the pre-transformation period. While the Hungarian rate has continuously risen in the new century, the East German one had its peak in 2004 (41.0) and has been declining again since then. During the last one and a half decades the divorce rate in Hungary has been higher than it ever was during the socialist era which does not – except for few years – apply to East Germany.

Finally, figure 2.10 clarifies that divorce rates in CEE countries were observably higher than in the countries of Western and Northern Europe. After transformation this difference diminished because the rates more or less converged. The divorce rate of (West) Germany was – apart from exceptional years – higher than the French and the Norwegian divorce rate. The general course of the French, the Norwegian, and the West German rates nevertheless evolved very similarly to each other.

Fig. 2.10. Crude divorce rates of France, Hungary, Norway, and Germany (separated)

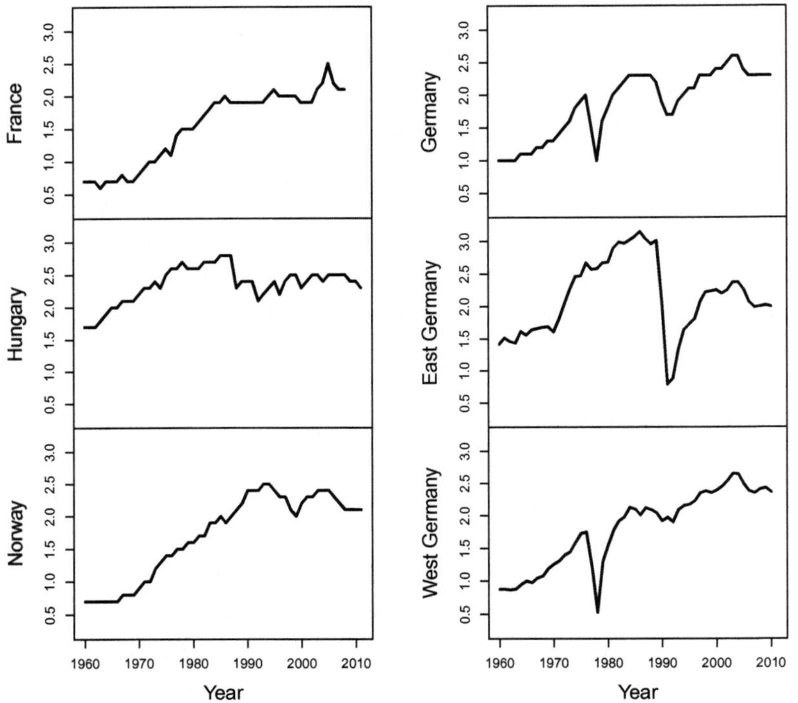

Sources: Eurostat 2012a, Federal Institute for Population Research 2012d.

Fig. 2.11. Crude divorce rates of France, Hungary, Norway, and Germany (integrated)

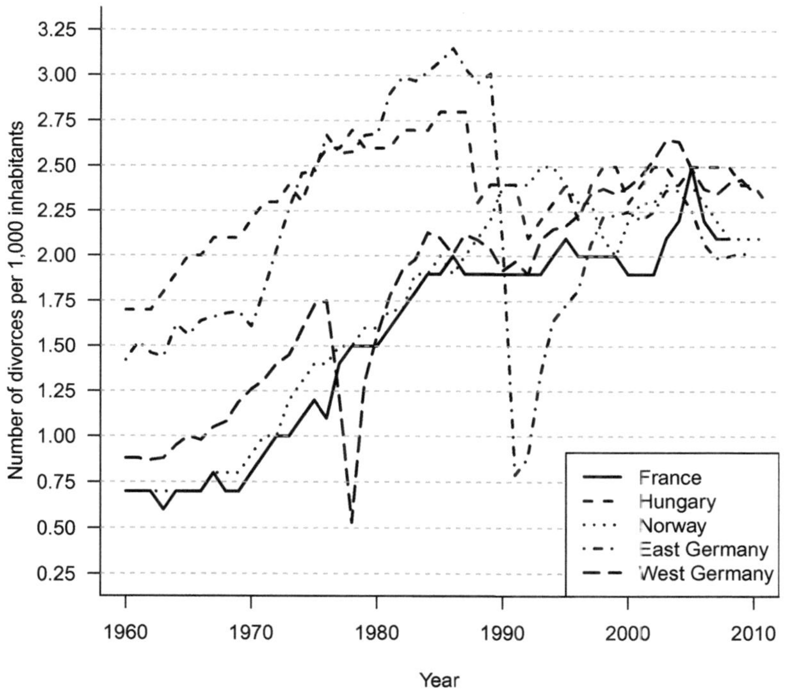

Sources: Eurostat 2012a, Federal Institute for Population Research 2012d.

3 Religion and Religiosity

Clear and precise definitions serve as arguments against an empiricist approach. Even if variables referring to religiosity have become rare in most data sets, their unreflected use has to be avoided to meet scientific requirements. Indicators of religiosity must be valid and reliable. Therefore, chapter 3 defines "religion" (3.1.1) and "religiosity" (3.1.2) and explains the multi-dimensional concept of religiosity. The second section deals with developments and factors that contribute to explaining diverging levels of religious vitality between the countries studied (3.2). The contexts within which religiosity takes place differ strongly. Therefore, it is important to compare them. The third section (3.3) reviews some studies analyzing the correlation between religiosity and fertility.

3.1 Definitions

3.1.1 Religion

The subsection can be subdivided into two parts. The first categorizes different definitions. Usually, they roughly belong to one of two main concepts of religion: either functional or substantive. The second part is concerned with the selected definition, a substantive one because it is more suitable in this context, and detailed explanations.

Finding an appropriate definition for religion has a long tradition in social sciences. A great many definitions already exist,[1] but the different scientific disciplines are still far from reaching agreement (e.g. Davie 2008: 19, Gabriel 2003: 112). Some even argue for abandoning the search for a definition and giving up the usage of the

[1] See e.g. the chronological overview of writings between 1873 and 2000 (Auffarth/Mohr 2006a: xxxiv–xxxv).

term "religion" in a scientific context (for details see Pollack 2003: 29). They criticize that it was coined in the modern Western world and furthermore is Eurocentric. In this respect religion cannot be suitably defined without impressing religion with a Western seal. Auffarth/Mohr 2006b write: "it has been formulated from the viewpoint of a Western-ancient-Christian vantage. More exactly: it is a concept of 'Christian object-speech', that is applied 'exclusivistically' within that speech (...)" (p. 1610). Religious science started to apply religion as a comparative concept of meta-speech in religious studies. According to Riesebrodt, this argument is not convincing as religion is not a linguistic phenomenon. Religion can rather be found in the behavior of humans (Riesebrodt 2010: 73).

As just mentioned, two kinds of concepts exist: substantive and functional definitions. The substantive method defines religion with regard to contents and tries to identify the characteristic traits that constitute religion as a delimitable subject area. It asks: What is the essence of religion? Which is the object of reference? For example, Max Weber 1922 implicitly worked from a substantive perspective. The most frequent point of reference is (the experience of) the "sacred" which demarcates the "profane".[2] In substantive definitions of religion the reference to "the godly", "God" or belief in the existence of a "transcendence" or a "transcendental power" is more specific (Gabriel 2003: 110–111). The reference may be monotheistic, polytheistic, pantheistic, even atheistic[3], etc. One example of a definition from the substantive point of view is "any shared set of beliefs, activities and institutions premised upon faith in supernatural forces" (Stark/Bainbridge 1985: 5). An early substantive definition originates from Durkheim: "A religion is a unified system of beliefs and practices relative to sacred things (...)"[4] (Durkheim 1965 [1915]: 46). Dobbelaere picked up the latter definition and altered it into: "(...) relative to a supra-empirical, transcendent reality"[5] (Dobbelaere 2004: 52).

[2] The "sacred" is not generally acknowledged as a scientifically suitable category. Sacredness definitely also depends on context, is subjective and hence a blurred category (Pollack 2003: 32).

[3] There seems to be no clear and precise definition of atheistic. In this context, atheism means, on the one hand, the denial of god or gods but not a complete denial of transcendence and things or events that exceed the material world.

[4] The rest of the definition is functionalist: "... that is to say, things set apart and surrounded by prohibitions – beliefs and practices that unite its adherents in a single moral community called a church" (Durkheim 1965 [1915]: 46).

[5] While the rest is also functionalist and more general than Durkheim's definition: "(...) that unites all those who adhere to it into a single moral community" (Dobbelaere 2004: 52).

In contrast, the functional concept specifies functions: religion is what fulfills those functions. The concept points to individuals' problems or situations that occur in the lives of humans and which can be solved with religion (Luhmann 1977: 9–10). What does religion accomplish? Kaufmann tried to establish an exhaustive list of functions (Kaufmann 1989: 82–88 and Kaufmann 2004 228–230):

1. the function to establish identity – religion helps to cope with fear and to pass through crisis situations;
2. the function to guide actions – rituals, values, principles, and norms offer orientation in exceptional situations;
3. the function to cope with contingency – to deal with and manage affliction, sorrow, harm, and strokes of fate;
4. the function of social integration and community building – it assures social cohesion;
5. the function to offer consistent principles of world interpretation;
6. the function of individual distancing from given social conditions – to be able to criticize injustice and unethical behavior (in society).

Kaufmann suggests to denote "something" as religion or religious if it performs more than one of the specified functions. It is not necessary to fulfill all functions simultaneously.

The functional definition proposed by Luckmann 1970 is known as one of the broadest definitions of religion and intends to encompass a widest possible spectrum of complexes, institutions, and social forms that fulfill "religious" functions. According to him, religion comprises all meaning structures that transform humans into socially and morally acting beings by transcending their biological nature through the human organism (Luckmann 1970: 47–53). Religion can be found everywhere where human behavior comprises actions that can be morally judged and where integration is accomplished in a meaningful manner. The function of religion is to involve the individual in a cosmos of meaning that transcends the single person (Luckmann 1970: 75; see also Gabriel 2003: 112 and Pollack 2003: 42–43). Functional definitions aim at broadening the definition beyond institutionalized forms of religion (mainly the institution "Christian Church"). This is in order to integrate alternative equivalents because no institution performs all functions the churches fulfilled in earlier times. In Luckmann's opinion, religion is an anthropological constant (Luckmann 1970: 41–50). That means, it is a precondition of existence and of the self; secularization, that is the loss of significance of religion and religiosity, is by definition excluded from happening (Pollack 2003: 6, Pollack 1996: 59). However, this is not the general view of functionalists (see e.g. Luhmann 2002: 126).

Substantive and functional approaches have benefits as well as shortcomings. Substantive definitions are accused of being restricted to the involvement of or reference to supernatural beings. Critics remark on not to use supernaturalism as a decisive feature when defining or identifying religion: "Such an emphasis is likely to exclude a whole range of activities or behaviour which – to the participants at least – take on the character of 'sacred' even if the supernatural as such is not involved" (Davie 2008: 20). The reference has the advantage to strongly correspond to historic religions (Pollack 2003: 32). A further point of criticism from the functional perspective refers to the impossibility of sociology as empirical science to make a statement on characteristic traits of religion since they are beyond the sphere of its competence (Gabriel 2003: 110).

Proponents of substantive concepts criticize various aspects of the functional approach. Religion is dogmatically credited with functions it neither always nor universally fulfills: "The functions of religion are as various as its different social and political conditions" (Riesebrodt 2010: xiii), i.e. religion does not have the same functions in all social systems. Frequently, the focus is on modern, Western societies although religion is of course a global phenomenon and cannot be restricted to the West. In fact, functional definitions do not explain religion but society since Luckmann claims that "religion is a necessary condition for society or the self and has a necessary function in maintaining them" (Riesebrodt 2010: 74). By arguing this way, religion advances to an indispensable precondition of human and social existence. The functional argument – religion constitutes and reproduces society – does not make sense from the point of view of the theory of action because it ignores the meaning of religious practices (Riesebrodt 2010: 73).

Functional definitions are rather unspecific and involve too many phenomena that can hardly be subsumed under the term religion. They also comprise other (non-religious) institutions, phenomena, and social forms fulfilling one or more "religious" functions (in modern, functionally separated societies) which cannot be understood as religion or religious according to the everyday understanding of religious adherents. The adherents' self-concept is ignored. This is the main point of criticism of researchers who prefer a substantive definition. The concept is not only too broad, it is also too narrow as it excludes several forms of religious practices and activities insofar they do not fulfill integrative functions or contribute to identity (see e.g. Spiro 1966: 95–96, Goody 1961: 151–152, 161, Pollack 2003: 43, Riesebrodt 2010: 112, Luhmann 1977: 9–10). In case "something" loses its religious function, it ceases to be religion. Religious contents and religious functions can consequently fall apart (Pollack 2003: 8–9). Arbitrariness dominates the definition hence while consistency is lacking.

The definition of religion selected as adequate in this work follows Riesebrodt who states:

> Religion is a complex of practices that are based on the premise of the existence of superhuman powers, whether personal or impersonal, that are generally invisible (Riesebrodt 2010: 74–75).

It is basically substantive but also takes parts over from interpretive sociology. All further explanations and information rely on Riesebrodt's theory of religion (2010). Interpretive sociology is an approach that has been rarely applied when it comes to theoretical statements about religion (Blasi 1998, Clarke 2009: 229–279). It assumes that an issue can only be understood if the researcher tries to consider and describe it from within. Therefore, it frequently emerges in anthropological and cultural studies (Pollack 2003: 37–39). Riesebrodt's social scientific definition draws on the one from Spiro 1966, but extends it by impersonal powers, claims universality, and convinces for several reasons. By its specific meaning – the reference to superhuman powers whose existence is the religious premise – religious and non-religious actions can be distinguished from each other. The powers are ascribed to influence human life and the natural environment. Furthermore, they elude direct human control. Riesebrodt 2010 argues that human beings have distinguished interactions with superhuman powers from all other forms of action at all times in history (pp. xii, 71, 75).

The definition demarcates religion from religiosity on the one hand and from religious traditions on the other. Religious traditions refer to the historical continuity of symbol systems (Riesebrodt 2010: xii). Christianity, Islam, Hinduism, Buddhism, etc. do not refer to a single system of practices but to traditions and continuous symbol systems that contain coherent systems of practices which intend to interact with superhuman powers (p. 14–15).

> To be precise, all religions in the traditional sense of the concept are actually religious traditions that have produced or contributed to a multiplicity of

religions in the empirical, historical sense of given complexes of practices (Riesebrodt 2010: 77).

In this respect religious traditions are more comprehensive than religions and also include ethnic and cultural elements. In a sociological perspective, religion is not a theologically constructed tradition, but an empirically given system of actions. Therefore, Riesebrodt criticizes the majority of substantive definitions for neglecting religious practices. His definition sidesteps the second argument mentioned above against substantive definitions: according to his concept, religion is indeed completely empirically measurable. However, it is not one of the usual substantive definitions because Riesebrodt does not specify the essence of religion to declare all of them being equal. Instead, Riesebrodt intends to make them comparable by revealing the structure of meaning that underlies all religions (pp. xii–xiii, 1). Finally, it is important to him to take account of the prevalent understanding of religion and the adherents' self-concept (p. 74).

Religious practices are meaningful, that is, they are "situated in a relatively systematic web of meaning". It is necessary that they are systematically interpretable (Riesebrodt 2010: 72). There are three sorts of practices: interventionist, discursive, and behavior-regulating practices. Interventionist practices enable to interact with or to gain access to superhuman powers with the aid of culturally specified means. That is, they vary between different (religious) cultures and traditions. There are four types of interactions with superhuman powers: (1) liturgies, prayers, vows, divination, sacrifices, chants, gestures, etc., (2) manipulation e.g. by wearing amulets or performing magical acts, (3) temporary interaction or even fusion with superhuman powers, e.g. mystical trance or ascetic ecstasy, and (4) activation of superhuman potential (Riesebrodt 2010: 75–76). The last two interaction types are mainly reserved for religious virtuosos. Discursive practices are the foundation of world interpretation and theology in a broad sense. They contribute to passing on and also to revising existing knowledge to following generations (Riesebrodt 2010: 75). Theologies therefore play a crucial role in the maintenance and reproduction of religion in the process of socialization.

Behavior-regulating practices comprise rules of conduct, codes, principles, and norms that have to be obeyed in everyday life with respect to the will of superhuman powers considering that the powers are able to sanction non-compliance. The forms of practices and cults, i.e. liturgies denoting the totality of ceremonies, rites, activities, and practices, are institutionalized. This means that rules exist regarding the communication of humans with superhuman powers. This is virtually a precondition to understand the meaning that underlies religious practices (Riesebrodt 2010: xii–xiii, 14, 116). The meaning of liturgies is contained in the promise of religion. Usually, religions claim to ward off harm and misfortune, to cope with crises, and they promise to provide salvation. In contrast to functionalist concepts, Riesebrodt is not concerned with functions of religion but its promise, one that is constant in historical periods and cultures irrespective of socio-political conditions (Hunt 2011: 76).

To conclude, religion has a social character. This is widely accepted by representatives of substantive definitions but mainly rejected by those of functional methods. The systematic coherence of religious practices may not only be perceived subjectively by the practicing individual but also by others, at least the community. The systematics has hence to be (socially) institutionalized to a certain extent.

3.1.2 Religiosity

As with religion, there are many definitions of religiosity. Riesebrodt defines religiosity as "subjective acquisition and interpretation of religion" (Riesebrodt 2010: 76). He comprehends "religious actions" as those whose meaning is characterized by referring to superhuman powers. Therefore, individuals can act religiously without practicing religion because religious actions do not presuppose the systematic coherence religion requires. Another definition is: "Religiosity is an individual trait that expresses the degree of agreement with the values, norms, and corresponding consequences of behavior specified by one's religion" (Kecskes/Wolf 1993: 272). These definitions of religiosity are, however, not satisfactory from a psychological point of view because the psychology of religion settles the definition of religiosity (see James 1925, Wulff 1991). Furthermore, most definitions ignore the adherents' subjective interpretations of religions which may even be contradictory.

Religiosity can be grasped as a personal construct that depends on two parameters: centrality and contents (Huber 2003: 17, 144, 193). Religious experience and behavior of an individual are determined on the one hand by the strength or centrality[6] of the religious construct within the personality and, on the other hand, by the theological contents and patterns of interpretation that are active within it. The

[6] Centrality means the centrality of theological contents (Huber 2003: 152). This will be explained later in more detail.

contents direct (religious) experience and behavior of individuals.[7] Huber builds a synthesis of two models of religiosity (p. 195): the personality psychological theory of Allport 1961 is the broad base for the theoretical framework and the phenomenological multi-dimensional measurement model of Glock and Stark operationalizes religiosity and measures it empirically (Glock/Stark 1965). They act on different theoretical perspectives and concepts but are complementary. Combining the models overcomes their theoretical and methodical shortcomings. Therefore, Huber applies another (non-religious) psychological concept as a consistent foundation of the framework which is based on Kelly (1955).

Following Kelly's concept of personal constructs,[8] he postulates that "a person's processes are psychologically channelized by the ways in which he anticipates events" (Kelly 1955: 46, 103). Processes are e.g. experiences, thoughts, perceptions, and behavior. Kelly describes everyday life as conducted by subjective theories or constructions of reality which can be understood as personal constructs. Their main function is to "anticipate and evaluate events by construing their replications" (Kelly 1955: 50, 103). This means that the constructs are based on past experience or observations. As "hypotheses" they are repeatedly tested against reality and adjusted when necessary. Amendments and reconstructions of constructs change future anticipations and can be understood as learning process.

The process of construing involves the interpretation of "something", i.e. a detail or part of reality (Huber 2003: 181). A construct defines a limited number of events and situations that can be construed by its means. Constructs can be e.g. physiological, ethical, or physical (Huber 2003: 181). A construct is religious when "something" refers to an ultimate reality or instance or authority (Huber 2003: 182, 190). This ultimate reality can be e.g. "God" in Abrahamic religious traditions. In this way, a

[7] They can hence be in large part explained by the effect that both parameters of the religious construct, which are closely linked with each other, vary (Huber 2003: 144, 194, 212). Effectiveness of theological interpretation schemes depends on the degree of centrality working in that construct (Huber 2003: 152).

[8] The psychology of personal constructs is a personality theory of which several exist. They can be grouped. Kelly's theory can be considered a cognitive personality theory (Boeree 2006). The underlying concept is constructive alternativism. It is the idea that "while there is only one true reality, reality is always experienced from one or another perspective, or alternative construction" (Boeree 2006: 3). A construction is "a perspective on [a small part of] the ultimate reality, and has some value to that person in that time and place" (p. 3). Constructions are helpful concepts of reality. "There are an infinite number of alternative constructions one may take towards the world" (p. 3). As experiences repeat, constructions are altered from time to time which is associated with a learning effect.

religious construct can be differentiated from all other constructs individuals use (Huber 2003: 183).

Religiosity as a personal construct depends on two parameters, the first one being "centrality". It embodies the significance of the religious construct of reality for an individual (Huber 2003: 144). The more central the religious construct is anchored within the personal ensemble of hierarchically arranged constructs, the more it determines individual experience, behavior, and other, subordinate constructs; and the less it is determined by other constructs (Huber 2003: 144, 187–188, 195). The sum of constructs builds a person's personality. The number of constructs that are subordinate to the religious construct increases with the centrality of the religious construct. This also means that the number of life spheres determined or at least influenced by religious constructs of reality rises. A personality in which the religious construct has such a central position can be referred to as "highly religious" (Huber 2003: 188). The more constructs are superordinate to the religious one, the more it can be assumed that an individual has a "non-religious" personality.

The basic idea of the religiosity definition originates from Allport 1950. According to his concept of intrinsic and extrinsic religiosity, religiosity is a value that may be differently anchored in the personality of an individual. If religiosity is a central value of a person, Allport refers to it as intrinsic religious motivation.[9] Religion plays a central role in the life of an individual. "(...) Perhaps the briefest way to characterize the two poles of subjective religion is to say that the extrinsically motivated person uses his religion, whereas the intrinsically motivated lives his religion" (Allport/Ross 1967: 434). It determines the self-perception, and directs and regulates behavior in everyday life. The difference between extrinsic and intrinsic religiosity is that in the latter case a functionally autonomous religious motivational system exists (Huber 2003: 51–52). Three features characterize a functionally autonomous religious motivational system: (1) religious self-perception, (2) strong influence on other (non-religious) life spheres, and (3) intense religious experience and behavior. They offer potential to derive indicators to find out someone's religious orientation. Functional autonomy means that motivational impulses assert themselves independent of external circumstances,

[9] Intrinsic religiosity is an ideal type of religious orientation and is characterized by the individual's aspiration to internalize religious or theological creed and realize these within their actions (Allport/Ross 1967). The process of internalization has already proceeded so far as that religious creed builds the most important motivational system within a personality and all other motives and motivational systems are subordinate to it.

that means irrespective of the surrounding frame and general conditions, e.g. in a country. The more intensely and frequently an individual expresses religiosity, the higher the probability that she or he is directed by a functionally autonomous religious motivational system. This is the point where Glock's model supplements Allport's model as it claims to involve all the important forms that religiosity can be expressed in (Huber 2003: 171). A religious individual wants to behave religiously and to express her or his religiosity, and these forms of expression are empirically measurable.

Allport refers to an extrinsic religious motivation if religiosity is a minor value in the personality of an individual. Religion does not play a central role in the life of this individual. His or her self-perception is determined by other values. Religious creed is – if at all – solely marginally anchored in personality. Even if it were activated, it serves other motives and motivational systems it is subordinate to. Extrinsic religiosity has more an instrumental or utilitarian character (Allport/Ross 1967: 434). Religious values merely direct behavior sporadically in everyday life. If an individual behaves religiously, his or her motivation is driven by other values. As experience and behavior differ in both quantitative and qualitative perspective according to whether an individual is intrinsically or extrinsically religious, it is reasonable to distinguish them systematically and to seek the motivational anchorage of religiosity (Huber 2003: 170). This is possible with the aid of Kelly's concept. A central position of the religious construct can be understood as a functionally autonomous religious motivational system (Huber 2003: 189). That is, intrinsically motivated religiosity can be expected when the religious construct constitutes one of the central ones. Experience and behavior are then influenced in a genuine manner and the influence is not restricted by superordinate constructs. An extrinsically motivated religiosity can be expected from the perspective of psychological constructs only if the religious construct has a subordinate status.

While the psychological models of Allport and Kelly build the theoretical framework, the sociological model from Glock and Stark helps to measure religiosity and to derive centrality from the religious construct empirically. It therefore offers an answer to the question whether an individual has a functionally autonomous religious motivational system. Glock and Stark regard religiosity as "commitment" that expresses itself – phenomenologically – in several forms (Glock 1962, Glock/Stark 1965, Stark/Glock 1968). According to them, religiosity is multi-dimensional. The model claims to specify all fundamental forms in which individuals can express religiosity.

They may be differently weighted in the existing religious traditions but do basically exist in each (Huber 2003: 92). Glock and Stark call them the core dimensions. They are simultaneously autonomous and mutually dependent (Huber 2003: 172, 175). However, in two cases religiosity seems to be one-dimensional: in the highly religious and in the completely irreligious case. In the first case all dimensions exhibit high intensities or frequencies, in the second case all dimensions show very low values and are hence (almost) perfectly correlated with each other (Huber 2003: 153, 156). Six dimensions of commitment can be distinguished:

(1) The dimension of belief or religious ideology: Each religious individual is expected to agree with certain belief statements that are usually not empirically verifiable. They refer to the existence and nature of (a) superhuman power(s) and vary by religion (Stark/Glock 1968: 14–15, 57–58; Huber 2003: 100, 122, 132).
(2) The dimension of ritual (worship): Ritual is one of two forms of religious practices and can be defined as "... set of rites, formal religious acts, and sacred practices which all religions expect their adherents to perform" (Stark/Glock 1968: 15). As it is a phenomenon of socially shared action patterns, this dimension integrates individuals into a social network that may serve as a social resource.
(3) The dimension of devotion (prayer): The second dimension of religious practice is similar to but also different from ritual in major respects. "While the ritual aspect of commitment is highly formalized and typically public, all known religions also value personal acts of worship and contemplation which are relatively spontaneous, informal, and typically private" (Stark/Glock 1968: 15). The definition already specifies the differences between the two forms. Worship therefore necessarily has a social dimension that requires several individuals to be executed. Prayer, in contrast, is somewhat more personal and can be carried out privately (Stark/Glock 1968: 81). But it is also a phenomenon of socially shared action patterns (Huber 2009: 30). However, it allows a greater flexibility in manner and frequency of execution as well as in its form.
(4) The dimension of religious experience: It considers that "the properly religious person will at some time or other achieve a direct, subjective knowledge of ultimate reality; that he will achieve some sense of contact, however fleeting, with a supernatural agency" (Stark/Glock 1968: 15). Religious experience can be feelings, perceptions, and sensations that involves some contact or "communication,

however slight, with a divine essence, that is, with God, with ultimate reality, with transcendental authority" (Stark/Glock 1968: 15).

(5) The dimension of religious knowledge or cognitive interest: It can be expected that religious individuals "possess (...) information about the basic tenets of their faith and its rites, scriptures, and traditions" (Stark/Glock 1968: 16). As there is a great variety of areas of knowledge, this dimension can also be – more broadly – understood as general cognitive interest as well as intensity and manner in which someone deals with religious matters and questions (Huber 2009: 22). Glock assumes that individuals with a pronounced knowledge are less religious with respect to other dimensions of religiosity and the other way round. Individuals who know little, show higher religiosity with respect to the remaining dimensions (Huber 2003: 111).

(6) The dimension of consequences for daily life (consequential dimension): Religious individuals are not only characterized by specific religious experience and behavior. It can be assumed that religious norms, attitudes, and behavior-regulating rules – if observed – "shape the way they lead their daily lives" (Huber 2009: 34). As opposed to the first five core dimensions, the scope of this dimension is less delimitable. Purity, dress or dietary laws can be relatively easily distinguished. But also a large variety of everyday life situations that are assumed to be influenced by religiosity can be subsumed under this dimension. As a result, this dimension encompasses a very broad and heterogeneous set of phenomena (Huber 2009: 34). The consequential dimension can be measured by variables that are frequent subjects of empirical research including (life) satisfaction and well-being, health, drug consumption, leisure time, socialization of children, coping with life crises, and dealings with key events in the family, like birth, marriage, or death. This also means that indicators of the consequential dimension are rather treated as dependents – as is the case in this work. Hence, a different character can be attributed to this dimension.

Beyond these dimensions, religious affiliation, i.e. the religious tradition an individual follows as well as religious socialization, measure religiosity. Religious affiliation can be understood as the base category of religiosity. Empirical research shows that parents are by far the strongest influencing factor on later religiosity (Huber 2009: 39). Moreover, each religious dimension mentioned above is also associated with religious socialization. This is principally a precondition for religiosity in adulthood, e.g. a deeper interest in religious matters or vital practice (Bisin/Verdier 2000, Bisin/Verdier 2010). Individuals who were not religiously socialized and educated can hardly pass on religious traditions, knowledge, and values to their own children. The correlation is very pronounced but far from being perfect: not all individuals who were raised religiously socialize their own children religiously (Pickel 2011: 187). Among other factors, it is the cultural and religious surroundings in which children are socialized that form future preferences.

A problem of Glock and Stark's model is that it does not consider the centrality of religiosity (Huber 2003: 145). A centrality index can however be easily derived from the intensity and degree of importance of the (equally weighted) first five dimensions of religiosity (Huber 2003: 144, 152, 174, 195–201).[10] The multi-dimensional structure receives a one-dimensional center by creating a simple additive index. It is a measure that provides information on the subjective importance of theological contents as well as the hierarchical status of the religious construct. It can be assumed that intrinsic religious motivation and centrality of the religious construct increase approximately proportionately (Huber 2003: 197). The higher the value of the index is, the higher the probability that the personality is functionally autonomous. This reconstruction of Glock and Stark's multi-dimensional measurement model to include the calculation of a centrality index leads to the integration of Allport's personality psychological approach. The procedure of measuring centrality enables to categorically differentiate intrinsic, extrinsic, and non-religious personalities in the sense of Allport. Huber refers to them – due to the alteration of the theoretical concept – as "highly religious" (the religious construct is functionally autonomous in that case), "religious" (the religious construct is functionally heteronomous), and "non-religious" (the religious construct is marginal; Huber 2003: 170–171).

In addition to centrality, the theological contents – what an individual exactly believes – is the second parameter the religious construct depends on. It determines the direction of experience and behavior (while centrality determines the strength). The contents of the construct cannot be measured by using the dimensional concept. Other methods have to be applied, e.g. a categorical mode, because theological interpretation schemes are not "increasable" like frequencies (Huber 2003: 131, 152, 168, 173, 202). There is a very great variety of possible contents that can be collected.[11]

---

[10] The consequential dimension is not part of the centrality index (Huber 2009: 19).

[11] Huber criticizes (p. 175) that neither Allport nor Glock considered the various, alternative possibilities of theological construct processes. This means that this aspect of individual

3.2 Factors associated with a nation's level of religiosity

Following on from the definitions of "religion" and "religiosity" this section focuses on factors contributing to explaining a nation's degree of religiosity.[12] Differences in the vitality of religiosity seem to be predominantly caused by three historical-cultural patterns that closely interact with each other (see e.g. Pickel 2003, Pickel 2009):

1. a country's level of modernization,
2. state-church relations, and
3. the dominating denominational cultural tradition.

Since the works of Max Weber, the degree of modernization has been closely associated with secularization. Different levels need to be distinguished in order to understand the relevance of religious traditions and the vitality of religiosity in a country. The effects of state-church relations can be well shown on the basis of the selected countries because they all differ in this respect. The third factor mainly concentrates on different traits between Protestantism and Catholicism from which the higher religiosity of Catholics can be partly derived. To conclude, possible explanations for the higher religiosity of Muslims are stated. Before discussing the three historical-cultural patterns, the concept of secularization which indicates the national degree of religiosity will be clarified. All subsections end with indicators that measure a specific factor. The last subsection compares all countries with each other and describes the patterns responsible for current societal religious vitality.

---

religiosity is not sufficiently considered as a central theme. But it should be since "for all religions it can be said that theology or religious belief is at the heart of faith" (Huber 2003: 128). One example, among many others, might be helpful: God is the central symbol or ultimate reality in Abrahamic religious cultures and traditions. But it does not suffice to merely ask for the intensity of belief in God. The question is still too general and requires further specification since God can be construed or interpreted differently. It is also possible that different notions of God contradict each other. The symbol can be specified by such attributes like omnipotence, justice, mercifulness, love, wrath, and jealousy. The individual notion of God hence depends on the attribute and the accompanying construction process (Huber 2003: 192). From those possibilities of construing theological contents it follows that orientating effects of the religious construct may lead in very diverging directions. For this reason, it seems advisable to operationalize and measure alternative religious contents (p. 193).

12 These factors determine not only the social relevance of religion but principally also individual religiosity.

3.2.1 Secularization

Statements on secularization – the decreasing relevance of religious institutions, religion and religiosity for society and individuals – have to distinguish three levels: the societal or macrolevel, the organizational or mesolevel, and the individual or microlevel.[13] Societal secularization, defined in a broader theoretical perspective, refers to

> the shrinking relevance of the values, institutionalized in church religion, for the integration and legitimation of everyday life in modern society (Dobbelaere 2004: 19, see also Luckmann 1970: 39–40).

In Luckmann's terminology, to draw on another definition, societal secularization is "a process in which autonomous institutional ideologies replaced within their own domain, an overarching and transcendent universe of norms" (Luckmann 1970: 101). Thirdly, it can also be conceptualized as

> a process of functional differentiation, i.e. a process of growing independence of societal spheres (such as politics, education, economy, and science), each developing its own rationale, which implies the rejection of the overarching claim of religion (Dobbelaere 2004: 27).

Before this process began "it may be said that nearly all the great social institutions have been born in religion" (Durkheim 1965 [1915]: 466).[14] The latter definition is most tangible. Societal secularization can occur as a latent or as a manifest process. As a latent process, it was the unintended consequence of actions that promoted functional differentiation. Religion became one subsystem alongside others. In contrast, laicization is a manifestly intended process (Dobbelaere 2004: 19–20). For example, socialism and communism can be understood as manifest actions to secularize societies.

Organizational secularization (mesolevel) can be described as the self-initiated modernization of religious traditions and institutions. On the one hand, this concerns the adjustments of teachings, beliefs, morals, and rituals. On the other hand, it affects

[13] However, this division ignores smaller geographical entities "below" the macrolevel where religious traditions can still be more powerful than in other regions.

[14] This refers to the extent to which subsystems such as the legal, the political, the education system, etc. are modern, autonomous or independent of the church and follow their own logic, values, and "laws".

structures that are subject to bureaucratization to ensure efficient procedures and not to waste resources. This is due to changes and developments in the world. It is equal to a decline in church orthodoxy (Dobbelaere 2004: 21, 35).[15] The need for such steps can be seen in the effort to prevent the loss of adherents.

Individual secularization can be defined as

> a decline in the extent to which people engage in religious practices, display beliefs of a religious kind, and conduct other aspects of their lives in a manner informed by such beliefs (Bruce 2002: 3).

It takes place when important transitions in the course of life – e.g. birth, marriage, and burial – cease to be sacralized, i.e. when fewer people participate in religious ceremonies at turning points in life. Affiliates pray less frequently, believe less in the truth of holy scriptures, and they are less integrated in the religious bodies (Dobbelaere 2004: 25). Furthermore, individual secularization includes the decreasing agreement between the attitudes, values, and conduct of adherents with the norms of their denomination. Normative guidelines lose importance in daily life. Altogether, it means a decline in individual religiosity, commitment, and cohesive force. Findings show that the several dimensions of religiosity developed differently. That means, processes of individual secularization do not affect all dimensions of religiosity simultaneously or equally strongly (Huber 2009). The decline in frequencies of church attendance can therefore not automatically be interpreted as declining religiosity in total. Perhaps it is just a shift from one dimension of religiosity to another. Usually, individual secularization is an inter-generational and not an intra-generational process (Dobbelaere 2004: 190). It does not happen within the same individual over the course of life. This does not exclude that the forms of expression change within a lifetime. One exception may be forced secularization, i.e. laicization.[16]

[15] Frequently it is argued that American churches have succeeded in keeping a central symbolic position and keeping their members actively participating in church congregational activities only by secularizing themselves internally (e.g. Berger 1969: 33–37). However, this is a case of circular reasoning: if it is not the church adherents that reduce their involvement, it must be the churches that secularize themselves.

[16] Casanova distinguishes three kinds of use of the term secularization (Casanova 1994: 211–214): it can firstly target a decreasing significance of religiosity, i.e. sinking relevance of religious practices and cohesive force of religious norms for actions in everyday life, political orientation and public order. Secondly, the term can aim at privatizing religion, i.e. retreat from the public to the private sphere. Thirdly, it can refer to a detachment or liberation of societal spheres from the control of the churches (institutional and constitutional especially separation of church and state). This differentiation received great attention but it remains

Societal secularization in particular, but also individual secularization can be thought to precede organizational secularization and insofar are a precondition. Several authors assume that the (aggregated) microlevel is associated with the social importance of religious traditions and religiosity (see e.g. Bruce 2002: 3, Dobbelaere 2004: 165–172, and Müller 2008: 64).[17] The methodological advantage of the distinction between different levels of secularization helps to understand why in one country the churches have a strong impact on policy-making and public opinion while religiosity of its inhabitants is weak, and in another country a strict state-church separation is associated with a high degree of religious vitality of its people.

3.2.2 Modernization

Max Weber 1930 [1904] was – alongside Émile Durkheim – first to postulate that the relationship between modernization and religiosity is probably tense. Progress and developments have contributed to the social decline of the significance of religious traditions and religiosity, as well as the stability and vitality of religious groups and practices. The level of modernization is still presumed to be the central indicator for secularization processes (Pickel 2009: 95–97).[18]

Not only secularization is a multi-faceted concept. Modernization is also a complex phenomenon. In general, modernization has often been equated with processes of democratization, industrialization, rationalization of economy including the emergence and development of a social welfare state,[19] urbanization, individualization, etc. But this list is rather unspecific and vague. Three types of modernization can be distinguished (Voas 2008): material, institutional, and ideological modernization.

unclear what e.g. "decreasing significance" really means, i.e. which of the three levels according to Dobbelaere is exactly referred to.

[17] These authors represent the secularization theory, while proponents of the individualization theory contest the association. They argue that the loss of significance of religious traditions merely takes place at the societal level and concerns the well-established churches while the individuals themselves remain religious. The kind of religiosity is rather diffuse, unstable, and subjective (see e.g. Luckmann 1970, Hervieu-Léger 1998, and Davie 2002).

[18] Several researchers on the sociology of religion have distanced themselves from simple causality statements regarding the association between modernity or modernization and religiosity. Popular ascriptions in this context are de-privatization (Casanova 1994), resacralization, de-secularization (e.g. Berger et al. 2005), re-enchantment, and individualization as the most advanced and powerful approaches against the secularization approach.

[19] This process contributed by and by to the loss of a variety of welfare tasks previously executed by the Church, such as care for the elderly, poor, orphans and widows (Vellenga 2003: 204–205).

"Material modernization is fairly straightforwardly economic and relates to the level, dispersion, and security of well-being" (Voas 2008: 32). He ascribes the least direct effect to material modernization and writes that becoming richer does not necessarily mean becoming less religious. Norris and Inglehart argue that human security – as another part of material modernization – determines the degree of religiosity very well. They argue that feelings of vulnerability to physical, societal, and personal risks are a key factor driving religiosity (Norris/Inglehart 2007: 33, 45). Their approach aims at explaining the great difference in the degree of religiosity between great parts of Europe and the USA, a country usually referred to as highly developed and modern. Religious commitment bestows security and keeps individuals grounded in an existence-threatening and insecure setting. Social security is not guaranteed by the state in the form of a social safety net and economic inequality is extremely pronounced.[20]

Institutional modernization, the second feature of modernization, is basically synonymous with functional differentiation. It has lead to a loss of power and universal interpretational sovereignty of the churches as well as a decline of the significance of religious norms whose progression is path- and nation-dependent. Finally, the third feature of modernization, the ideological one, "is a matter of the degree to which authority has been displaced by individualism and a scientific and democratic world view has taken hold" (Voas 2008: 32). In his law of three stages, Auguste Comte postulated in the 19th century that the scientific world view will completely replace the religious (first stage) and metaphysical (second stage) world views. The third feature also comprises early processes of individualization. Traditional family ties and local or rural communities began to weaken at the time of urbanization and industrialization. One consequence was growing individual empowerment (Voas 2008: 35).

Church-related religiosity has decreased in the course of the last decades. The Christian churches have been suffering from the loss of members. In Germany, where Christians of any denomination are official, church tax paying members, this is especially verifiable. But while secularization theorists link the decline of church-related forms of religiosity to the social decline of religiosity in modern societies generally, proponents of functional definitions come to another conclusion (e.g. Davie 2008: 3). In their opinion, religion merely change their social *gestalt* and turn to private,

[20] In less developed countries where the majority of inhabitants subsist on agriculture there are a lot more factors that threaten existential security.

non-institutionalized forms and practices of religiosity.[21] The explanatory power of the individualization theory is lowered by survey results in which self-identification as religious is correlated with the degree of religiosity (Gabriel 1996: 8, 11). Moreover, alternative forms of religiosity can be more frequently found in countries where church-related religiosity is also pronounced (Pickel 2011: 179). The individualization approach can hence not refute the correlation between modernization and secularization.

To conclude, the level of modernization can be compared across countries on the basis of their position in ranking of the Human Development Index (HDI). This is a prosperity index made up of indicators reflecting per capita income, life expectancy, and level of education. Of course it it not the most appropriate index to discriminate between European countries as they do not differ greatly in a global perspective. In the HDI, Norway ranked 1st between 2001 and 2006, and then reclaimed this position from 2009 through 2011 (United Nations Development Programme (UNDP) 2010). France and Germany are almost equal: both states are among the 15 most modern countries in the world (United Nations Development Programme (UNDP) 2009). Prior to transformation East Germany already had a relatively high socioeconomic development degree compared to other countries of Central and Eastern Europe, that means also compared to Hungary that can be understood as the least modern of the five countries of importance in this work. In 2010, Hungary ranked 36th (United Nations Development Programme (UNDP) 2010; 43rd in 2009). Per capita income in most of the 19 Hungarian counties is much lower than in the neighboring countries in the West – it amounts to almost US$13,000 while it is more than US$42,000 in France and Germany (The World Bank 2011). Life expectancy in Hungary was and still is considerably lower: in 2009 men's life expectancy at birth was 70.3 years (78.0 in France, 78.0 in Norway, 77.8 in Germany) and women's was 77.2 years (83.8 in France, 83.0 in Norway, 82.0 in Germany). Infant mortality rates and child poverty rates in Hungary were only slightly higher than in France, Germany, and Norway (Eurostat 2010a, OECD 2008). Finally, educational attainment of the population older than 25 in Hungary (36.5% had less than upper secondary, 48.9% had upper secondary or post-secondary non-tertiary and 14.7% had tertiary education) was lower than in Norway (14.5%, 53.8%, 31.7%) and Germany (21.5%, 57.1%, 21.4%), but higher

21 See especially Luckmann 1970 as a protagonist of the individualization approach. See also Davie 2008 who coined the slogan "believing without belonging" to characterize the current situation of religion, and Hervieu-Léger 1998 are further representatives.

than in France (42.6%, 35.9%, 19.8%; United Nations Development Programme (UNDP) 2009).

3.2.3 The political situation and state-church relations

The second factor that exerts an impact on religious vitality is the political situation, especially in cases where governments are anti-religious. A Marxist-Leninist-materialist ideology involving scientific atheism refuses and combats all kinds of religious traditions and religiosity as nonsense, contrary to state doctrine, and progress impeding (Knauft 1980: 83, Tomka/Zulehner 1999: 35). This was the case in most countries of Central and Eastern Europe (CEE) between 1949 and 1990. Christians were disadvantaged, stigmatized, socially segregated, and persecuted. The strength of repression as well as the degree of anti-church measures varied between the countries (Martin 1978, Pickel 2011).

Apart from totalitarian systems, other forms of church-state relations influence religious vitality: a strict separation of church and state and cooperative forms of relationships (e.g. concordat or state church) between them. Cooperative forms of legal organization seem to prove more favorable for religious vitality than a rigid separation (Pollack/Pickel 2009). For example, McCleary/Barro 2006 find that the presence of a state church raises religious participation and beliefs.

The strength of repression of the SED regime in the former GDR was intense and very successful in fighting religiosity. Various anti-clerical measures were implemented. In the GDR the goal of annihilating religiosity was pursued more systematically and more perseveringly than in most other socialist states (Jagodzinski 2000: 55). Public day care for children was emphatically promoted from an early stage in their life onwards. The political regime usurped children's socialization or nationalized it by special programs. They undermined intrafamily (religious) socialization to a large extent. This expanded the state's influence on children's attitudes and values (Jagodzinski 2000, Knauft 1980). The party succeeded in stopping the intrafamily process of handing down religious practices, knowledge, traditions, and values from the older to following generations to the greatest possible extent. Moreover, the SED prevented religious communication in intermediate (leisure or youth) groups. The consequence was accelerated – because actively promoted – secularization which is usually assumed to be a slow, continuous process (Dobbelaere 2004). In the case of East Germany one can assume that (individual) secularization is irreversible – the religious foundation has been destroyed sustainably. Christian teachers were forced to educate their pupils in materialist ideology and to request them to take part in the *Jugendweihe*, the secular rite replacing Christian confirmation in the GDR. Christians, and this was also the case in Hungary, also suffered from discrimination in the education systems. The consequence was their lower educational achievements as they were barred from attending higher educational facilities. In Hungary many – mainly old, educated – citizens were disadvantaged and persecuted (Tomka/Zulehner 1999: 35).

Socialism and its inherent church hostile ideology left marks on the behavior, attitudes, and in the minds of the citizens (Martin 1978). This can be substantiated by the absence of mass church re-entries (of older generations) or baptisms (of younger generations) after the system's breakdown. For many older citizens the question of re-entry did not arise due to far-reaching alienation. Maybe they left the church years before because of political pressure. However, the indoctrination of ideology led, by degrees, to the perception that religious ideas and imaginings are suspicious and absurd (Pollack 2000: 43–44).[22] In younger generations the lack of religious socialization in the family and the anti-church socialization outside of the family are unambiguously against baptism.

After 1990, the legal arrangement between state and church of West Germany was transferred to East Germany. Here, an additional reason can be held responsible for further church exits after transformation, namely the introduction of a church tax for members (Pollack 2000: 27). On the whole, the characteristic "without religious affiliation" means something very different in East and West Germany. In the West, the arrangement can be described as cooperative (Wick 2007: 3–27). This form of cooperation also includes religious education as a normal subject in schools.

---

[22] One reason why the regime was very successful in fighting religiosity was that at the end of World War I, the tradition "*cuius regio, eius religio*" ended (Gabriel 2003: 117–118). The ruler of a territory prescribed which denomination the population living in his territory had to follow. This tradition impeded the rooting of the Christian belief in the population (Gabriel/Kaufmann 1988: 32). After the civil revolution of 1848, freedom of religion became the first civil freedom which caused religion's privatization. The path to extreme de-churching, as in the GDR, was partly predetermined. First, the state stopped supporting the church. Secondly, the state turned to a church-hostile system that discriminated and stigmatized Christianity and excluded it from public life. Consequently, it may not be surprising that religiosity experienced a radical breakdown in regions where anti-church policies lasting 60 years (1934–1990) met the lack of anchoring of Christianity in folk culture.

In France, state and church are legally and institutionally separated (*laicité*).[23] *Laicité* is one of the basic principles of the French Republic and fixed in the constitution (see e.g. Schwartz 2007: 15–16).[24] The strict separation was the consequence of the French Revolution and of a Catholic Church experienced as too overpowering. This was symbolized e.g. by the additional ascription of an absolutist monarch "by the grace of god" (Vellenga 2003: 200, Wick 2007: 29–35). Official membership, church taxes, and religious education as a school subject do not exist.[25] The (Lutheran) Church of Norway was a state church from the time of the Reformation and until 2012. The state officially recognizes and strongly financially supports it. However, other religious groups are also subsidized. Traditionally, every citizen of Norway became a member of the Church of Norway upon birth (Fraser 2012).

3.2.4 Denominational characteristics and dominant cultural tradition

In countries with a Catholic cultural tradition, religiosity proves to be higher than in those with a Protestant or Orthodox tradition (see e.g. Martin 1978 and Tomka 2006). In Hungary, Catholics are in a religious perspective more observant than Lutherans, and even more than Reformed Christians (Tomka 2006: 48). "The more rigorous the criterion of religiosity, or the narrower the group to which 'religiousness' is applied, the higher the rate of the Catholics in comparison to Protestants" (Tomka 2006: 49).

[23] The relevant law was passed in 1905, amended five times, and it revoked the concordat enacted in 1802 (Fath 2007: 51).

[24] *Laicité* and *laicisme* have to be differentiated. While the first term is free of ideology and denotes the process of secularization, namely the emancipation of polity from the churches, the latter is an ideological concept and the independence of the state from the churches has the connotation of being militant, anti-clerical, even anti-religious (Dobbelaere 2004: 13). *Laicité* is linked to the three components freedom of conscience, equality of secular and religious orientations, and neutrality which is an objective description of the independence of the state from religious traditions and institutions. The state ensures the free exercise of religiosity, does not privilege and financially support particular denominations (Schwartz 2007: 16–19, Fath 2007: 49, Grosser 2009: 60, Bischof Stenger 2009: 69). However, it promotes the maintenance of churches built before 1905 while the church has to finance its newer churches and the salaries of its priests on its own (Grosser 2009: 58). Religious education in public schools does not exist; theology cannot be studied at state universities. In contrast, more than one sixth of all French pupils attend Catholic schools and there are far more applications than places. However, the wording of the law and social practice have to be distinguished. The separation is no long practiced that extremely: the presence of the church and theology in public life has become established, e.g. in ethics commissions or in the media (Nientiedt 2009: 126, Kranemann/Wijlens 2009: 9).

[25] Confessional state schools have not been allowed since 1904.

It seems to promote attachment and commitment to religious tradition and the church. Higher religiosity and a stronger cohesive force among Catholics have also been documented empirically (Müller 2008, Müller 2009). Therefore, the factor "cultural path dependency" has to be added to secularization approaches.

Protestantism possesses traits that may weaken religious activity (Graf 2007: 104–107). Weber linked the advent of capitalist societies by modernization processes to "the disenchantment of the world" (Weber 1919: 17). Where humans had previously resorted to magic to explain and interpret the world, now they turned to technology, knowledge, and calculation (Gerth/Mills 1958: 139). In Weber's opinion it was Protestantism, especially John Calvin's exegesis of scriptural predestination and the ascetic or Puritan work ethic that promoted the emergence of capitalism – provided that the material, economic, and social conditions were right (Weber 1930 [1904]). The Puritan work ethic arose from the observance of the predestination doctrine. By enabling modernization processes connected with ascetic work behavior that has gotten more and more self-evident, it rid itself of its religious legitimation. This process led to the modern economy's detachment from its religious roots (see Knoblauch 1999: 18–28). Independent of the extent of accordance with Weber's theory, it is acceptable to ascribe to Protestantism a higher degree of internal rationalization. While in subsection 3.2.2 secularization was described as a consequence of modernization processes, this explanation further specifies that modernization processes happened earlier in regions with a Protestant cultural tradition.

A second trait weakening religious vitality is the stronger anchorage of Protestantism in contemporary societies than Catholicism, which can also be grasped as a "this-worldliness" reference. Moreover, there is no strict delimitation towards the "external", the secular world outside of the church (Graf 2007: 86–87, 102). At the organizational level the degree of secularization is higher (Dobbelaere 2004). The more conservative and other-worldly religious teachings and theology are, the higher the commitment of the affiliates, which is (however) due to self-selection (Iannaccone 1994, Olson/Perl 2001).[26] The Catholic Church is more conservative from a theological perspective and prescribes affiliates' behavior both explicitly as well as

[26] Evangelical sects in the USA deliver good evidence of this (e.g. Assemblies of God, Southern Baptist). When the main church gets too "adjusted" to the secular outside world to remain attractive for mainstream affiliates, sects with strict rules come into existence. Above-average committed affiliates then sort themselves into one of these new sects while the boundary between internal and external mainstream church becomes more and more indistinct (Berger 1963). In Europe, where religiosity is much lower, Protestant sects do not exist

by general behavior-regulating practices much more strongly than the Protestant churches do. It is not only that the Catholic affiliates are more committed: since the time of the Reformation the Catholic Church has been better at keeping its sheep together. The avoidance of internal pluralization and disputes partially prevented further secularization (Dobbelaere 2004: 36–37, Graf 2007: 85–86).

Thirdly, from a theological perspective, in Catholicism the church is the mediator between God and the affiliates. The importance of the church in Protestantism is much lower (Graf 2007: 79, 88–93). It is not an institution that mediates salvation. Luther prioritized the pious individual over the church as an institution. A decisive difference between Calvinism and Catholicism is "the complete elimination of salvation through the Church and the sacraments" (Weber 1930 [1904]: 104–105, Kippenberg 2009). Protestants are much more bound by their own conscience in central questions of life. They are not required to celebrate mass on Sundays and partake in significant religious ceremonies to receive the sacrament of Eucharist. Protestantism is lacking the extensive social character of Catholicism, it is much more individualized as can be seen, for example, in its basic principles established by Luther *sola scriptura, sola fide, sola gratia, solus Christus, soli Deo gloria*, (Graf 2007: 90–92, Goujon et al. 2007: 244). The reference expressed in *sola scriptura* is associated with a critical attitude towards institutions (Graf 2007: 89, Huber 2003: 134). Church traditions are not endowed with normative orientational power in Protestantism.

Fourthly, Protestant and Orthodox churches are organized in the form of national or regional churches while the official residence of the Pope and the *Curia Romana* are situated outside of the single countries and therefore outside of government's possibility to encroach and to interfere. This structure eases independence of any national political situation. Protestant and Orthodox churches, on the contrary, can defend themselves less well against interference (Pickel 2011: 186, Tomka 2006: 51). Transnationally, the Catholic Church was more successful in coping with persecution than the Protestant churches were. Associated with the organizational structure is the synodal principle and the flatter hierarchy (Graf 2007: 85). An institution that is tightly organized and has a steep hierarchy is better able to communicate its doctrines and norms (McQuillan 2004). Moreover, it can protect itself better against secularizing influences than an institution with a grassroots democratic organization.

---

to a noteworthy extent. Church exits are much more probable than the emergence of a new sect or (church or sect) conversions.

Further reasons contribute to explaining the uneven de-churching of European societies and point to a historic path. Diverging ways of de-churching can be traced back to the building and development of religious mentalities a long time ago. Christianization of the Germanic peoples in Northern Europe in general happened usurpingly. This was not the case in Southern Europe. There, Christianity was basically adopted peacefully (Höllinger 1996: 133–138, Gabriel 2003: 114). These differences in religious mentalities still continue to have an effect in the present. Denominational differences in mentality in pre-industrial times can also be explained by the diverging way of dealing with traditions based on popular piety (Gabriel 2003: 115). In Catholicism, various interconnections between popular piety and the Church occurred, which strongly met the magic demands of the rural population and lower classes in urban areas. Protestantism was imprinted by urban middle classes and their interest in education and a rational arrangement of life conduct. They were distant to all forms of magic. Protestantism with its specific piety remained alien to the rural population and urban underclasses. Higher religiosity and stronger attachment to the Catholic Church can also be found here. Processes of de-churching already started in pre-industrial times, e.g. in Protestant towns (Gabriel 2003: 118).

Modernization processes were followed by the establishment of a Catholic subsociety due to the Catholics' – politically, socially, economically, educationally, numerically – deprived status compared to the Protestants in Central Europe comprising roughly the German-speaking areas (territory of pre-war Germany, Switzerland, the Netherlands). It consists of a great variety of very different associations, organizations, clubs, and initiatives such as Catholic labor unions, cooperatives, newspapers, kindergartens, insurances, etc.[27] that correspond to the similar interests of Catholics who felt not only deprived but also discriminated against and the interests of their Church ignored (Pollack 1996: 65, Gabriel/Kaufmann 1988: 45).[28] This Catholic subsociety constituted a numerical minority within a Protestant, culturally hegemonic, greater society in the emerging nation state in the middle of the 19th century (see Blaschke 2006: 267 and Gabriel/Kaufmann 1988: 34–36). The Church was able to mobilize the religious masses. Practices and participation in church activities were very intense and moreover much more intense than in Protestant communities (p. 45). Researchers document that adherents of religious minorities are more committed

[27] The formation of such organizations was enabled in 1848 and actively used since then. These associations, clubs, and initiatives took care of for their clients' social needs.

[28] This fight of confessional classes culminated in the *Kulturkampf*.

than adherents of majorities (see e.g. Adsera 2004 and Adsera 2007 for Spain). The superstructure of the sub-society was built by the Catholic view of life. Ideology, philosophy, as well as church norms, principles, and attitudes acted as answer to and code of conduct for all religious issues and the religious sphere exceeded everyday life situations and permeated the whole lifestyle. Hence, the intense activity rate rested upon close interrelations between the Catholic Church and other spheres of life (Pollack 1996: 66). Here, secularization processes could not happen because one feature of modernization (Voas 2008) – institutional modernization, i.e. functional differentiation – did not take place.

Social relations within the sub-society were closely interwoven and cemented by several memberships and activities in Catholic organizations, associations, groups, etc. One important stabilizing factor of the Catholic sub-society and its networks was communication. The interaction density was high. This considerably contributed to the transmission and internalization of church views, opinions, and practices.[29] By interacting with each other, the Catholics mutually confirmed and encouraged each other in their behavior and attitudes (corresponding to rules and norms of the Catholic Church). Interactions with non-Catholics were confined to a minimum. The homogeneous and closed sub-society sharply delimited itself against the modern, secular-civil, "degenerated" environment (Gabriel/Kaufmann 1988: 36). Catholicism, sub-societal structure, and rigorous demarcation from Protestantism created a unique identity. It was a social system according to the definition of Luhmann 2005 (pp. 15–19) and exerted pressure to adapt (McQuillan 2004). The Catholic sub-society experienced its heyday at the time of the turn of last century.

After World War II, extensive migration movements took place resulting in confessional mixtures, the expansion of interactions between the two main confessions, and the emergence of an ecumenical consciousness that surmounted Catholicism as the primary trait of identification (Gabriel/Kaufmann 1988: 37). Another change happened: the division of Germany led to numerical parity amongst Catholics and Protestants in the Western part. This strengthened the Catholics and removed their minority status. These and several further factors forwarded processes of disintegration

[29] Pollack found a significant reason for why religion has such an outstanding position in the everyday life of Americans in the close net of voluntary associations and unions. In combination with the argument that a lack of existential security promotes religiosity (Norris/Inglehart 2007; see subsection 3.2.2) a great part of the higher level of religiosity in the United States becomes explainable.

of the Catholic sub-society starting in the middle of the 1960s. They accelerated the decrease of individual religiosity and the strict observance of moral guidelines and general norms set by the Church (Pollack 1996: 69).[30] The birth cohorts focused on in this work (1930–1962) were socialized by parents who were part of the sub-society – conditional on their being Catholic. A continuing influence of the sub-society on the behavior of the relevant birth cohorts can hence be assumed.

Catholics are today still disadvantaged in a socioeconomic perspective. Catholics earn 5% less than Protestants due to lower educational achievements. Martin Luther promoted education of girls so that they could also read the Bible (see Becker/Woessmann 2008 and Becker/Woessmann 2009).[31] Gabriel and Kaufmann attribute the still visible educational deficiency of Catholics against Protestants to the secularization process at the begin of the 19th century when 18 Catholic universities on German territory closed due to expropriation by Napoleon (Gabriel/Kaufmann 1988: 33).

Catholics in Hungary have lower educational achievements than Protestants (Tomka 2006: 46–47). However, educational and demographic differences also exist between Lutherans and Reformed Christians. The Calvinist population is above average in age while their educational attainments lag behind those of the Lutherans "who have an urban and middle class basis" (Tomka 2006: 46). More Lutherans have completed tertiary education and work in white-collar occupations.

Now the selected countries will be assigned to a cultural tradition. Hungary is often pointed to as having a Catholic cultural tradition, but Tomka 2006 declares this to be incorrect with respect to history. Before World War I, Hungary was much larger: territories of most of its neighboring countries belonged to the Hungarian state territory. Half of the population was Orthodox or Protestant. Today, within the present borders, the proportion of Protestants is much lower and the number of Orthodox Christians is negligible. While the German territory was confessionally segregated until World War II, this was not the case in Hungary. Catholics, Protestants,

[30] Some further factors include: achievement of political influence and finally equality, rise of general prosperity that increasingly – but not completely – obliterated socioeconomic differences between the two confessions, educational expansion (Gabriel/Kaufmann 1988: 43–44, 55).

[31] Becker and Wössmann claim that the higher literacy of Protestants in Prussia in the 19th century causally explains the prosperity gap between Catholic and Protestant regions then as well as the earlier industrialization and rationalization. The wage gap may still be traced 500 years back to Martin Luther.

and Orthodox Christians coexisted peacefully. "Denominational plurality became [a] key notion of Hungarian identity (...) with substantial Protestant contributions to Catholic culture and political life" (Tomka 2006: 44). Molnár 2006 expounds why Calvinism but not Catholicism corresponds to the characteristics of an ethnic religion of Hungarian nationals living abroad, sometimes for decades, mainly in neighboring countries. Calvinism is perceived as the Hungarians' religious tradition by the autochthonal populations that are mainly affiliated to Orthodox Christianity. This is also true for the self-perception of the Reformed Protestants. Religiosity was higher among the Reformed Protestants than among Catholics. However, "their religiousness is rather community or public-based, than personal piety" (Molnár 2006: 85–86). Community life of the Reformed Protestants is more similar to the structure of the Catholic sub-society on German territory than community life of the Catholics themselves.

France has a Catholic cultural tradition but can be characterized as one of the exceptional cases when it comes to the significance of religiosity and religious traditions in countries that are shaped by Catholicism. This is due to history, especially the developments triggered in the time around the French Revolution (Casanova 2003: 19; Casanova 2007: 323–328; Kranemann/Wijlens 2009: 10; Nientiedt 2009: 138). "Overall levels of church disengagement had advanced furthest in France, Britain, and the Netherlands" (Norris/Inglehart 2006: 34). West Germany is mixed from a denominational perspective, with a Protestant influenced North and a Catholic imprinted South. Affiliates of both religious traditions live in the geographical middle. As homeland of Martin Luther, Eastern Germany had an unambiguously Protestant cultural imprint which is however fading. Therefore, it would also be right to characterize that region as secular. Norway is straightforwardly a Protestant country with a Lutheran state church which does not need to be elaborated in detail. Christianity outside the Church of Norway consists of small minorities of free, evangelical churches and sects as well as Catholics.

Finally, it can be said that the characteristics of the Catholics or the Catholic sub-societal structure basically correspond with the situation and the characteristics of Muslims in many European countries today. These include: (i) lower socioeconomic achievements (compared to the average population), (ii) deprivation, (iii) the high richness of details of prescriptions, proscriptions, rules, and norms guiding daily life and behavior-regulating practices. They are recorded in the Qur'an and the Hadith,[32] (iv) their minority status (life in the diaspora), and (v) social control in combination with a close (family) network. The above list does not rule out differences, for example the absence of a hierarchical authority or a centralist organization. In addition, there is no religious leader like the Pope (see e.g. Glock/Stark 1965, Olson/Perl 2001, Morgan et al. 2002, Alesina/Giuliano 2007, Breuer 2008, Hubert/Althammer/Korucu-Rieger 2009, Riesebrodt 2010). While due to the processes described above the Catholic specificities have begun to weaken, the pronounced religiosity of Muslims – mostly migrants – is still a current matter.

3.2.5 Factors associated with a nation's level of religiosity in comparative perspective

Now the factors will be summed up in comparative perspective. In East Germany, a very unfavorable combination of the factors treated can largely explain the low religious vitality. This comprises the high proportion of citizens not affiliated to a religious denomination, who do not believe in superhuman powers or exhibit cognitive interest in religious questions, as well as the low proportion of church attendees. The country exhibits a rather high socioeconomic level of development, which has accelerated church exits after system breakdown. Eastern Germany has a Protestant cultural tradition which may have additionally eased the struggle of the regime against the Church. Obviously, the Protestant Church was too weak to effectively defend itself against repression. However, a traditionally low attachment to the church since the 19th century has been discussed controversially (Gabriel 2003: 114–115). Finally, the share of Muslims is very small, which also reduces religious vitality.

In Hungary, a country with a rather mixed denominational cultural tradition, and a somewhat lower socioeconomic level of development, revitalization of religiosity – as opposed to East Germany – has been observable. Due to the inertia of processes, it did not however happen immediately after transformation. The section has shown that the factors introduced and the developments considered are not independent of one another. These interactions may even have had their own effects on religious vitality, either weakening or strengthening it. This matter makes the identification of the isolated impact of the single factors difficult.

[32] The Hadith comprise the Sunnah of the prophet Muhammad. The Sunnah is his important actions and teachings. It includes his specific words, habits, practices, and silent approvals (Ruthven 2001: 107).

France has a very high socioeconomic level of development and a Catholic cultural tradition. The latter principally results in a higher level of religiosity, but France is an exceptional case in this perspective. State and church are strictly separated. The proportion of Muslims is higher than in the other countries. The level of modernization in West Germany equals that of France; it has a mixed cultural tradition and the state-church relations can be characterized as cooperative. The proportion of Muslims is only slightly lower than in France but higher than in the other three countries. Finally, the level of modernization is highest in Norway. The share of Muslims does not exceed 1% (Statistics Norway 2012h). The country has a pure Protestant cultural tradition. These facts level down religious vitality. The Church is a favored institution because the Lutheran Church of Norway was a state church. This should raise the religiosity level but as will be seen later, it does not apply to this country. The constellation of these factors can be summarized in the statement that all the people of all five countries have a rather low religious commitment.

3.3 Review of the literature on the effects of religiosity on fertility

In the USA, a wealth of scientific research with regard to the – pronounced – effects of religiosity on fertility behavior can be found due to high religious vitality and religious pluralism with a low rate of unaffiliated people, many exclusivist as well as ecumenical Protestant groups, a considerable share of Catholics, and a small share of Mormons. A high proportion of individuals is engaged in a church community. Religious affiliation itself already generates high fertility variance. Such impressive results cannot be expected for Europe. Nevertheless, existing studies document a positive correlation between religious affiliation, religiosity, and fertility. Some are summarized in the following.

Adsera concludes from the 1985 *Spanish Fertility Survey* (SFS) that family sizes of married practicing and non-practicing Catholics hardly differed (Adsera 2004, Adsera 2006). This changed until 1999. For that year she discovers that fertility of younger non-practicing Catholics (the majority among the younger generation) converged to the fertility level of unaffiliated persons, while fertility of practicing Catholics was noticeably higher. For this reason, she identifies religious practice as a distinct trait for birth behavior. Continuously growing Evangelical and Muslim minorities have the highest fertility. Furthermore, Adsera provides evidence that marriages that are composed of two practicing Catholics have their first and third child faster. Couples with diverging religious affiliations have fewer children than homogamous unions.

Based on the 1998 Spanish and Italian samples of the *International Social Survey Programme* (ISSP), Brañas-Garza and Neuman find evidence for effects of parental church attendance when the daughter was 12 years old on her later family size (Brañas-Garza/Neuman 2006 and Brañas-Garza/Neuman 2007). The mother's effect is surprisingly negative while the father's one is positive. The results indicate that fertility preferences are already shaped in childhood and remain stable even if the daughter's frequency of church attendance decreases with rising age.[33]

Heineck investigates the correlation between religiosity and fertility with the help of the 1996 Austrian *Family and Fertility Survey* (FFS) and concludes that both women's religious affiliation and religiosity positively influence the number of children born (Heineck 2006). Transition rates to a third child are – unexpectedly – higher for non-Catholic than for Catholic women. Nor do the latter have a higher overall fertility. The most decisive factor is that a women is not unaffiliated. Likewise, based on the FFS, Philipov and Berghammer analyze the impact of different religiosity indicators on the desired, intended and realized number of children of women between 18 and 39 years for 18 European countries. All in all, a positive impact can be confirmed whereas the authors measure a stronger effect of the indicators on the desired number of children rather than on actual behavior. Catholic and Protestant women are very similar to each other. With regard to the desired and intended number of children, women attending church at least once a month differ considerably from those with a lower frequency (Philipov/Berghammer 2007).

Berinde's findings come to the conclusion that religious activity – measured dichotomously with "high" and "low" activity – does not influence the transition risk for a third birth for Swedish mothers born between 1949 and 1963 by employing the *Swedish Family and Working Life Survey*. She traces the lack of an effect back to the highly secular environment. Moreover, mothers are well enabled to reconcile family and work (Berinde 1999).

Frejka and Westoff infer from analyses on the basis of the *World Values Survey*, *European Values Survey* and the *National Survey of Family Growth* that fertility dif-

[33] The findings are not unproblematic and may be biased because of the high selectivity of the (small) sample used. It is limited to Catholics married to each other; their parents are all Catholics as well.

ferences between American and European women are partly caused by the dissimilar extent of religiosity (Frejka/Westoff 2006). Moreover they find that differences between women in the USA aged between 18 and 44 years can be detected independent of the selected religiosity indicator, while only the "importance of religion in daily life" shows significant results for European women. Frequencies of attending religious services remain without a significant effect except for Southern Europe.

Goujon and her colleagues calculate shifts in population composition of the Austrian population in terms of fertility rates varying by religious affiliation between 2001 and 2051 based on the 2001 census allowing for a large variety of influencing factors and imponderables (Goujon et al. 2007). They arrive at the result that the proportion of Catholics will fall from 75% to below 50% while the proportion of Muslims in the total population will rise from 4% to about 14–18% (due to their higher fertility and immigration) and will be about one third among minors. Furthermore, the proportion of the religiously unaffiliated will increase from 12–34%. This however cannot be a consequence of their – low – fertility (their fertility rate totaled 0.9 children in 2001), but results from the inter-generational non-transmission of religious values, omitted baptisms, and church exists.

With the aid of the *German Family Panel (pairfam)* (wave I), Hubert found that frequent worshipers aged 35–37 years have more children than rare attenders. Religiously affiliated individuals are more fertile than their unaffiliated peers. Both results hold for women as well as men. Catholics and Protestants do not differ from each other controlling for public practice. Muslims most often have large families and are most rarely childless. Couples whose wedding was accompanied by a religious ceremony are not expected to have more children than couples that exclusively celebrated a civil wedding. Marriage by itself is associated with a higher number of children compared to unmarried respondents (Hubert 2011).

4 How Religious Affiliation and Religiosity Affect Fertility

The following chapter theorizes the association between individual religiosity and completed fertility in order to be able to explain the expected effects. Section 3.3 has already summarized studies that analyze the influence of religious affiliation and religiosity on birth behavior. The findings document a positive impact. The theoretical approach tries to take account of a variety of factors that matter in the context of fertility behavior and decisions. 4.1 presents the mechanisms that are usually applied to explain the affinity for a higher number of children as well as higher birth rates among affiliates across religious traditions. Section 4.2 summarizes denomination-specific behavior-regulating practices. They may influence fertility behavior as one major secular consequence of religiosity.

Section 4.3 combines religiosity with an economic approach. The first part (4.3.1) introduces the basics of the economic theory of the family. The second part (4.3.2) integrates religious affiliation and religiosity of both spouses into the economic approach and discusses its implications. It thereby takes account of possible disagreements within the couple resulting in lower fertility. Marital stability is assumed to be of decisive importance for the fertility outcome. But as stability not only depends on the religious composition of a couple, section 4.4 gives an overview of some characteristics promoting or endangering marital stability.

To start, figure 4.1 illustrates diverse determinants of fertility (and religiosity). It summarizes all the associations, developments, and traits this work deals with. Most of the characteristics involved but not yet elaborated will be addressed in this and the two following chapters. Some points have already been mentioned in the preceding chapter. The figure also presents the main hypothesis of this work: religious affiliation and religiosity have a positive impact on completed fertility. There are both direct and indirect mechanisms which will be clarified in detail later in this chapter. Indirect mechanisms are mediated by marital stability and hence the religious composition of a marriage. Therefore, including indirect mechanisms expands the perspective from the individual to the couple-based one. The main hypothesis will be particularized in sections 6.2.3 and 6.2.4 after the data employed and the operationalization of the indicators have been introduced.

Fig. 4.1. Determinants of completed fertility (and religiosity)

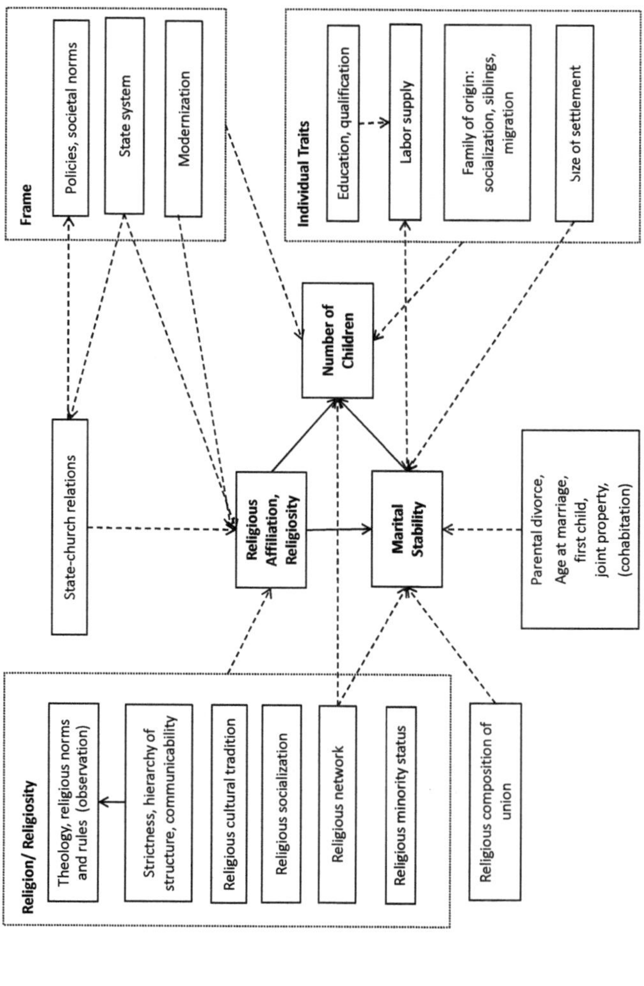

4.1 Explanations for the direct influence of religiosity on fertility

Two branches of approaches explaining the number of children across affiliates of different religious groups can be distinguished (Goldscheider 1971). One branch argues that variance in fertility between religious groups is caused by socioeconomic differences. Goldscheider calls the association between socioeconomic traits and religious traditions the *characteristics approach*. This means that the higher fertility of Muslims, for example, could be ascribed to their deprived socioeconomic status or lower educational attainment (see e.g. Morgan et al. 2002). One can argue against this approach on the basis of the human capital theory (see subsection 4.3.2). If a woman sees it her task to be mother and housewife it will – according to the theory – be indeed rational to limit her market-specific investments in schooling and training as they do not pay off to a reasonable degree. Hence, it is problematic to negate the causal link between socioeconomic traits and religious norms.

The second branch explaining fertility differentials based on religious traditions is called the *particularized theology approach* and seeks to explain diverging birth rates with differences in norms, teachings, and doctrines (Goldscheider 1971). Most religious traditions approve of a high number of children and specially appreciate marriage and family. But: this rather explains existing fertility differences between the affiliated and the unaffiliated but does not sufficiently help to discriminate the varying fertility levels between adherents of different denominations. Behavior pushing fertility is thereby encouraged by denomination-specific norms and rules. For instance, more affiliates of one denomination refrain from doing an action because it has been declared a sin in comparison with affiliates of another denomination in which this is not the case.[1] Section 4.2 deals with denomination-specific norms, principles, and attitudes.

However, the pure existence of norms and rules is not necessarily sufficient to influence behavior (or no longer). For that reason, further conditions have to be fulfilled (see McQuillan 2004, Tomka 2006): The stricter teachings and doctrines are

[1] There is has been documented empirically by Blume/Ramsel/Graupner 2006 (pp. 16–17). More religious persons refrain from actions that have been declared a sin than non-religious individuals. The authors document the accuracy descriptively: only 17.7% of respondents who declared not to be religious state that they refrained from an action because it has been defined as a sin by their denomination while this applies to 30.3% of moderately religious, 50.9% of religious and 68% of the very religious respondents. These actions can be pre- or non-marital sex, promiscuity, use of contraception, abortion, etc. They refrained from it because they were afraid of punishment or other consequences.

formulated and the better they can be communicated, e.g. by a religious institution whose internal structure is hierarchically organized, the better the possibility to impact the behavior of affiliates. There are further factors that increase the probability that affiliates behave in line with their church, their religious tradition or holy scripture. A religious socialization as a precondition for religiosity in adulthood (Bisin/ Verdier 2000, Bisin/Verdier 2010) has already been mentioned. This transmission from parents to their children is explained with imitation and adaption processes. This means that a religious socialization influences a higher affinity for children which again raises the probability to effect behavior in adulthood.

Although probably not all behavior-regulating practices are completely obeyed at all times, one can assume that (very) religious individuals comply with the rules and norms to a larger extent than those with a functionally heteronomous religious construct.[2] The probability rises with the degree of self-identification with a certain religious tradition, belief, church, community, religious leader, scripture, etc. (Berggren 1997) which promotes conformity and the correspondence of the adherents' values with religious norms. Of special importance is the identification with other affiliates. Religious networks mean social capital or resources and consequently social integration (Heineck 2001). The network may be closer, the more committed the affiliates are within the congregation, especially if it is a religious minority. Activities comprise groups that study holy scriptures, regular meetings about any topic, voluntary work organized by the church, and many more.[3] Network members serve as role models supporting as well as confirming each other in their actions and behavior. Therefore, it is a combination of individual religiosity and religious networks – whose affiliates share similar values and attitudes – that gives vigor, strength, and confidence.[4] Furthermore, a deep trust in superhuman powers and the promise of religion takes from the adherent the uncertainty the birth of a(nother) child may be associated with. The decision to have a child is an irreversible event and accompanied by many changes. This may lead to the decision of non-religious persons to decide against a child, even if affinity is equally pronounced.

[2] See explanations on this term in subsection 3.1.2.

[3] See details in subsection 3.2.4 that elaborates on the effects of networks on behavior.

[4] This is of course not restricted to religious networks.

4.2 Denomination-specific behavior-regulating practices

Subsection 3.2.4 has contributed to explain why Catholics exhibit higher religiosity levels than Protestants, and why Muslims are more religious than Christians. These explanations have been derived from a variety of traits, specific characteristics, and historical events. Now, denomination-specific behavior-regulating practices with respect to sexuality, relationships, and fertility will be addressed that contribute to explain higher fertility levels among Muslims followed by Catholics then Protestants, and implicitly also unaffiliated individuals.

Rules are particularly strictly formulated by the Catholic Church. According to Catholicism, it is an obligation to have and raise children within marriage:

> Married couples should regard it as their proper mission to transmit human life and to educate their children; they should realize that they are thereby cooperating with the love of God the Creator and are, in a certain sense, its interpreters. They will fulfill this duty with a sense of human and Christian responsibility (Ecclesia Catholica 1994: 2367).

The decision against children allows priests to refuse solemnizing the marriage. However, the married couple is allowed to space the births for the sake of the children's well-being (Ecclesia Catholica 1994: 2368). Divorces are prohibited ("what therefore God has joined together, let not man put asunder" (Ecclesia Catholica 1994: 2364)). If the (first) marriage is valid, it is indissoluble and a church re-wedding is impossible (Ecclesia Catholica 1994: 1650). Marriage is one of the seven sacraments of the Catholic Church. According to Canon law, the first marriage can only be annulled in a few cases. Among these are defective matrimonial consent, e.g. one spouse refuses to have children but this was not known to the other spouse at the time of the marriage ceremony (Libreria Editrice Vaticana 1983: Cann. 1095–1107). Catholics who (civilly) marry a second time, risk being penalized. Generally, they are not allowed to receive the Communion or to take part in the Eucharistic mass as long as the first spouse is alive. If they are employed by the Church, they risk being dismissed. The more religious a Catholic and the higher the individual importance of the religious network is, the lower the probability of exposing oneself to these consequences.

Further differentiated positions with respect to gender roles, including the division of labor, and the autonomy of women exist: "God gives man and woman an equal personal dignity" but created them different in function (Ecclesia Catholica 1994:

2334, 2335). This is the complementarian – as opposed to the egalitarian – view. Another fertility-promoting factor is the prohibition of any form of contraception and abortion: "each and every marriage act must remain open 'per se' to the transmission of life" (Ecclesia Catholica 1994: 2366).[5] Clear positions are formulated regarding the entry into sexual unions, and the non-acceptance of sexual activity outside of marriages ("Carnal union is morally legitimate only when a definitive community of life between a man and woman has been established. Human love does not tolerate 'trial marriages'" (Ecclesia Catholica 1994: 2391)). Teachings and doctrines are not only strictly formulated by the Catholic Church. They can also be very well communicated due to the hierarchical organization with the Pope as the head and the bishops as "regional voices". In the age of mass media this is a specific advantage. Moreover, religious education (outside school) in the form of Communion classes takes place early in the life of (Catholic) children. They are about eight or nine years old whereas Confirmation classes for Protestants start some years later. These may be decisive years in the life of young affiliates.

In comparison, prescriptions made by the main Protestant churches are delimited.[6] Protestants are allowed to divorce and to celebrate church re-weddings. The foundation of this possibility is a merciful God who forgives mistakes, e.g. the choice of the wrong partner (Goujon et al. 2007: 246). Marriage is not a sacrament but a secular matter. The church ceremony is merely the benediction of a previous civil marriage. However, these positions on divorce do not have a long tradition, and indissolubility is nevertheless aimed at. To dissolve a marriage is a sin, but humans are assumed to be sinners. Contrary to the Catholic Church, the Protestant churches do not explicitly forbid extra-marital relationships and births. These issues are subject to the Protestants' own conscious and their individual interpretation of the Bible. The same applies to the use of contraception. Sexual intercourse is an expression of love and physical affection and insofar does not only serve procreation (Evangelische Kirche in Deutschland 2004).[7] This stance clarifies that the Lutheran Church approves the use of contraception. Apart from the latter, there are no universal binding clerical teachings on many family topics (any more).

[5] However, bishops in Germany are currently (first quarter of 2013) discussing whether the morning-after pill would be acceptable in case of extreme hardship, e.g. after rape, but only if the pill prevents fertilization and not if it aborts a zygote.

[6] Free churches that are often especially conservative in some respects are excluded from the following statements.

[7] The Catholic Church has only recently revised its position on this point.

The possibility to exert influence on its affiliates is lower for the Church and its church leaders. The church hierarchy is flat and there is no central, supranational authority (see 3.2.4). In the Protestant Church the egalitarian view dominates. Men and women are not only equal in dignity, but also equal in their roles. Leadership in the church is also possible for women. Accordingly, a gender hierarchy created by God is rejected (Evangelische Kirche in Deutschland 2004). Positions on current issues remain indistinct in contrast with a hierarchically organized and stronger visible Catholic Church with thoroughgoing and unequivocal points of view that are repeated again and again, today especially via mass media.[8]

The Qur'an is unambiguously family-oriented and appreciates a high number of children. However, the book emphasizes that maintenance and well-being of the children have to be assured and are of higher importance than mere quantity (Morgan et al. 2002: 518). The main sources of Islam, Qu'ran and Sunnah, regulate questions with respect to family life in great detail and exactly dictate behavior (Breuer 2008: 9). In many Islamic countries, established law is arranged in conformity with sharia guidelines and has hardly been changed over several hundred years. Most Muslims living in Europe originate from those countries or were born to parents who were socialized in Islamic countries. Muslims pass on a high family orientation from generation to generation, and this is realized in the form of large families. To have many children is often ascribed to Islam by the Muslims themselves (Borooah 2004: 563–565). Marriage can moreover be understood as a general norm – celibacy does not exist in Islam – whereas the unmarried state is undesired because human beings are considered as sexual beings (Breuer 2008: 7, 40–41). This is a fundamental difference compared to the Catholic understanding. Sexual intercourse itself is therefore exclusively allowed within marriage. This point of view equals the Catholic position. It may also be practiced without the intention to procreate but not continuously because procreation is one of the main goals of marriage (Breuer 2008: 47).

From this follows that non-permanent means of birth control are not prohibited. To plan the spacing of births is unproblematic. The Qu'ran recommends a breastfeeding period of two years and according to Mohammad breastfeeding during pregnancy is not permitted. The motivation for using contraceptives is very important. It is not acceptable if it is for personal interests such as gainful employment (Breuer 2008:

[8] It should be added that this is a "German impression" and Germany is a country in which the proportions of Protestants, Catholics, and unaffiliated individuals are balanced.

48). The duties as wife and mother must not be neglected and always have the greater significance (p. 104). With respect to the reasons for controlling births, scholars and imams – who are often neither theologians nor scholars of Islamic law – have no uniform point of view. As already mentioned, Muslims usually have more children than affiliates of other religious traditions. They regard a higher number of children as ideal and abstain from the use of contraceptives more frequently when they already have their desired number of children (Morgan et al. 2002: 515). The non-use of contraception is also qualified with demography and the goal of a quantitative dominance of Islam.

Divorces are not forbidden per se but are the thing most reprehensible in the eyes of God according to a statement made by Mohammad (Goujon et al. 2007: 246). However, divorce is only permitted in exceptional cases, a last-ditch expedient. At marriage, usually a contract is signed (Ruthven 2001: 135, Breuer 2008: 22–23). Husband and wife can file for divorce in case the other spouse infringes or breaks elements of the contract. Matters contradicting fundamentals of an Islamic marriage cannot be part of the contract. It is, for example, not permitted to exclude children. A divorce has negative consequences for the social standing of a woman. Her possibilities to request divorce are moreover restricted.[9] The male spouse receives custody of his children if they are at least seven (sons) or nine (daughters) years old (Ruthven 2001: 135). In case a male Muslim out-marries, that means he marries a Christian or Jewish woman, his wife cannot include bringing up the children in Christian or Jewish belief into the marriage contract. The children of a Muslim father are automatically Muslims and must be educated as Muslims (Breuer 2008: 32, 64). That is the reason why a Muslim woman should not enter into an inter-marriage unless her future spouse converts to Islam. She is obliged to marry a Muslim (Ruthven 2001: 136).

In contrast to the Catholic Church, artificial insemination, especially in vitro fertilization, is regarded positively because parenthood enjoys such great importance (Breuer 2008: 53). The Catholic Church refuses the cold act of how a new life comes into existence ("morally unacceptable") – namely without the actions of a married couple (Ecclesia Catholica 1994: 2364). To adopt an abandoned child is accepted according to the Catholic Church (Ecclesia Catholica 1994: 2379) but prohibited under

[9] She loses the dowry usually paid at marriage. If the husband files for divorce, she is allowed to keep it (Ruthven 2001: 136).

Islamic understanding. Parenthood can only be biological parenthood (Breuer 2008: 54).

Islamic law allows a man to be simultaneously married with up to four women on the condition that he treats all of them equally and is able to maintain them because he is obliged to provide for his wives and children. The tolerance of polygamy dates back to times in which wars led to a shortage of men. No woman should remain unmarried or unprovided for. Since polygamy is not allowed in any country in Europe, in Turkey (since 1926), and Tunisia (since 1956), it has become a rarity which is also the result of a greater gender balance in modern times (Breuer 2008: 35–38).[10]

Islam does not have a strict religious hierarchy and is principally not comparable with the Christian form of organization because Islam is not an institutionalized religious tradition, i.e. it is not structured in the form of institutions (Ruthven 2001: 18–22).

4.3 Religiosity within an economic approach: the indirect influence of religiosity

The approaches introduced in sections 4.1 and 4.2 contribute to explaining denomination-specific fertility differences and why the religiously affiliated, especially Muslims and Catholics, have on average more children than unaffiliated individuals. However, they do not sufficiently acknowledge societal developments that have occurred, e.g. increasing divorce risks and improved educational perspectives that resulted in further behavioral adjustments, namely lower fertility, presumably also among the affiliated. In subsection 3.1.2 it has made clear that from Allport's postulation of functional autonomy it follows that its motivational impulses prevail independent of concrete external circumstances. This means that highly religious individuals should be excluded from the statement. This section sketches in a first step basics of the economic theory of the family and, secondly, integrates religiosity. The partner perspective will be emphasized. Fertility decisions are usually made within partnership although both partners have a veto and can withhold approval.

[10] From the perspective of the economic theory of the family, which is addressed in the following section, it can be said that if the sex ratio equals unity, monogamous unions are the most efficient marital form, whereas polygamous unions are encouraged when the sex ratio significantly differs from unity (Becker 1973: 820). In this respect, the Islamic arrangement is, according to Becker, efficient and also explains why polygamy has strongly decreased in importance.

4.3.1 The theory of time allocation and fertility

The economic theory of the family uses neoclassical microeconomic theory to explain family behavior, e.g. the division of labor between spouses. As well as having stable preferences, individuals are assumed to behave rationally, i.e. to make the utility-maximizing decision subject to both time and budget constraints. The total utility of a household is a function of leisure, market goods, and commodities. Commodities – that are both produced and consumed by the household – are (in)tangible goods and services which are comprised of a combination of market goods, time, and environmental inputs. They can usually not be purchased. Therefore, they do not have market prices but shadow prices equal to the cost of production (Becker 1965: 497, Becker 1981: 7–8). Commodities comprise "children, prestige and esteem, health, altruism, envy, and pleasures of the senses" (Becker 1981: 8), but also "recreation, companionship, love" (Becker 1973: 816).

Both men and women subdivide their time into three uses: paid market work, unpaid homework, and leisure. Paid work is used to purchase market goods while homework is needed to create commodities. Leisure is the only time use that is not transferable (Beblo 2001: 2). The time allocation of household members is determined by the goal of achieving the highest feasible utility given the preference structure of the household. Hence, income is a function of the intrafamily allocation of time and earnings potentials (Mincer 1963, Becker 1965).

A couple is assumed to merge their resources (i.e. to move together) if both expect that their utility from joint production will exceed the combined utility from remaining single (Becker 1973: 815–822). They substitute market relations by a favorable internal organization, the division of labor, assuming that complementarity between spouses is the major gain from living together. It results in mutual dependence. Unless the partners differ in their relative work abilities or have young children, there are nonetheless further economic gains as well as non-economic benefits from their decision to move into a joint household and to form a family. These comprise economies of scale, externalities in consumption, quasi-public goods, pooled risks, and institutional factors (see for details e.g. Blau/Ferber/Winkler 2002: 41–43).

The theory assumes that time allocation depends on the comparative production advantage of the single household members. Each individual specializes in the activity that he or she can do more efficiently (Becker 1973: 829–831). They may then exchange their output or pool all resources. "If time is spent working in the marketplace, the wage rate has to equal the shadow price of household time, otherwise the marginal value of working time would be less than the marginal value of household time" (Becker 1981: 7), or "the allocation of time would be optimal if the marginal product of working time equaled the marginal product of household time" (Becker 1981: 15). Therefore, a household member replaces homework by market work when the value of a time unit falls below the value of the wage rate.

All time units are valued with a price which varies between the members of a household. The family member whose time has the lower opportunity costs compared to the wage rate should do the (unpaid) housework. Even today, women on average earn less (see statements on the gender wage gap in subsection 5.2.3). Additionally, due to gender-specific socialization (especially common in older birth cohorts), women are more experienced in household tasks. This means that as well as their lower earnings prospects women are ascribed to have a production advantage in homework. Therefore, the traditional division of labor with a husband earning money and a wife producing commodities (doing the homework and caring for and rearing the children) should achieve the highest efficiency gains (Becker 1981: 14–37).[11] Additional investments in specific human capital again raise efficiency. Therefore, these are exclusively effected in activities where they pay off. Men anticipate that their duration of employment lasts longer, so they invest more in market specific human capital while women anticipate childbearing and employment interruptions (or a shorter working life) which altogether encourages their investments in homework-related human capital.[12]

The relationship between fertility and income is based on the assumption that children are a normal good. Thus, "demand" rises with income.[13] A growth in non-labor income without any change in the wage rate reduces working time and increases the

[11] This especially applies to the time period when the children are young and the demand for household production is most pronounced.

[12] Becker assumed that all women will find a partner. But of course this assumption is not very realistic. Moreover, even if a woman anticipates being a mother and housewife in later life she will attend university if she attains the entrance qualification due to the pool of men with good income prospects being able to provide for a family. Section 5.2 will show that income prospects depend on branch and field of study. Furthermore, the public sector is a good way to combine a job and family so that labor market oriented investments will pay off although the woman has children. Policies in many countries have been adjusted to the increased labor force participation of women and support their commitment with public child care (see section 5.1). Finally, technical progress has contributed to a decrease in the time needed for housework.

[13] The demand for inferior goods falls as income increases.

demand for most goods and household time (Becker 1981: 7). Reality has been contradicting this prediction, however (Ahn/Mira 2002). Three alternative explanations have been developed to keep the assumption: (1) the access to means of family planning (e.g. Schultz 2008, Adsera 2008), (2) the quality of children (e.g. Becker/Lewis 1973), and (3) the price of time (Mincer 1974).

Means of family planning are the improvements to and accessibility of reliable contraception since the 1960s. The costs have been affordable since then. This development reduced the monetary and psychic cost of limiting births, and promoted women's employment investment by reducing the pregnancy risk while allowing women to remain sexually active (Schultz 2008, Adsera 2008). The quality of children implies a quality-quantity trade-off. The consideration of a consumption good's quality was not part of the traditional household theory. It is not merely the number of children that contributes to maximize utility but also their quality (Becker/Lewis 1973, Becker/Tomes 1976). This means that expenditures per child for education, health, leisure activities, etc. increase with income. If the income elasticity of demand for child quality sufficiently exceeds the income elasticity of demand for the quantity of children, rising income leads to higher costs per child and fewer births.

The third explanation refers to the women's price of time. Originally, the price was fix. Due to educational expansion, whose causes are treated as exogenous factors in the economic theory, tertiary education has become more widespread (see subsection 5.2.2). According to human capital theory, education (schooling and training) is a time investment in human capital[14] of individuals that ought to increase the returns from employment (Mincer 1974, Mincer/Polachek 1974). An upward change in the price of a time unit boosts the price of time allocated to unpaid child rearing and care; it increases the opportunity costs of an employment break. Opportunity costs also comprise increases in the wage an individual had experienced without employment interruption, e.g. because of missed long-term employment chances, foregone earnings after the re-entry due to possibly reduced working hours, and acquired human capital that has become obsolete. While the quality of a child refers rather to the direct child-related costs, this explanation turns to the indirect child-related costs.

[14] Human capital "embodies a set of skills that can be 'rented' out to employers. The knowledge and skills a worker has – which come from education and training, including the learning that experience yields – generate a certain stock of productive capital" (Ehrenberg/Smith 2009: 279). Individuals can undertake three major kinds of labor market investments: education and training, migration, or search for a new job. To only consider the time investments or educational attainment an individual has, is restrictive but the usual procedure.

The total effect of a wage rate increase has to be subdivided into two parts. The substitution effect is a shift towards an extension of paid work because opportunity costs of unpaid homework (and leisure) rise. The income effect reduces working time because the same income can be earned in a shorter time interval (Lewis 1972). If the substitution effect outweighs the income effect, which is usually assumed by the theory, the total effect is positive. Vice versa, the total effect would be negative (the income effect is greater than the substitution effect then). In this case, the time excess can be used to expand leisure and/or homework. The assumption underlying these statements is a simultaneous decision of time allocation and the number of children. Keeping leisure constant, a positive total effect leads to less time for the production of commodities, mainly children. Data show that the total effect varies by gender.

For women, the total effect is positive resulting in higher income and fewer children. Reasons for wage rate increases are given in section 5.2. An increase in men's earnings would augment the demand for children as does non-labor income on the condition that he is not involved in child-rearing activities as time provider (Del Boca 2002). In reality, the total effect for men is apparently zero. Despite wage increases labor supply has by and large not changed significantly during the last decades.[15] Principally, considering lowered fertility, men's time allocation has shifted towards an expansion of leisure time (Beblo 2001: 99–104).[16] An important factor able to explain gender-specific effects is women's and men's different working behavior. Men usually work full-time, and can principally not further expand the time already spent in the labor market (or only in the form of – unmeasured – overtime) while women were either not employed at all or at most part-time.

4.3.2 The implications of religiosity

The assumption that a household maximizes one joint utility has been criticized as not realistic because the head of the household does not control all resources and cannot decide alone on their distribution (see e.g. Blau/Ferber/Winkler 2002: 43–49, Althammer 2000: 2–4, Ott 2001: 130–132). The decision on the allocation of income and time to various commodities is easy to make if both have the same tastes and

[15] In the longer run, working hours have fallen.

[16] Section 5.1 reports political measures cushioning the opportunity costs for women as well as influencing the time allocation decisions of men. The consequence of higher wage rates may then even be childbearing supportive because services, support, and hence time can be bought (see Ermisch 1989).

preferences. Then both would opt for the same combination of goods and services to be shared. The assumption of homogeneous preferences is however not reasonable. If the partners' tastes differ significantly, the question arises as to how they will decide on the combination of commodities to be produced and consumed. This will be discussed in the following.

A marriage is assumed to dissolve when the utility expected from remaining married falls below the utility expected from separating and becoming single or re-marrying (Becker/Landes/Michael 1977: 1142). Marriage-specific capital consists of investments that are made during a marriage. It is assumed to be worth far more within the marriage than outside of it (Becker/Landes/Michael 1977: 1152). The prime example of marriage-specific investments is the bearing and rearing of children. Children are "a source of psychic income or satisfaction, and, in the economist's terminology, children would be considered a durable consumption good" (Becker 1960: 210). Parents devote much time and energy to nurturing and educating their children, to bringing them up and to transmitting values. While they provide considerable satisfaction to their parents within the current marriage, their value drops when the marriage breaks up and may lower the parents' chances to attract alternatives. They can be an obstacle to form and maintain a successful new relationship with another partner.

In fragile relationships, the spouses refrain from investing too much time and money in marriage-specific capital because they anticipate the divorce risk (Becker/ Landes/Michael 1977: 1142). This means they restrict the number of children. The woman extends her labor supply to "acquire insurance" against the potential negative shock of divorce (Bargain et al. 2012: 17) and spends less time with unpaid child rearing. She concentrates her commitment on market-related capital accumulation to preserve her employability to care for herself in case the relationship splits up, rather than investing in housework-specific skills. The male spouse has an interest in limiting his investments as well. If the marriage breaks up, he will be confronted with the need to pay alimony for the children and – depending on the divorce law – also for his ex-wife (Blau/Ferber/Winkler 2002: 48). He risks losing contact with his children.[17] Mostly, it has been the mother who received sole custody of the children although

[17] Bodenmann et al. 2006 as well as Knoester/Booth 2000 analyze barriers and attractors of divorce. Especially men reported the presence of children to be a major barrier. Many worried about losing contact to their children.

this has changed now in many countries.[18] Once the investment has been effected, marital-specific capital may decrease the probability that a couple will dissolve its marriage by increasing both the attractiveness of the current marriage and the costs of leaving it (Becker/Landes/Michael 1977: 1152, Waite/Lillard 1991: 930).

Women and men are inclined to ensure a high marital stability ex-ante. Before however, it must be clarified why a couple should marry at all if all economic and non-economic gains seem to be already available for cohabiting couples. Apart from norms that for a long time made it impossible for unmarried couples to live together, feelings of obligation are higher. It has already been mentioned that the fragility of unmarried unions is higher than of married ones so that marriage itself can be interpreted as a stabilizing factor. According to Becker's theory of marriage, the efficiency of commodity production depends on the composition of the spouses and on the quality of their match (Becker 1973: 823–836). This raises the issue of assortive mating. Negative assortive mating refers to traits that are substitutes and positive assortive mating is used for traits that are complements. Religious affiliation is a complementary trait for which the mating of likes is ideal (Becker 1973: 827). In general, Becker assumed that negative assortive mating is optimal only with respect to specialization skills and earning capacities (p. 815).

If a man and a woman meet in the marriage market, both have an interest in ascertaining that the other is an eligible match for an everlasting, high quality marriage.[19] In addition to many traits that decide about a suitable match, religious affiliation and religiosity serve as a mutual "signal" for otherwise unobserved characteristics that simultaneously affect fertility and divorce decisions, namely one's preferences, even early in the establishing phase of a relationship (Coppola/Di Cesare 2008, Lillard/Waite 1993). While some decades ago, it was acceptable to take for granted the affiliates' agreeing with the norms of their religious tradition and observing the rules, today this is no longer self-evident. But it can be assumed that the more central the religious construct is anchored within the personality of a spouse-seeking individual, the lower will be the probability to out-marry, that means to marry someone with another religious affiliation or another – lower – level of religiosity. The unwillingness to compromise regarding this special matter should increase with individual religiosity.

[18] For some years joint custody has now become the rule.

[19] As the search for a compatible mate can be defined as competition, a marriage market supposedly exists. All individuals try to get the best mate "subject to restrictions imposed by market conditions" (Becker 1973: 814).

This decision however depends on the opportunity to be able to find such a partner and hence on the (local) marriage market and the availability of suitable partners. In diaspora, the chances may on the one hand be lower because selection is restricted. On the other hand, out-marriage may be unacceptable to the religious network and the parents. It has to be added that religious couples are assumed to marry directly rather than to cohabit in advance so that the first stability step linked to higher union obligation is better reached compared to non-religious couples.

Religiosity in a partner perspective also comprises correspondence regarding religious spirituality. Religious intimacy can take place within marriage and need not be looked for outside of it. Therefore, religiosity also strengthens marital companionship (Lehrer/Chiswick 1993: 386). Religiosity can moreover be interpreted as a proxy for joint tastes, interests, goals, and priorities with respect to a large variety of topics and matters, e.g. a general world view, allocation of time and money, recreational activities or the socialization of children (Lehrer/Chiswick 1993). To share these and to have a joint social network reduces the potential of conflicts and disagreements in (daily) life.[20] Finally, if behavior-regulating practices possess major importance for the spouses – especially with reference to indissolubleness – they may be deeply committed to marriage (Call/Heaton 1997: 383).[21] All these aspects increase both marital quality and stability beyond the mere religious norm of the prohibition (Catholics) or impossibility (Muslims) of divorce.

The religious composition of a union is significant with respect to the divorce risk and spousal mutual confidence. As opposed to Becker's claim, the mating of likes cannot automatically be regarded as optimal. Homogamy is merely efficient if both spouses are religiously affiliated to the same or similar religious traditions and moreover religious, but not if they are unaffiliated and irreligious. High marital stability can especially be assumed if both spouses are religious Catholics or Muslims (see Lehrer/Chiswick 1993 and Lehrer 1996). The mutual expectation of observing the rules and principles of Catholicism or Islam increases the willingness to invest more in marriage-specific capital. The woman is more inclined to quit gainful employment

20 As specialization gains have decreased due to technical progress, social similarity has gained importance.

21 Even if marital quality is no longer sufficiently high, many couples decide to remain married. To get divorced is not only a couple-based decision. A social network that strongly opposes divorces must also be conceded influence. Otherwise stigmatization and marginalization or even exclusion from the network may be the result. Many couples are not prepared to accept such pronounced social costs of dissolution.

at least temporarily or to strongly restrict her labor supply (conditional on her having been employed at all) to give birth to the desired number of children and to rear them (at home). Her giving up her participation in the labor force is equal to a restriction of market-specific investments. The husband in turn delivers on his promise by sharing the economic resources with her (and the children). He keeps up the relationship and does not take advantage of his relatively improved bargaining position – he now commands a larger share of the economic resources – to claim a larger part of the commodities produced jointly. Due to his continuous employment, his bargaining position improves relative to her position. It can be argued that with the marriage a long-term agreement has been entered into which will not been broken by either spouse. Both of them cooperate by realizing the desired number of children. This does however not exclude disagreements about the timing of family formation. Sequential non-cooperation can occur, although the couple agrees upon general life goals.

Other unions are composed either of spouses who both do not have a religious affiliation or of religiously heterogamous spouses, which both raise the divorce probability. To start with the "religiously" homogamous case of two unaffiliated partners, the composition can principally not be characterized as ideal because priorities, interests, and views are undetermined at the time the man and the woman get to know to each other in the marriage market (Lehrer/Chiswick 1993, Lehrer 1995, Lehrer 2004). Unaffiliated individuals may have a clear affinity for children and desire several of them – but this cannot be derived from a theoretical point of view. Long-lasting spousal cooperation cannot be automatically guaranteed by either spouse. The risk that one spouse breaks the agreement is elevated. Therefore, even if an unaffiliated couple has the same affinity for a higher number of children as in a homogamous couple in which both spouses are religious Muslims or Catholics, the probability to finally realize more children is higher among the latter. In the end, homogamy among religious couples leads to the result that desires and realization will accord in more marriages than in marriages composed of two unaffiliated spouses.

A religious inter-marriage enforces compromises and entails potential for conflict, for example with respect to the realizable number of children. If childbearing desires do not accord, the spouses have to bargain about fertility. In the worst case, the result diverges from the desired number of both spouses. Furthermore, daily quarrels due to diverging views, interests, life goals may be exhaustive in the long run. Both points lead to a "bargaining effect" whose magnitude depends on the precise religious composition of a union (holding other characteristics constant, Lehrer 1998: 246). The bargaining effect can be regarded as an additional reason why religious – especially very conservative – minorities prefer to intra-marry. Intra-marriage then entails less conflicts and the sharing of more commonalities.

Depending on the precise religious composition of the inter-marriage, the anticipation of a high divorce risk discourages at least one partner from investing too much into a relationship perceived as fragile. From that point a "marital (in)stability effect" follows (Becker/Landes/Michael 1977). It implies that inter-marriages lead to a lower number of children than intra-marriages. First, a shorter marriage duration can be assumed, reducing the years of exposure. But beyond that almost tautological reason, fertility will, secondly, be lower because it is restricted (due to the perceived dissolution probability) even while the marriage is still intact (Lehrer 2004: 708–709).

The case of homogamous unions has already been clarified. In the "affiliated case" the bargaining and marital stability effects work in the same direction promoting a higher fertility. In the "unaffiliated case", the marital stability effect is negative while the bargaining effect remains undetermined. Thus, fertility will be lower – always compared to the case of a homogamous union composed of two (religious) Catholics or especially two Muslims. The case of Muslims cannot be separated from the fact that they or their families originate from (Islamic) countries with a much lower level of (material, institutional, and ideological) modernization. In this respect, Catholics and Muslims should not be equated when considering fertility levels. Muslims (should) have a higher fertility, but it can also be assumed that their fertility behavior approaches the behavior of the autochthonal population, the longer they have already been residing in Europe.

Now, the marital stability and bargaining effects will be estimated for different constellations of compositions. If one spouse is Catholic and the other one is unaffiliated, both effects are negative for the Catholic while only the bargaining effect is negative for the unaffiliated spouse. Hence, fertility of the unaffiliated spouse will be higher than it would have been if she or he had married an unaffiliated partner. It is acceptable to suppose that the woman has the higher risk when she gives up gainful employment for a longer time. The (unaffiliated) wife gains more security that her spouse will provide for her and the children in case the man is the Catholic part of the union. Therefore, not only the religious composition of the union in general should be decisive. Also, the gender perspective should be taken into consideration.

A heterogamous union comprising a Catholic and a Protestant should only lead to slight effects. Fertility of the Catholic can be supposed to be somewhat lower and that of the Protestant to be somewhat higher compared to a homogamous – Catholic – marriage. The marriage of a Muslim to a non-Muslim leads to lower fertility from the perspective of the Muslim due a relatively strong bargaining effect. Furthermore, the marital stability effect also has a negative sign. The magnitude of the effects is associated with individual religiosity. Finally, these effects should result in higher labor market commitment of unaffiliated women, followed by Protestant women, especially if the husband is not a religious Catholic. Labor market commitment of Muslim women – especially if it is considered that they principally are not allowed to out-marry – should be lowest.

There is one case in which a heterogamous marriage should lead to higher fertility than a homogamous union. This outcome should apply if the heterogamous union involves at least one religiously affiliated spouse while the homogamous union is composed of two unaffiliated spouses. To conclude, both the bargaining as well as the marital stability effect influence fertility in inter-marriages and finally lead to a lower number of children compared to intra-marriages. This is however only valid, when the latter are religiously affiliated – both spouses are either Catholics or Muslims – and it is especially valid when they are both religious.

4.4 Determinants of marital (in)stability

It has just been argued that marital stability has an influence on fertility as well as the labor supply of women.[22] People marry although they are aware of the fragility of their union due to its unfavorable religious composition (Lehrer 2004: 709). The reason is that marital stability and the quality of a match depend on a wide range of factors of which religiosity is only one (Lehrer/Chiswick 1993).[23] In this section, a summarizing overview of stabilizing as well as destabilizing traits is given (figure 4.1 mentions only some of these traits).

With respect to religiosity, studies show that divorce is notably more uncommon among Catholic couples than among unaffiliated and Protestant couples (Diek-

[22] Empirical results confirm this postulate (see e.g. Coppola/Di Cesare 2008, Meggiolaro/Ongaro 2010, and Thomson et al. 2012).

[23] A further point is the absence of a perfect marriage market so that sorting is usually not optimal.

mann/Engelhardt 1995, Call/Heaton 1997, Hall 1997, Wagner/Weiß 2003, Bodenmann et al. 2006, Kraft/Neimann 2009). Beyond intra-marriage – measured solely by religious affiliation – the researchers confirm that religious commitment, a church wedding, religious beliefs as well as regular attendance of religious services lower the divorce risk.[24] Call/Heaton 1997 found several religiosity indicators provide evidence for an effect on marital stability. The indicator "church attendance" had the greatest effect. If only one spouse attends religious services regularly, slight gender differences in favor of the woman can be observed. The total effect is however notably smaller compared to regular attendance of both spouses. Homogamy in case of non-religiosity destabilizes a marriage (Kraft/Neimann 2009: 27). Empirically, indicators of religiosity document a more significant result than only affiliation.

The difference between the high utility that is expected from marriage at its beginning and the low utility at the time of its dissolution is the result of uncertainty leading to deviations between expected and realized utilities in the course of the marriage (Becker/Landes/Michael 1977: 1142). It seems to be a natural consequence to conclude that uncertainty in a couple composed of two religious spouses, ideally two Catholics or two Muslims, is very low. The increased probability of divorce can – among other things – be explained by decreased rates of religious and affiliated individuals, a reduced binding power of religious norms as well as processes of individual secularization caused by the developments described above. From these processes follow increased proportions of heterogamous marriages resulting in lower fertility – also for the religiously affiliated insofar as they enter into a heterogamous marriage.

The significance of children is frequently discussed in the context of divorce studies. While this work argues that couples are reluctant to invest in a relationship they recognize as unstable (anticipation argument), many studies argue the reverse: joint children reduce the divorce risk (for the USA: White 1990 who reviews literature on divorce determinants, Waite/Lillard 1991, and Lillard/Waite 1993, based on a meta-analysis for Germany: Wagner/Weiß 2003, based on a meta-analysis for Europe: Wagner/Weiß 2006). Studies report the greatest stabilizing effect for the first child whereas childless marriages have the highest risk of dissolution. The stabilizing influence of children seems to diminish with their rising age or with increasing marital

[24] The importance of a church wedding ignoring religious affiliation has also been documented by Brüderl/Kalter 2001. The same applies to the indicator "religious beliefs" whose importance has been attested by Knoester/Booth 2000.

duration; two time series whose effect cannot be clearly separated. Children from preceding relationships – only one spouse is the biological parent of the children in the current union – boost the risk of dissolution. This finding is in accordance with economic theory as presented in the preceding subsection. These results indicate that the anticipation argument is stronger. Another study has shown that Catholic marriages are not more stable in the early years than other marriages. Rather, the "Catholic effect" increases with marital duration (Wagner 1993: 383).

A very young age at marriage has also been shown to endanger marital stability (Lyngstad/Jalovaara 2010 in a literature review, Wagner/Weiß 2003 in a meta-analysis), as apparently older age also does (Lehrer 2008 for the USA). The level of information about the other spouse is limited at the time of union formation, the quality of the match is uncertain and the search duration is rather short. As time passes, the spouses gather new information on the quality of the match as well as on outside options and alternatives. White 1990 cites literature suggesting that poor role performance is a factor. Young people tend to be less mature and make less forward-looking decisions (Lyngstad/Jalovaara 2010: 259). Wagner and Weiss report that the time period between getting to know to each other and the start of the relationship is also important (Wagner/Weiß 2003: 39–40). Lehrer 2004 comes to the conclusion that Catholics in the USA marry later. They want to ensure that the selected future spouse is appropriate because divorce is excluded (p. 718). It can be assumed that the strong rise in age at marriage reported above has inhibited an even more intense increase in the divorce rate. The u-shaped curve of dissolution risks dependent on age, Becker and Lehrer suggest, means that women with unfulfilled desires to have children hear their "biological clock tick" and become pregnant within a match that is not optimal (Lehrer 2008: 10).

Parental divorce increases the later divorce risk of their children, a phenomenon which is well known in the literature as inter-generational transmission of divorce. It significantly contributes to explaining the rise in divorce risks and hence rates over time (see e.g. Bumpass/Sweet 1972, McGue/Lykken 1992, Wagner 1993, and Amato 1996). The risk of divorce for a spouse with divorced parents is twice as high as for a spouse from an intact family of origin 20 years after marriage (Diekmann/Engelhardt 1995: 220). Considerable differences by gender exist in their study: the effect of transmission is rather weak for women, but extremely strong for men. The risk for men with divorced parents to divorce is three times higher than that of men from complete families (p. 221). Other studies report a higher risk of 50% for both sexes together (Wagner/Weiß 2003: 50).[25] Diekmann/Engelhardt 1995 mention further traits that might explain the pronounced gender differences: men with divorced parents marry earlier on average and they have fewer children. Another trait is the lack of religious attachment (pp. 224–225). Put simply, Catholic parents produce – with a high probability – Catholic children and their attitudes towards marriage and divorce are transmitted during socialization. This applies more strongly to girls. Moreover, men less often enter into a homogamously Catholic marriage but tend to marry more often unaffiliated women resulting in a marriage composed of two unaffiliated partners. A meta-analysis of European longitudinal studies shows that the lower the divorce barriers are, the weaker the association between parental divorce and the divorce risk of their offspring (Wagner/Weiß 2006).

Joint property strongly decreases the divorce risk. It can be understood as a major marriage-specific investment. Children with divorced parents more rarely acquire joint property (Diekmann/Engelhardt 1995: 223, Brüderl/Kalter 2001: 415–417). This can be interpreted as reluctance to invest more in the marriage due to the anticipation of divorce.[26] The divorce rate is higher in urban than in rural areas. In towns the acquisition of property is more expensive and fewer people can afford to buy an apartment or even a house. Moreover, in urban areas the opportunities for meeting a better partner are greater (Brüderl/Kalter 2001, Kraft/Neimann 2009).

During recent decades the prevalence of (premarital) cohabitation has steadily risen – starting to spread out in urban areas first – and today is the usual way to

[25] The literature proposes four main hypotheses to explain transmission, namely a stress hypothesis, a socialization or learning hypothesis, a socioeconomic deprivation hypothesis, and a hypothesis about the inheritance of personality traits (Wagner/Weiß 2006 and the literature quoted there). According to the stress hypothesis, parental divorce acts as a pull factor inducing the children to leave home early and marry at a young age (Diekmann/Engelhardt 1995: 216–217). The socialization hypothesis points to the conditions for growing up including the transmission of attitudes towards marriage and divorce. The children learn by observation, including how to solve problems within a relationship (Diekmann/Engelhardt 1995: 217). Children of divorced parents may view marriage dissolution with greater acceptance which may increase their readiness to end an unhappy union (Lehrer/Chiswick 1993: 387). The socioeconomic deprivation hypothesis refers to the economic consequences of a divorce. In a one-parent family, mostly with the mother, financial resources are scarce and socioeconomic circumstances are often difficult, which also makes the children leave home and marrying early. For an explanation of the hypothesis about the inheritance of personality traits see McGue/Lykken 1992.

[26] In this case the counterargument would be also reasonable. In this respect, similar arguments can be advanced for children and for joint property.

start co-residence. A significant reason for cohabitation is the need to learn about the potential spouse and to insure against future shocks. Though the level of (premarital) information about the partner is high, cohabitation seem to be associated with an elevated risk of later divorce compared to relationships where co-residence directly began as a married couple (see e.g. White 1990, Hall 1997, Andersson 2003, Brien/Lillard/Stern 2006, Lyngstad/Jalovaara 2010). Wagner/Weiß 2006 come to the conclusion that in European countries where more rigid marriage norms prevail, cohabitation has a stronger effect on marital instability than in countries where marriage norms are weaker. In the former, cohabitants are a more selective group that rebels against well-established norms than in the latter mentioned societies that are characterized by a weak institutionalization of marriage and where liberal attitudes towards cohabitation prevail (p. 484). This result is not confirmed by Andersson, who also analyzes European data and reports that the excess instability of unions that began with a cohabitation is evident regardless whether cohabitation is the typical way to start a union in that country (such as France and Norway), or whether direct marriages dominate (such as Hungary) or both modes of entry into a union are common (e.g. Germany). In all countries Andersson involves in his investigation, the level of dissolved unions after 15 years was at least twice as high. Researchers hold selectivity processes responsible for the rather unexpected positive link. Partners who do not cohabit before marriage might also be reluctant to divorce: "the kinds of people who choose to flout convention by cohabiting are the same kinds of people who flout normative marital behavior, have lower commitment to marriage as an institution, and disregard the stigma of divorce" (White 1990: 906). Direct marriage in combination with a lower risk of dissolution is linked to unobserved, stable characteristics, such as a strong attachment to religion or conservative family values (Lyngstad/Jalovaara 2010: 261). One study has however provided evidence that the negative effect of cohabitation diminishes if the duration of the relationship is modeled (Brüderl/Kalter 2001).

The increased occurrence of divorce is frequently traced back to the increased labor force participation of women and ultimately their income (Becker/Landes/Michael 1977). The risk rises with working hours. Full-time employment shows the highest risk (see e.g. the review of studies in White 1990; see also Jalovaara 2003, Böttcher 2006, Kalmijn/Loeve/Manting 2007, Kalmijn 2007). Referring to the couple perspective, a husband's high income and socioeconomic status lowers the probability of marital disruption. A wife's high income destabilizes a marriage and especially endangers it if her income exceeds her husband's (Kalmijn 2007). Knoester/Booth 2000 confirm that dependence on the spouse keeps a marriage intact.[27] Böttcher 2006 concludes in her empirical analysis that while labor supply was positively connected to the divorce risk in East as well as West Germany before unification, the effect size was stronger in the West. She relates this to the more traditional frame within which gender roles are rather complementary than similar or egalitarian. In countries where the rate of employed women is pronounced, the effect seems hence to be weaker (Kalmijn 2007: 244). This points to a micro-macro association and the frame within which actions take place.[28] The literature offers the following explanations for the correlation. One reason for the higher divorce risk is seen in an underinvestment in marriage-specific capital indicating the argumentation presented above. Employment strengthens the economic position of women which brings independence and lowers the benefits of specialization (Kalmijn/Loeve/Manting 2007: 159). Similar gender roles are assumed to lessen marital cohesion due to the lack of mutual dependency (Becker/Landes/Michael 1977, White 1990: 905). It also reduces the costs of leaving a troubled marriage. Causality may also be reversed, but this line of argument has already been presented.

Effects of educational achievement and the educational composition of a couple on marital stability are equivocal. Jalovaara 2003 and Kraft/Neimann 2009 review literature and show that all kinds of results exist. In general, there seems to be no clear evidence that either a certain level of education or educational homogamy – and hence positive assortive mating – stabilize a marriage. Their own analyses come to the conclusion that two medium- or two highly-educated spouses have a lower divorce risk than two low-educated spouses. A repeating but also not uniform result seems however to be that a woman's higher educational achievement compared to her husband's enhances the divorce risk. A positive consequence of higher education for marital stability may be the higher age at marriage which is due to the longer time spent in educational institutions (Bumpass/Sweet 1972).

The divorce risk varies with marital duration (Peuckert 2008: 171). The most pronounced risk manifests between the 5th and the 9th year of marriage with a mode in the 5th year. Since the late 1980s the risk of late divorce around the 19th year

[27] An increase in wage rates of women (relative to men) should already entail a lower incentive to marry at all (Becker 1973: 822).

[28] This issue will be addressed in section 5.1.

of marriage has grown (Peuckert 2008: 176). While earlier the probability of a late dissolution declined, the share has now increased to 20% of all divorces (in Germany).

Finally, sometimes changes in divorce laws are considered in divorce studies as a non-individual or non-couple-based factor. Reforms of divorce laws mainly took place in the late 1970s, shifting them from mutual consent requirements to unilateral divorce, and the results of the studies are ambiguous in many countries (for Europe: Smith 2002, Fella/Manzini/Mariotti 2002, Kneip/Bauer 2009, González/Viitanen 2009; for the USA: Friedberg 1998, Wolfers 2006). Unilateral divorce law allows a spouse to seek divorce without the consent of the other spouse. Figure 2.8 shows the dramatic outliers (around 1978) in the West German curve at the aggregated level. The turning point in the East German curve rested on the legal passage from a liberal divorce law with high divorce rates to the West German law including the "separated from bed and board" period of one year with a lower rate. Kneip/Bauer/Reinhold 2011 find on the basis of data for several Western European countries that unilateral divorce law increased the risk of marital dissolution by about 20% and would have been even higher without self-selection into marriage. Kneip/Bauer 2009 conclude that *de facto* unilateral divorce practices led to a sustainable increase in the divorce rate. They cannot document long-term effects for legal rights to unilaterally divorce. González/Viitanen 2009 find with the aid of a panel of 18 European countries that the shift from fault to no-fault legislation was followed by strong and permanent increases in divorce rates whereas the shift from bilateral to unilateral divorce law merely had temporary effects on divorce rates. They estimate that reforms account for about 20% of the rise between 1960 and 2002.

Teachman 2002 has examined whether the determinants of divorce are invariant across historical time. He finds that the effects of major sociodemographic predictors of divorce have not varied over the course of time. Consequently, anything that diminishes the real or perceived gains to marriage constitutes a risk factor for marital disruption. Although Teachman uses US data, this is an important result as he refers to marriages concluded between 1950 and 1984. This result does not contradict the finding that developments in religiosity, female labor supply, and parental divorce have contributed to a rise in divorce risks.

Several characteristics that promote or endanger the stability of marriages can be reconciled with the economic theory and some of them are associated with religious affiliation and religiosity. It has been reasoned that marital stability positively influences fertility. Another position in the literature, however, is that the consequence of union disruption is not self-evident. On the one hand, a separation does lead to a discontinued fertility history which may result in lower completed fertility. Lillard/ Waite 1993 think that having experienced a separation can reduce the chance or the desire to enter into a new relationship and the confidence in its stability, which in turn lowers the probability of a (further) child. On the other hand, many people who enter into a new partnership prove their commitment by having a new child which would indeed have the opposite effect (Billari 2005). Klein 2003 discovered that a third or fourth child is rather born in a new partnership while a second child is more often born within the same partnership as the first one. According to that finding, higher order births are a step-family phenomenon. This is however conditional on dissolving the first marriage early, namely during the childbearing years. It simultaneously lowers the probability to have more children in the first marital union unless age at first marriage and childbearing are low, which has well-known consequences. Moreover, the opportunity to be able to decide in favor of another child depends on re-partnering. Finding a new partner incurs search costs, at least in the form of time – but only if the new partner was not the reason to leave the first marriage.

5 The National Frame and Individual Characteristics: Further Determinants of Fertility Behavior

The economic theory just presented usually neglects non-individual and non-couple based factors. Behavioral changes are "simply" traced back to changes in relative prices and surrounding conditions which constitute the frame. Couples make fertility decisions within a certain frame (Strohmeier 2002) and therefore the following section 5.1 focuses on it in more detail. In a national perspective, this frame is composed of policy results (laws and regulations), social norms, political and historical events, etc. The frame not only influences demographic behavior but also reacts to demographic developments and changes. It could hence be called an "interacting frame". The first part of section 5.1 compares French, Hungarian, Norwegian, and German policy-making motives and results, and discusses the impact of the churches on policy-making (5.1.1). A (much shorter) second part (5.1.2) presents the impact of socialism on families during the transformation period around 1990 in Hungary and East Germany, which had short-term as well as long-term implications for demographic behavior. Of course, further factors are important in the context of fertility decisions, insofar the section merely presents a (restrictive) selection. The first section closes with some study results clarifying the effects of the frame on fertility (5.1.3).

Section 5.2 changes the level from the nation back to the individual. It discusses some important traits and factors associated with fertility. These play a decisive role in the theoretical approach and re-emerge in the empirical analyses. The traits considered are gender (5.2.1), education, and closely related factors such as qualifications (5.2.2), and female labor force participation (5.2.3).

5.1 The interacting frame for fertility decisions

5.1.1 Family-related policies

Family-related policies comprise all fields that concern family issues, e.g. decisions made in the family context: "family policies can be defined as an amalgam of policies directed at families with children and aimed at increasing their level of well-being" (Gauthier 2002: 456). Explicit family policy refers to all political measures explicitly justified by the objective to promote families or to shape (family life) normatively (Kaufmann 2002: 429–433). It requires institutional autonomy, e.g. in the form of a dedicated ministry, and measures that concentrate directly on issues concerning families and not only on individuals who may be family members. Implicit family policy involves measures reasoned by other motives or measures with other objectives that may also affect family life. These measures can relate to, for example, the labor market, or social, educational, and tax policy. Family policy may also be characterized as family-related policies. Motives and effects have to be differentiated when political measures are assessed. While the legislature prioritizes motives over effects, the effects are of higher importance for the addressees and researchers analyzing them (Strohmeier 2002: 325).

A typology of (seven) arguments motivating political interventions has been compiled by Kaufmann (2006: 426–428). (1) The institutional motive forefronts the institution family as a value in itself that is worth preserving. (2) The natalist motive aims at influencing the birth rate by restricting or promoting births. (3) The eugenic motive refers to the quality of populations. (4) The economic motive tries to secure and advance the level of human capital in a population. (5) The socio-political motive focuses on the reduction of poverty and (economic) discrimination of families. (6) The gender motive targets the reduction of disadvantages for and discrimination of women. (7) Finally, the children's welfare motive is geared to secure the rights, to meet the needs and to raise the well-being of children. On the one hand, political measures intervening in the family sphere deal with more than one motive. On the other hand, it may happen that they follow one motive while contradicting another one. The overall goal of family policy is to enable families to fulfill a range of functions that are necessary to maintain a population and can exclusively be performed by families (Lampert/Althammer 2007: 383–385). In the following cross-country comparison, the natalist as well as the equality motive are of special interest. All countries concentrate on the well-being of children although realizations diverge across nations and are embedded into the specific, national path-dependent policy systems.

With regard to the motives and goals, four kinds of intervention can be distinguished (Kaufmann 2002: 433–436): (i) Legal intervention comprises measures referring to the legal status of family members, e.g. in family, labor or social law. (ii) Economic intervention involves measures that directly impact the economic resources of families. (iii) Ecological intervention consists of measures changing the environment and hence opportunity structures for families, e.g. infrastructure, social services, housing policy, etc. (iv) Individual-related interventions embrace measures aiming at the improvement or recovery of family members' abilities and capabilities, e.g. in the education, social, and health systems. National family(-related) policies are the result of a large variety of determinants of moral and legal traditions, social state concepts, gender roles, overall concepts of family, state-church relations, the organization of fulfillment of state tasks as well as fiscal frame conditions (Gerlach 2010: 358).

During the 1950s and the 1960s in most Western European countries including France, Norway, and the Federal Republic of Germany, both labor force participation rates of women and divorce rates were low. In addition, lone parenthood and separation had a low incidence while marriage rates and fertility were high – compared to the following decades. Policies stabilized this demographic pattern. After this period, demographic behavior changed and moved to the center of the political agenda – earlier in some countries, later in others. The marginalized position of family issues in general was reversed as they moved up the political agenda.

In West Germany, the socio-political and the children's welfare motives have long been the only ones for family policy-making, even though the country has a dedicated ministry which was founded in 1953. Compensating families for child-related costs and hence distributive considerations were foregrounded for a long time (Schratzenstaller 2002). The fairness of income distribution was an important goal (Strohmeier 2002: 325, 355). The economic intervention and hence monetary instruments were the dominant measures to support families (e.g. child-rearing allowance, child-related tax allowances but also joint taxation with full income splitting for married couples[1]). Family policy was, however, not successful in reducing child poverty

[1] This means that spouses' incomes are added together and divided by two. Income tax then has to be paid on the two separate incomes. In a progressive tax system this has a tax reducing effect and the savings increase as the difference between the two initial incomes

and inequality (Bundesministerium für Familie, Senioren, Frauen und Jugend 2006). It cannot be characterized as sustainable if this term is defined as increasing births, effectively fighting child poverty, and improving the participation of mothers in the labor market to enable them to make their own provisions for old age and health care (Gruescu/Rürup 2005).

Policy instruments did not comprise pro-natalist elements for historical reasons. The promotion of female labor force participation by reducing incompatibilities between the family and the job has hardly occurred. Social developments, such as women's improved educational attainments followed by their steadily rising labor supply as well as career and employment orientations have been ignored (Dorbritz 2008: 590–591). No steps were taken to actively encourage individual female autonomy, to curtail opportunity costs, and to enable reconciliation of family and work. Finally, the perception of high poverty rates changed the alignment of family policy and enhanced the significance of this neglected field of policy (Ministerium für Generationen, Familie, Frauen und Integration des Landes Nordrhein-Westfalen 2006: 11). Until the end of the 1980s, family policy was also shaped by the Federal Constitutional Court. It repeatedly had to refer to constitutional violations, e.g. with respect to justice towards families (Althammer 2000: 39–43, Gerlach 2010: 292–295). The coerced choice to decide between motherhood and employment has probably contributed to rising childlessness, especially among highly-educated women and in certain social settings (Strohmeier 2002: 356). Over time, this has led to a normalization to a childless environment and growing acceptance of childlessness, which in turn results in a decline in the desired number of children. The paradigm change of family policy at the end of the 1990s and its practical implementation some years later came very late and was not able to influence fertility quickly – long-term effects may be positive, however (see e.g. Salles/Rossier/Brachet 2010 and Hoem 2008). Nevertheless, in principle there was no alternative to the adoption of a modern family policy.

France is another example of a country with an explicit family policy.[2] In France, family policy is very active, has a long tradition dating back to the end of the 19th century, and has steadily been taking a central position in social policy (Kaufmann 2002: 430). Family policy comprises a comprehensive assortment of measures "based on

rises. In fact, joint income taxation with full income splitting is not a family promotion measure but mirrors the spouses' individual ability to pay (Althammer 2000: 33–34).

[2] Bundesministerium für Familie, Senioren, Frauen und Jugend 2006: 43 and Ministerium für Generationen, Familie, Frauen und Integration des Landes Nordrhein-Westfalen 2006: 40.

varying ideological backgrounds" (Toulemon/Pailhé/Rossier 2008: 505). These reflect struggles and discussions between politicians and social groups. Family policy-making has traditionally had a strong pro-natalist orientation. This also has historical roots: France was the first country worldwide that experienced an extreme birth decline already in the 1870s – known as the first demographic transition – and was therefore especially sensitized (Köppen/Mazuy/Toulemon 2007: 83–84).[3]

Until 1994 a clear three-child policy was pursued. The country counts among the very few (developed) countries that do not pay any child benefit for the first child (*allocations familiales*). Apart from child benefit there is a large variety of other benefits payable to parents (*Caisse Nationale d'Allocations Familiales* (CNAF)). Because of the long-standing three-child policy, large families have enjoyed many privileges, monetary incentives, and support. This may be a reason why the proportion of women born in 1960 who have three children is still higher than the proportion who have only one child (Köppen/Mazuy/Toulemon 2007: 92). Income tax benefits (*quotient familial*) depend on the number of children.[4] If there are no children, the tax system is similar to the German one (joint taxation with full income splitting). The only difference is the inclusion of couples who have entered into a *Pacte civil de solidarité* (Wrohlich/Dell/Baclet 2005). The dependence on the marital status was abolished in 1996. Before that date, only married couples were entitled to full income splitting. This legal adjustment contributes to explaining the high rate of extramarital children (Köppen/Mazuy/Toulemon 2007: 86). Almost at the same time, namely after 1994, the political goal of promoting births decreased in significance: since then families with two children have also been supported.

At the same time, the gender equity motive started to gain importance. Principally, this is a convergence toward the policies of Northern Europe, e.g. Norway. Reconciliation of family and employment had already been possible, but the ideological

[3] Among other triggers, this early experience is regarded as a driving factor for the nation's explicit pro-natalist policies (van de Kaa 1987: 5). For a different argumentation see Veil 2007 who refers to the *Ancien Régime* that followed the doctrine of the association between a people's productivity and the numerical increase in a population.

[4] Baclet et al. 2005 compare the distributive effects of state family promotion in Germany and France. The alignment of the family components in the income tax system lead to the conclusion that families with low income benefit more in the German than in the French system. In France, tax allowances are differentiated by the number of children which results in a stronger tax relief in France relative to Germany for families with high income.

preconditions were different.[5] Mothers are basically free in deciding for or against employment. If they decide in favor of employment, they receive – dependent on income and the number of children – financial support towards the cost of public child care for children aged under three (*complément de libre choix du mode de garde*). If they stay at home with their children or work at most part-time, they are financially supported by a high home care allowance (*complément de libre choix d'activité*) until the child is six months old. If the family has more than one child, the time period is extended until the child's second birthday (Veil 2005, Veil 2007).[6] Only non-working mothers qualified for the child-rearing allowance (*allocation parentale d'education*, payable until the child's third birthday), however until 1994 only for the third and higher order children. After 1994, parents were already entitled to it from the second child on. In 2004, the child-rearing allowance was replaced by the two kinds of *complément*, paid from the first child on. This explains the employment-related reactions of mothers. The parent that stays at home for longer than the period of paid maternity leave is not paid income compensation. A small lump sum is paid to parents on the birth of their child. Beyond these instruments, there is a monthly basic allowance for child care (*allocation de base*) that is means tested (Veil 2007: 30–31). One part of increasing gender equity is the involvement of fathers in child-rearing. For more than a decade fathers have been allowed to share unpaid leave for two years with the mother. And since 2002 fathers are entitled to take paid leave for 14 days.

The country has a comprehensive and subsidized system of day care with long opening hours for children of all ages (Toulemon/Pailhé/Rossier 2008, Letablier 2002, Veil 2007).[7] The *école maternelle* was established in 1881 and is attended by almost

[5] The republican state with its principle of universalism behaves neutrally towards, among others, the behavior of individuals comprising the category "gender" (Veil 2005: 6). This means that the opportunities for reconciling family and employment rested on the gender indifferent view but not on the gender equity motive.

[6] This has resulted in a selection effect: lower educated women, women with a high risk of unemployment or working on fixed-term contracts are provided with a monetary incentive to select themselves out of the labor market and to bring up their children at home (see e.g. Toulemon/Pailhé/Rossier 2008: 531–532). Opponents fear this might negatively influence the future achievements of these children who should rather be cared for in public nurseries. Stay-at-home mothers do not pay contributions toward their old age pensions. In contrast, proponents of this arrangement strive for the maintenance of a traditional way of family life.

[7] The number of places in public child care facilities (*crèche*) has continuously grown since the early 1980s. In 2002, 9% of the under threes were cared for in a *crèche*, 18% by registered childminders or home helps (18%). One fourth of small children attended preschool facilities or were cared for by a relative, neighbor or a non-registered childminder (Letablier 2003: 247).

all children aged three and older, traditionally full-time. In 2002, a third of the two-year-olds also attended an *école maternelle* that already prepares them for school and is free of charge. In 1960, the corresponding rate totaled 10% of all preschoolers. The expansion of maternelles already started somewhat earlier and rose in parallel with the labor force participation of women, who usually work full-time. In general, school in France is equivalent to full-time school (Gottschall/Hagemann 2002, Veil 2002: 29). The country tries to ensure social equity by providing high quality public child-care to do justice to the republican principle of *egalité* (Letablier 2003). Parents' income should not decide on children's development. In this respect, however, French family and education policies are not successful to the desired degree. Social origin significantly affects school achievement although to a lesser extent than in Germany (OECD 2010).

Norway numbers among the social-democratic, universalistic welfare states (Gerlach 2010: 366–369). Social rights are granted to individuals (and not to families) independently of their civil and family status. These countries are characterized by a high degree of redistribution, defamilialization, and decommodification (Esping-Andersen 1990, Esping-Andersen 2002). Decommodification is the level to which an individual can maintain herself or himself without market income. A high level of decommodification strongly reduces financial insecurity. Defamilialization is the degree to which individuals (independent of their gender) are able to generate their own income (Blum/Rille-Pfeiffer 2010: 28–29). Family policy in Norway has mainly been implicit, but the country has a long tradition of extensive social policies directed at individuals. The family as a social unit is not protected by the constitution (Rønsen 2004a: 278). Norwegian social policy is not driven by pro-natalist motives but is nevertheless assumed to positively affect fertility behavior (Frejka/Calot 2001: 136). Equality in general is one of the major objectives for policy-making, which includes gender equality. This goal aims at minimizing the conflicts between child-bearing, child-rearing, and employment, especially for women but also includes the involvement of men in family tasks. The result has been a high female labor force participation rate (it rose especially during the 1970s) with many women working long part-time,[8] and reluctant behavior on the part of men regarding family commitment. These results are called "gender equality light" (Rønsen/Skrede 2010: 327).[9]

The Norwegian welfare state today is the result of a longer development. In the 1950s and 1960s, it was a different kind of state. At that time, the dominant family model was a male breadwinner and a female homemaker and carer, as was the case in many European countries (Rønsen 2004b: 145). Traditional patterns of fertility and gender roles were typical for couples born between 1930 and the early 1950s while the new patterns characterize increasing shares of couples born later (Lappegård 2000). Since the middle of the 1980s, policies have striven to promote the dual-earner/dual-carer model (Skevik/Hatland 2008: 89).

A universal right to paid (parental) leave is granted by the National Insurance Act of 1956. Initially, the benefit period for entitled women was short (12 weeks) and the level of income compensation was low (Rønsen 2004a: 278), but extended stepwise. The benefit and job guarantee period were expanded in 1977.[10] Also fathers got the right to share the leave, except for the three weeks before and the six weeks after the birth. This time period was still reserved for the mother (statutory maternity leave). In addition, fathers are entitled to two weeks of unpaid paternity leave immediately after the birth. Traditionally, most fathers have taken these two weeks of paternity leave (but not more). The benefits were raised substantially to cover 100% of previous income for most employed women in 1978 (Rønsen 2004a: 279).[11] Further extensions did not happen until 1987 when the benefit period was prolonged several times. By 1993 maximum leave was 52 weeks at 80% income compensation or 42 weeks with 100% (Rønsen 2004b: 147). These arrangements were still in force in 2004. Hence, if women decide not to remain out of the labor market for long, their loss of income is low. Altogether this means that the instrument of income compensation was

[8] "Long" part-time means between 20 and 35 hours of work per week while "short" part-time is less than 20 hours of work per week.

[9] It evokes concern among researchers. Even if the Nordic states are often presented as a positive example, high fertility is often widespread among women trained for female-dominated jobs. The labor markets are strongly gender segregated, horizontally and vertically. In the hierarchy of jobs, the great majority of women are to be found in lower positions. They are frequently employed part-time. Men rarely work less than full-time, undertake much less homework, and in spite of gender-neutral leave policies rarely take parental leave longer than the time reserved exclusively for them (Rønsen/Skrede 2010: 327–328).

[10] After the period of paid parental leave, parents are entitled to a period of unpaid leave. In Norway, the right to leave in association with job security until the child is one year old, was introduced in 1977 (Rønsen 2004a: 278).

[11] They were made taxable and subject to pension payments.

introduced very early and the current situation has existed for a long time, especially compared to most other countries.

Women who are not entitled to leave – it requires a certain length of employment during pregnancy in order to acquire eligibility for benefits[12] – have received a tax-free lump sum on the birth of their child since the late 1980s. Due to the fact that very few fathers have used the opportunity to share parts of the common parental leave period, an amendment was passed in 1993. After that year, four weeks of the extended leave period have been exclusively reserved for the father ("daddy quota") to encourage their commitment to child care (Rønsen 2004a). Three years after its introduction, almost 80% of entitled fathers made use of the quota. In addition to the usual leave period, parents can do time banking since 1994, which is an alternate way to take parental leave (Skevik/Hatland 2008: 100–101). After a shortened employment break, a reduced number of weekly working hours and a reduced benefit level for a longer than the usual time period are combined. This arrangement prevents an income loss for the parent who wants to reconcile child-rearing and employment.

(Subsidized) childcare facilities for preschool children were expanded at the end of the 1970s. "The 1975 Day care Institutions Act marks the beginning of modern policies for publicly sponsored childcare in Norway" (Skevik/Hatland 2008: 94). Before 1975, day care institutions were uncommon. In 1973, the coverage rate among preschoolers was below 5%. The Act established the principle that day care should be available to all parents who are in need of this service. This ambitious aim had not yet been reached in 2005, but had resulted in a strong expansion especially in the 1980s and the first half of the 1990s. In 2005, almost half of all one- to two-year-olds and about 70% of all one- to five-year-olds attended day care institutions (Skevik/Hatland 2008).[13] Due to parental leave, children younger than 12 months are exclusively cared for in the family. In combination with paid leave, the provision of public and private child care lowers the indirect child-related costs. It contributes to defamilialization and hence to more gender equality.

A relevant percentage of parents care for their children mainly at home. Since 1998, families who have children aged one or two years are supported by a home

[12] Before 1977, women had to be employed for the last eight months out of ten prior to the birth. After that year the length was reduced to six months out of the last ten.

[13] In 1980, one fifth of all preschoolers attended day care institutions. Ten years later the proportion had risen to 36%, and in 2001 the proportion amounted to 54% (Rønsen 2004b: 148).

care allowance. The amount roughly corresponds to the state subsidy for a child care place. To take advantage of the allowance, attendance hours must be less than full-time (33 hours a week). Part-time attendance is associated with a reduced allowance (Blum/Rille-Pfeiffer 2010: 9). A great majority of the eligible parents make use of the home care allowance: in 1999, shortly after introduction, the proportion was 75%. The allowance led to a temporary stagnation in the rise of the proportion of one and two year old children in public day care (see figure in Skevik/Hatland 2008: 95). The generous home care allowance in combination with unpaid leave while the job position is guaranteed generates freedom of choice for women of children even before they are three years old. In Norway the home care allowance was extremely controversially discussed prior to its introduction (Skevik/Hatland 2008: 104). Evaluating studies show that the instrument affects parental behavior far less than opponents feared. Employment orientation and use of public child care remained pronounced.[14]

It seems reasonable to compare family-related policies in Norway, France, and West Germany before moving on to East Germany and Hungary. The differences in the arrangement of family-related policies can, among other things, be traced back to nation-specific historical experiences, the development of a central state, and diverging state-church relations (Gerlach 2010: 363–369, Bahle 1995: 47, Fix 2001). The design of social policies in Norway has been strongly influenced by the Protestant Church and left-wing governments. In countries with a Protestant state church, equality was established early as an important goal for state actions. Social policies developed an individualistic alignment and comprised interventionist-egalitarian measures (Bahle 1995: 49). Detachment of traditional – Catholic – views on marriage and family occurred fastest where, among other things, a Protestant state church in association with a strong monarchy existed. Compatibility of childbearing, child-rearing, and paid employment for both sexes is fostered to promote equality. The fertility outcome and the high level of state support are similar in Norway and France, although the kinds of support, the ideological background, motives, and justification for state interventions differ quite strong.

According to the principle of subsidiarity, family is mainly regarded as a private matter; and according to the principle of solidarity, families have to be enabled to perform their tasks such as child care. In Germany these principles have been realized

[14] The reason for the diverging reactions towards the home care allowance may be the different labor market situations, but also different employment orientations in Norway and France.

by financial subsidies and monetary benefits but much less by direct interventions.[15] They reinforce the traditional gender role model with the husband as breadwinner and the wife as homemaker and carer with derived entitlements. This led to Germany's usual classification as conservative welfare state.[16] In France in contrast, care for children as well as childhood in total is seen as being a state responsibility and a public task (Letablier 2003: 247). It is considered a right of the child to be publicly cared for. Hence, the state intervenes in the family and undertakes tasks that in Germany are traditionally left to the family (Letablier 2002, Toulemon/Pailhé/Rossier 2008: 537, Gottschall/Hagemann 2002: 15). The French procedure is widely accepted by the population. The state regards itself as expert in educating and bringing up children while denying parents this competency. This understanding resembles the socialist one. It permits the conclusion that the French and West German population's understanding of policy-making and state paternalism differs fundamentally. France features some characteristics of a conservative welfare state but also has a high child care coverage rate which is rather a sign of defamilialization.

In the FRG, legitimation for political activities and the arrangement of social policies were derived from and are in accordance with Catholic social teaching (Fix 2001). Ideas of marriage and family have moreover been based on Catholic norms and reflected in their alignment. Representatives of the churches brought their strong influence to bear on the writing of the Constitution in 1948 and 1949 (Sontheimer/Bleek 2005: 32) which is a result of the German system of corporatism. Family matters have – of course – always been one of the churches' main concerns. They are still very active and comment on current social topics, are integrated into state committees, and act on the formation of the public opinion. In France, the strong presence of the state in the educational system – mainly the institution of the *école maternelle* that represents a republican-laicist comprehension of early child education – also has historical reasons. A strong central state that developed early was particularly keen to diminish the influence of the Catholic Church in the family sphere and the educational system and to take over control of them. Therefore, the educational system

---

15 One can argue that family was never a purely private matter due to the benefits paid to and support for families (Althammer 2000). To consider family as a purely private matter would completely ignore the fact that individuals have to care for children while others do not.

16 Further characteristics of a conservative welfare state are: medium decommodification and medium to high level cash support (including employment-related state supports), and long leave and limited child care facilities; Esping-Andersen 2002, Blum/Rille-Pfeiffer 2010: 21).

is the result of a struggle between state and church (Köppen/Mazuy/Toulemon 2007: 84–85, Toulemon/Pailhé/Rossier 2008: 536, Gerlach 2010: 363–368, Bahle 1995: 47). An important reason can be found in diverging moral concepts of state and church. The start of this process goes back to the end of the 19th century – the republican, secular educational system was already established in 1881 – years before 1904 when *laicité* was legally anchored in the French Constitution (Veil 2002: 29). One special state interest was to educate offspring in being loyal republican citizens.

In socialist societies, family policy was often reduced to population policy. The (pro-)natalist motive dominated the arrangement of public policies.[17] The decline of fertility (e.g. in the 1950s in Hungary or during the 1960s in the GDR) happened unexpectedly and contradicted all theoretical and ideological assumptions of the political leaders. Population growth was regarded as the predominance of socialism over capitalism (Besemeres 1980: 260–262). In Hungary and the GDR monetary and non-monetary measures were various, generous, frequently expanded, and usually based on the number of children. This pattern is obviously similar to French family policy before 1994. France was the country outside CEE with the most aggressive pro-natalist policies (van de Kaa 1987: 51, Spéder/Kamarás 2008: 647–651). From 1972 onwards (the time after the first deep drop of the fertility rate in the GDR) several policy measures were implemented. They were explicitly directed towards increasing fertility and encouraged early family formation, higher order births as well as the reconciliation of employment and family (Kreyenfeld 2004: 278–279, Huinink/Kreyenfeld 2004: 2).

The *Babyjahr*, a paid leave which offered a relatively high level of income replacement can be considered a birth promoting measure. It was introduced in 1976 and granted from the second child on. Employed mothers with three or more children (3+) were allowed special leave and to reduce their working hours (Kreyenfeld 2004: 278–279). The percentage of extra-marital births already rose considerably in the 1970s. Especially the *Babyjahr* – among other socio-political measures – was a decisive incentive to stay unmarried because unmarried mothers were already entitled to it from the first child on (Kreyenfeld/Konietzka 2004: 17). Even after the extension to married mothers in 1985, the percentage of children born out of wedlock did not stop rising.[18] Larger families were given priority access to housing (Frerich/Frey 1996:

[17] For Hungary see e.g. Spéder/Kamarás 2008 or Frejka 2008b: 149–151; for the GDR see e.g. Frerich/Frey 1996: 412–423, Kreyenfeld 2004: 282.

[18] It even went on rising after unification, i.e. after the legal adjustment to West Germany.

427–428). In Hungary, where a severe housing shortage existed, it was similar: in 1973 special housing support was introduced. Families with at least three children were given council flats at low rents within a short time period (Spéder/Kamarás 2008: 648). The "marriage loan" in the GDR gave couples who married the possibility to apply for an interest-free loan usable for furnishing (Cromm 1998: 477). That loan could be "paid back" by bearing three children. The first child redeemed one fifth of the sum, the second one a further 30% and the third one the last 50% of the amount. Direct child benefits also rose with parity. The Hungarian arrangement differed merely in content from the East German one, but the idea was the same: a certain share of a bank loan, awarded to purchase housing, functioned as a kind of a baby bonus and did not have to be paid back if the couple gave birth to children within a certain time after having been granted the loan. The proportion of the loan not to be paid back depended on the number of children born (Oláh/Fratczak 2004: 217).

Institutional child care was expanded earlier than in France or Norway. At the beginning of the 1970s, already one third of all children younger than three years attended public child care in the GDR. This percentage rose to 70% by the middle of the 1980s (Kreyenfeld 2006: 3). Comprehensive coverage for 3–6 year olds was reached in the 1980s. Opening hours of child care facilities were very long (Kreyenfeld 2004: 279). In Hungary, the development of a network of *crèches* and kindergartens started already in 1953. Universal child care fulfilled a second purpose. It enabled state control of child-rearing to prevent children's exposition to influences that were not in line with the socialist, materialist ideology (e.g. Christian values). After 1990, the situation in East Germany changed fundamentally because availability was restricted due to the adjustments to West Germany. Nevertheless, the level of provision (especially of *crèches* and nurseries) remained much better in the Eastern part of the Republic – until now. In the 1990s, the ratio was still ten times higher and almost all child care facilities were full-time places in contrast to the West German part-time places (Kreyenfeld/Konietzka 2004: 27).[19] Since the turn of the millennium, East and West Germany have been treading a new family political path as already mentioned above.

Since the 1950s the dual-earner principle with two full-time employed partners was widespread and actively supported by public policies in socialist societies (see e.g. Oláh/Fratczak 2004: 217, 230). While the integration of women into the labor market was pronounced, leading positions were reserved for men (Schwartz 2005:

[19] In 2006 for only 3% of all children under three could be cared for institutionally in the West, while the value was 40% in the East (Haan/Wrohlich 2009: 8).

79–80). Family work was solely the responsibility of women (Oláh/Fratczak 2004: 218), which also reflects the policy's perspective: leaves, allowances, and benefits were mainly, partly exclusively, addressed to mothers. Women did not have the choice of whether to stay at home to care for their children or to work in the labor market – female labor force participation was rather a social obligation and an economic necessity. Moreover, the role model of the working mother was even anchored in the constitution. Article 24 guaranteed the "right" to work, which in 1961 was replaced by the "right and duty" to work. By this means, women (and men) were pressed into the labor market. Furthermore, social benefits and support were closely connected to individual employment (Kreyenfeld 2004: 278, Frerich/Frey 1996: 175). Hardly any derived entitlements existed. Policies, ideology, behavior, and attitudes in the GDR regarding female employment greatly differed from the FRG. But it should be remembered that completed fertility was just 0.2 children higher in East Germany than in the West. Early family formation resulted in a faster replacement of a woman's cohort, however.

In Hungary, non-pecuniary, pro-natalist measures were temporarily drastic. Between 1953 and 1956 abortion[20] and access to contraceptives were extremely restricted (Spéder/Kamarás 2008: 603, 614, 648). These restrictions left observable marks on the time series of the TFR.[21] The baby boom of the mid-1950s was presumably attributable to this policy while the cohort fertility rate did not change its course. This does not necessarily mean that all steps the government took were non-effective. But it seems as if births were merely brought forward so that a timing effect is observed. After 1956 – between 1954 and 1962 the level of fertility decreased by 40% – the right to induced abortions was deregulated and adjusted to the liberal Soviet law. The TFR fell to one of the lowest levels worldwide in subsequent years. The government of the GDR legalized abortions and provided free access to reliable contraception in 1972 (Obertreis 1986: 300–302). The very liberal abortion legislation in combination with the limited availability of modern and efficient methods of contraception in most socialist countries led to the so-called "abortion culture" which characterized the nature of birth-regulating behavior during the socialist era in CEE (Stloukal 1999). Abortions were socially accepted. In Hungary and the GDR however, the situation

[20] In Norway, France, and the Federal Republic of Germany abortion has been exempt from punishment since the middle of the 1970s (Toulemon/Pailhé/Rossier 2008: 524, Coppola/Di Cesare 2008: 122, Frejka 2008a: 79–80).

[21] This has been shown in the figures 2.1 and 2.2.

was favored, i.e. modern contraception was easier to obtain. Abortion rates were hence lower.[22] Laws changed after the transformation. This especially applies to East German legislation which was adjusted to more restrictive West German laws. The abortion rates dropped subsequently (Frejka 2008a: 80).

Significant fluctuations characterized Hungarian family policy after 1990. After system transformation family policy became the center of political struggles in Hungary. Depending on the political wing of the governing parties – either conservative or socialist (Spéder/Kamarás 2008: 650–651), alignment, extent, and target groups of benefits varied. This political course provoked uncertainty and unreliability. Family policy and levels of child-related support became highly unpredictable. In general, a process of refamilialization started after the system transformation (Blum/Rille-Pfeiffer 2010: 29, 34). Provision of public child care facilities has been reduced since then and today hardly exists at all (in 2006, the coverage rate amounted to only 8%; Blum/Rille-Pfeiffer 2010: 39–40). The basic principles of support for families changed often and profoundly. Moreover, high inflation during the 1990s devalued benefits: in 1997, their value amounted to no more than 40% of the 1990 value. The fluctuations mainly affected families with higher income because in some legislative periods (when left-wing parties governed) measures were means tested and much less generous (e.g. employment-related child care benefits were abolished) and in other periods (temporarily, in conservative legislative periods) measures were universal and expanded. Between 1990 and 1995, from 1998 to 2002 and from 2010 onwards, Hungary had a conservative government. In the periods in-between, the country had left-wing governments (Aassve/Billari/Spéder 2006: 136).

5.1.2 Socialism and the transformation

The processes accompanying the regime collapse of the systems in Central and Eastern Europe around 1990 as well as the interactions between single processes resulted in great and rapid changes in family behavior and in adjustments of life course plans to the new conditions (Frejka 2008b: 140). Some behavioral changes partly had their starting point before 1990. This applies to, for example, out of wedlock births, the spread of cohabitation, and marriage behavior. However, the upheaval

---

[22] Only in Hungary and in East Germany were modern contraceptives, such as the pill and the intrauterine device, used to a noteworthy extent since the 1970s (see e.g. Oláh/Fratczak 2004: 216).

provoked further huge reactions in the fertility and divorce rates in East Germany and the fertility rate in Hungary.[23] The causes partly differ between East Germany and Hungary although the more vigorous reactions occurred in East Germany.

The collapse entailed a profound transition process from a society built on totalitarianism, socialism, and planned economy to a society built on liberal democracy, capitalism, and market economy. The entire societal and institutional system was transformed (Frejka 2008b: 140). Legislation, especially in East Germany, underwent drastic changes after unification.[24] Uncertainty about the future, sudden personnel cutbacks and unemployment rates (as a consequence of the recession), inflation[25], university enrollment rates, inequality, and poverty rates rose while real wages and consumption capabilities sank (the latter only in Hungary; see e.g. Aassve/Billari/Spéder 2006, Kreyenfeld/Konietzka 2004). Lifelong employment guarantees ended. Before the transformation, economic stability, employment security, and a reliable family policy existed and the population was accustomed to them. After the end of the socialist era, the market economy forced the closure of inefficient industries (Aassve/Billari/Spéder 2006: 129–130). In East Germany, education-specific unemployment rates developed and female labor force participation decreased (Kreyenfeld 2006: 7).

After unification, selective migration processes started. More women from East Germany, especially well-educated ones, migrated to the Western part of the Republic – East Germany exhibits the most unfavorable female to male ratio in all of Europe (Peuckert 2008: 95–96). Values, norms, and attitudes seem to have changed, but until today this can apparently not be substantiated. As previously mentioned, the transformation resulted in a range of policy changes. Although, they vary between East Germany and Hungary, they seem to have had an impact on family behavior in both cases (Aassve/Billari/Spéder 2006: 129). In Hungary, transformation led to

[23] See figures 2.1 and 2.9.

[24] This is especially obvious when considering the divorce rates: in Hungary, the decline merely lasted a few years before the rate disproportionately rose again. The previously higher rate of East Germany plummeted and did not recover until 2010. This sharp drop in East Germany was among other things the result of a completely new divorce law, and the introduction of a separation year prior to divorce as a consequence of the adoption of West German law (Dorbritz 2008: 563). The very liberal socialist divorce legislation was completely repealed. The only temporary decline in Hungary was caused by modifications of laws referring to families that made divorce procedures more cumbersome and time-consuming (Spéder/Kamarás 2008: 629). Frames in East Germany were hence subject to stronger changes than in Hungary.

[25] Inflation is a sign of the hardship and uncertainty many families endured during this period (Aassve/Billari/Spéder 2006: 148). Inflation only rose in Hungary.

discontinuities as well as a lack of reliability. With respect to East Germany, the people had to accept adjustments to a completely different frame, legislation and practice (Kreyenfeld 2006: 5). The German unification contract stipulated the substitution of the legal and political system of the GDR by the West German one. One effect the transformation apparently had on family behavior was the delay in family formation of higher-educated individuals due to the introduction of means-tested benefits in combination with difficult economic conditions.

After the transition process was completed – and temporary concomitants such as recession, rampant inflation, and high unemployment abated – fertility did not return to pre-transitional levels. This can be traced back to several long-term impacts the changeover had, such as catching up on educational expansion, enduring change to values and attitudes, as well as increased labor productivity and efficiency (Aassve/Billari/Spéder 2006: 129, 148–149). It is, however, questionable whether temporary processes really influenced cohort fertility. The slump was – at least in East Germany – mainly caused by the abrupt rise in childbearing age – towards an adjustment to West European levels (Kreyenfeld 2004: 277). Persons born prior to the early 1960s were only marginally affected by the transformation (Hoem 2008). As mean age at birth was very low in the socialist countries, even the youngest cohort (1960), that were 30 years old at the time of the transformation, had almost completed their fertility before 1990 (Kreyenfeld/Konietzka 2004: 8).

5.1.3 Effects of policies on fertility

In the following, some empirical results with respect to the effects of policies on fertility will be presented. Effectiveness of family political interventions to raise fertility are often weak, inconclusive, ambiguous or even contradictory (Neyer/Andersson 2007: 3). This may be due to theoretical and methodological difficulties. Neyer and Andersson argue that effects can only be properly assessed under the condition that the impact of policies on individual behavior is studied. Microlevel studies come hence more frequently to the conclusion than macrolevel analyses, that family policy indeed has an impact on childbearing behavior (Neyer/Andersson 2007: 3). Salles/Rossier/Brachet 2010 point to the time horizon – either short-term or long-term – that has to be distinguished with regard to the measurement of pro-natalist effects of policies and to interpret ambiguous results of various analyses.[26] Long-term effects are more difficult to evaluate. Moreover they "depend more on a favorable context to families than on specific family policies" (Toulemon/Pailhé/Rossier 2008: 541). It has proven difficult to link specific policy measures introduced in single countries to durable and substantial fertility increases.

Effects interact with dominating attitudes towards maternal employment. Effects of policies seem to be weaker if the general opinion is that mother's employment harmfully affects her child's development – as in West Germany (Salles/Rossier/Brachet 2010: 1082–1085). Before acceptance has not been reached, broad availability of institutional child care will not change fertility and employment decisions – least of all in the short run. This acceptance probably contributes to higher fertility in France and Norway.[27] Hoem 2008 adds that "national fertility is possibly best seen as a systemic outcome that depends more on broader attributes, such as the degree of family-friendliness of a society, and less on the presence and detailed construction of monetary benefits" (p. 249). Such a family-friendly culture has to be developed. It is a long-term commitment and goes far beyond family policy alone. He advocates a broad coordination of several policies such as economic, employment, housing, gender, and core family policies to establish conditions that raise the well-being of families and the desire of the younger population to enter into parenthood and to rear children (Hoem 2008: 256; see also Neyer 2003 and Neyer/Andersson 2007). Generous monetary benefits alone are unlikely to succeed in escalating the fertility level significantly in the long run. Nevertheless, they seem to be effective in countries that generally behave supportively to families and their requirements (Del Boca/Pasqua/Pronzato 2008: 8). As mentioned above, the Norwegian fertility rate started to re-increase at the end of the 1980s. Norwegian researchers trace this back to family-related reforms (e.g. Lappegård 2000, Frejka/Calot 2001: 168, Rønsen 2004a:

[26] Family policy can hardly be expected to have quick effects on the birth rate as the example of Germany demonstrates. In 2007, there was a changeover from child-rearing allowance, a fixed sum paid for utmost 24 months to mothers working less than 30 hours a week, to parental leave benefit, an income-related replacement income for the duration of 12–14 months. It was associated with the hope of improving reconciliation of work and family especially for highly-qualified women and of promoting births. But the TFR has remained roughly stable in subsequent years. Long-term effects remain to be seen (Salles/Rossier/Brachet 2010).

[27] The acceptance is also high in East Germany leading to a high female labor force participation rate and a low level of childlessness. Fertility is not high however due to a low desired number of children. Acceptance is hence a major but not the only factor that explains fertility.

273). The reforms and legislative changes involved not only – but also – monetary matters such as the increase in child allowance and extended duration of paid leave at childbirth.

A complete evaluation of family policy, especially in cases where measures are extremely various, is difficult to realize and faces methodological difficulties.[28] It is relatively common in empirical research that fertility-promoting impacts of single measures are studied in isolation, such as the availability of child care.[29] Haan/Wrohlich 2009 cannot attest a correlation between the local provision of subsidized institutional child care facilities for children younger than three years and fertility at the population level in East and West Germany. However, subgroup analysis shows large and significant effects on the likelihood of first births as well as on the fertility of highly-qualified women. Moreover, it has positive effects on employment.[30] Hank/Kreyenfeld 2002 find for West Germany that access to informal care arrangements observably raises the transition probability to motherhood, but cannot discover any statistically significant impact of institutional child care coverage.[31] They trace this result back to (infra-)structural deficiencies such as very limited opening hours and strongly restricted availability. The authors' analyses are based on data from the German *Socio-Economic Panel* (GSOEP) for several years (1984–1999). Later Hank/Kreyenfeld/Spieß 2003 expand their estimations to East Germany where the extent of provision of crèches and day nurseries is far higher and find that regional availability of institutional child care facilities positively influences the transition to motherhood.

Evidence based on individual level Norwegian data indicates that there may be a slightly positive effect of increasing the availability of public child care on the probability of a third birth. The effect is not linear as it is more pronounced at low availability rates (Rønsen 2004a). Women with a high level of education respond most strongly to the expansion of public child care. The results of Björklund 2006 for Sweden, which has many similarities with Norway, suggest that the expansion of policy instruments raises the fertility level and diminishes the spacing of births.

28 A complete evaluation of German family policy instruments has however just been concluded. It took several years to accomplish this huge project.

29 This is a measure at the focus of current interest due to the more pronounced childlessness of well-qualified women in (West) Germany (see e.g. Hank/Kreyenfeld 2002, Schrage 2007, and Haan/Wrohlich 2009.

30 Their analysis is based on a sample of married and cohabiting women for the period 2000–2007 employing panel data from the GSOEP.

31 If the respondent's parents live nearby, first birth risk increases by roughly 20%.

Del Boca 2002 shows in a study that the availability of child care and part-time work both increase the probability of working in the labor market and having children in countries that suffer from a shortage of both. Another study by Del Boca/Pasqua/Pronzato 2008 explores the impact of policies and labor market characteristics on women's decisions regarding work and childbearing with the aid of data from the European Community Household Panel. They estimate the two decisions jointly. The availability of public child care, and the arrangement of parental leave schemes, family allowances, and labor market flexibility causes significant differences in the fertility and female labor force participation rates in a variety of European countries. Environmental effects vary by educational level. Child care and parental leaves have a larger impact on the fertility and participation decision of women with a lower educational level while well-paid part-time opportunities and further labor market arrangements more strongly influence women with a high educational level.

The child care allowance reform realized in 1994 in France affected the employment behavior of mothers. The reform extended child allowances to the second child (Toulemon/Pailhé/Rossier 2008: 531–532) as described above. It led to a large decline in young mothers' participation in the workforce. The activity rate of mothers with two children of which at least one was under three rapidly decreased: within three years from 69% to 54%. Predominantly women with lower qualification, poor work conditions or insecure jobs took parental leave but had preferred to remain employed under different conditions.

Gábos/Gál/Kézdi 2009 investigate the effects of child-related benefits and pensions on fertility by using aggregate Hungarian time series data from 1950–2006. Their results indicate moderate but robust effects. According to their estimates, an increase of 1% in child-related benefits brings about a rise of total fertility by 0.2%, while the same increase in pensions would decrease fertility by 0.2%. The magnitude of both effects increases with birth order, but it is more robust for child-related benefits. The results of Aassve/Billari/Spéder 2006 (also) for Hungary suggest that the introduction of means-tested benefits had an adverse impact on individuals in the highest income decile. After means testing was abolished in 1998, their estimates no longer show a significant negative impact on persons with higher education. Oláh/Fratczak 2004 study the transition to motherhood in the first co-residential union in a dual-earner context during the era of state socialism (1960–1989) in Hungary. Their results indicate that women's employment does not reduce the propensity to become a mother if the work-family balance was facilitated by policy measures.

When citing effects of policies and policy outcomes, it is obvious that if people have no desire for children they cannot be reached by family policy. Beyond the enormous variety of supportive measures for families, the French and Norwegian policies may have contributed to positive attitudes towards families in general, which again may have influenced the desired number of children. Not all people who do not wish to have children remain childless and vice versa. In the latter case, desired temporary childlessness turns into undesired childlessness. With rising age, conception becomes more difficult and is fraught with increasing health risks for the woman and the unborn child. Another reason for undesired childlessness is the absence of a stable relationship. Analyses based on the GSOEP show that 50% of childless women and about two thirds of childless men either did not have a partner nor were they cohabiting shortly before concluding their reproductive period (Schmitt/Winkelmann 2005: 11–13). Again, policies must be non-effective.

5.2 Individual characteristics associated with fertility (behavior)

5.2.1 Gender

In general, women's fertility seems to be higher than that of men (see e.g. Rendall et al. 1999 or Schmitt/Winkelmann 2005). Assuming that the numbers of women and men in fertile age are approximately equal, this should not be the case. Some explanations for this phenomenon can be considered. First, there may be difficulties in the collection of data. Until recently, it was – e.g. in France and Germany – not possible to conclude the exact number of children a women had given birth to from civil registration data (Gerlach 2010: 62). It was even less possible to find out the number of children a man had (biologically) fathered. Female respondents were only asked about the number of children born within the current marriage (Germany) or current relationship (France) and not about the actual birth order of the newborn child. In the German *Microcensus* only the number of children living in the household of a respondent has been collected, but this shortcoming has fortunately been remedied. As children mostly live with the mother after a union breaks up, the number of children a man has must hence be lower. Men's statements may not be reliable which is why they were simply not asked. In France, a 1% sample is thus drawn within each census and delivers precise information about individual fertility history (Toulemon/Pailhé/Rossier 2008: 514). The gender-specific divergence gap could not be completely closed by carrying out this step, however. The data set used in this work (GGS) collects all children women and men have, independent of the child's place of residence.

Secondly, a small percentage of men neither acknowledges paternity nor even knows about their fatherhood because the relationship ended before the pregnancy was ascertained. Or a relationship with the mother has never existed (Köppen/Mazuy/Toulemon 2007). Hence, unmarried men under-report the number of children they have fathered in surveys. Thirdly, the fertile period is more difficult to delimit. A small proportion of first-time fathers is older than 50 years (Köppen/Mazuy/Toulemon 2007: 97). This slight fuzziness will be accepted in the empirical analyses. A final reason why the indicator "gender" must not be neglected in fertility analyses is its interaction with several other indicators such as educational achievement, occupational position, or income – and maybe religiosity. Thus, men should not be ignored.

5.2.2 Education and qualification

Demographers have explained declining birth rates, increased childlessness, and postponed family formation with education and its related domains such as qualification, occupational position, field of education, and career orientation as some of the core factors. Especially women have benefited from the expansion of educational systems starting in the 1960s in many countries in Europe. However, the higher educational achievement, occupational position, etc. are, the higher the (country-specific) probability to remain childless. A higher proportion of women with tertiary education remains childless or postpones family formation compared to women with a lower educational attainment. This can be regarded as a stylized fact: "High income switches from having a positive to a neutral fertility effect, while the fertility effect of education is negative for as long as this relation has been measured" (Skirbekk 2008: 154). Skirbekk adds that studies describing how education relates to fertility were firstly published early in the 20th century. This matter has gained societal importance as more and more women attain higher levels of education. In all world regions the fertility depressing effect of education is much more pronounced for women than for men in all periods (Skirbekk 2008: 158).

The education-fertility link is also true for countries with low proportions of childless individuals such as France (Köppen/Mazuy/Toulemon 2007: 93–94), Norway (Kravdal 2001, Rønsen 2004a, Lappegård 2000), and Hungary where the education system had not been considerably expanded before the system transformation (Spéder/Kamarás 2008: 653 and Aassve/Billari/Spéder 2006: 129). Moreover, it applies not only to developed but also to developing countries (Population Reference Bureau 2007 and Skirbekk 2008). Merely the national fertility levels differ. The correlation is very close in West Germany, a country that also has the highest rate of childless women (Statistisches Bundesamt 2009b: 27). The negative effect of educational achievement on completed fertility seems to be stronger in countries where gender inequality is pronounced and where caring for children and occupational commitment are irreconcilable with each other (Andersson et al. 2009: 327). The strength of the association between completed fertility and educational achievement depends, e.g. in Norway, on the decade. The link was stronger for women born in the 1930s and 1940s, but weaker for women born in the 1950s, which is partly due to compatibility efforts of policy-makers who decreased child-related costs (Kravdal 2001).[32] One exception of this almost systematic linkage is East Germany where no significant connection between education and fertility seems to exist (Statistisches Bundesamt 2009b: 27, 30).

This statement depends on the indicator used and is not true for the age at first childbirth. Cohorts that had their childbearing period during the socialist era also differ with respect to age at first childbirth by education. Women with the highest school achievement were three years older than their peers with the lowest attainable school leaving certificate when they had their first child (Kreyenfeld 2006: 20). The age difference in West Germany for the same cohorts was more pronounced. East German cohorts of childbearing age during the time of the transition diverged even more strongly with respect to education than the respective West German cohorts. Women with lower education had their first child pre-transitionally, while women with higher education delayed it until the time after the upheaval.

Hoem/Neyer/Andersson 2006a and Hoem/Neyer/Andersson 2006b analyze the link between fertility and field of education for women born in the second half of

32 The author mentions a variety of possible reasons, e.g. "Another possibility (...) is that the selection into education may have changed over time. Only 6% attained the level corresponding to at least a Bachelor's degree in the 1941–45 cohorts as compared to 17% in the 1956–57 cohorts" (Kravdal 2001: 210).

the 1950s. The researchers use Swedish data, but it seems plausible to transform the conclusions at least to neighboring Norway (see also Rønsen/Skrede 2010 including the literature cited there). The countries have many similarities (Andersson 2004: 156, Andersson et al. 2009: 314). Hoem, Neyer, and Andersson found that field of education is a more essential indicator to predict childlessness than mere educational achievement. This especially applies to the fields teaching and health care where the proportions of childless women are far below average for all levels of education. The exclusive consideration of educational achievement suggests that all women who have attained a certain qualificational level have equal opportunities to make use of this education. This is definitely not true. In many cases field of education is linked to specific occupations, a certain sector or branch of the private or public economy. These occupations, sectors, and branches differ in their opportunities regarding income prospects, employment stability, working conditions, opportunities to work part-time, etc. Nevertheless, the level of childlessness does rise with the level of education within single fields of education. Hoem, Neyer and Andersson cannot yet clarify the causality question. It may be that family-oriented women select themselves into fields of education preparing for occupations and branches that enable compatibility.

Köppen/Mazuy/Toulemon 2007 try to find answers to the question of which traits characterize individuals (in France) who remain childless. They detect that childlessness does not only vary by the level of education but also by occupational status (p. 94). A higher percentage of female employees in managerial positions (*cadres*) than blue-collar workers, self-employed women, or those who have never been economically active remain childless. A high occupational position is often associated with a high workload, strong work commitment, and high opportunity costs in case of a job break. The lowest rates of childlessness can be documented for women who are economically active in agriculture and manage their own farm. Most influences from industrialization and urbanization – which lead to today's dominating type of family, the nuclear family – are not applicable to those women. Living and working coincide, which strongly facilitates reconciliation of family and work.

In France and Germany, the level of education of a woman positively affects a second birth (Köppen 2004 and Köppen 2006). The impact weakens in Germany but not in France after the level of education of the (male) partner is held constant. This can also be interpreted as a still prevalent *male-breadwinner* principle in combination with still existing incompatibilities between family and employment in Germany.

A not insignificant percentage of relationships are homogamous with respect to education. This explains why no significant differences between highly-educated women and men can be found. In contrast, lower educated women have a higher transition rate to a first child than their male counterparts (Schmitt/Winkelmann 2005). This provides additional evidence for the *male-breadwinner* principle. Men with low income in precarious employment or economically insecure jobs more often have lower educational attainments. Furthermore, these men are disadvantaged in the partner market.

In comparison with lower educated women, a higher share of women with tertiary education lived without a partner shortly before concluding their fertile life stage. Additionally, this proportion has risen during recent decades. The great majority of these women is childless (for France: Robert-Bobée/Mazuy 2005, for Germany: Duschek/Wirth 2005). Therefore, the higher childlessness among well-qualified women is not only caused by their educational level but also by interactions between education and marital status. That means higher shares of low-educated men and highly-qualified women are single. Women still tend to marry socially upwards which does not contradict the fact that a certain proportion of unions is homogamous with respect to educational attainment. Unions where both partners have a high educational level and those in which the woman has the higher achievement level remain childless more frequently (Wirth 2007: 188). In fact, the probability to have a child is lowest in the latter case. In France, no significant differences for men of different educational levels can be found (Köppen/Mazuy/Toulemon 2007).

5.2.3 Female labor force participation

The expansion of vocational training and the educational system since the 1960s resulted in rising female labor force participation rates. Both these developments are closely interconnected but also have their own facets (see e.g. Del Boca/Pasqua/Pronzato 2008 and Kreyenfeld et al. 2007). Labor supply of well-qualified women is higher than of their less educated peers. These social changes could be observed in most developed countries but exhibit remarkable national variety which again differs in its outcomes for fertility. The tense relation between labor supply and fertility (as well as marital stability) has also been discussed theoretically in the preceding chapter. Greater labor market integration of women makes up a fundamental part of the gender revolution and the changed gender roles and is related to the reduction or abolition of gender-specific education barriers as well as improved career opportunities (Daly 2005: 383). The entry of more and more women into the labor market in developed countries has not only been facilitated by educational expansion but also caused by increased income prospects and the growth of the tertiary sector. Women's share is higher here than in the secondary sector. The emphasis in activities that require physical strength declined due to the successive shift from manufacturing towards services. This technological transformation augmented the demand for activities where women have a comparative advantage and it raised the relative wages of women (Galor/Weil 1996: 375, Adsera 2008: 288, fundamentally Willms-Herget 1985).

Nevertheless, the gender wage gap is even today still large in France (17.1%), West Germany (25%), Germany altogether (23.2%), Norway (17.2%), and Hungary (17.5%). The German gender wage differential is one of the highest in the whole EU. In contrast, it is small in East Germany (6%; data for 2008; Eurostat 2012e, Statistisches Bundesamt 2010a). The gaps have been reducing during recent decades which means they were even larger before (see e.g. Blau/Kahn 2000). The values mentioned are unadjusted wage gaps.[33] That means, wage differentials do not account for gender-specific work behavior and characteristics that are partly able to explain them. Women more often work part-time and a certain proportion of part-time jobs does not correspond to the qualifications of their holders. (Older) employed women are on average still less educated than (older) men. Women have less work experience due to employment breaks. They work in smaller enterprises, choose worse-paid occupations and less career-oriented subjects of study, and they fill lower occupational positions (see e.g. Holst/Schimeta 2011). Finally, women are more frequently employed in worse-paid branches: rather in the tertiary than in the industrial sector (see e.g. Mincer 1974, Blau/Kahn 2000, Weichselbaumer/Winter-Ebmer 2005, Christofides/Polycarpou/Vrachimis 2010, Livanos/Pouliakas 2009). However, some points of this list require further explanation. Depending on the measurement, the gender wage gap cannot completely be explained by the characteristics mentioned. The rest must be traced back to differences in productivity that are due to unobserved factors or to discrimination (Ehrenberg/Smith 2009: 396–406).

[33] "The unadjusted gender pay gap (GPG) represents the difference between average gross hourly earnings of male paid employees and of female paid employees as a percentage of average gross hourly earnings of male paid employees" (Eurostat 2012e).

Female labor force participation rates differ depending on how "participation" is defined. According to Eurostat, the reported rates refer to one hour of paid work within a certain week. Therefore, it is a rough indicator because it ignores the extent of working hours.[34] In 2009, participation rates of women were highest in Norway (78.6%), followed by Germany (67.8%) and France (65.5%). They were lowest in Hungary (55.1%; Eurostat 2012c). In 1997, rates had been much lower in Germany (58%), France (57.4%), and Hungary (50%), but not in Norway (76%). This points to an earlier development in Norway: the labor force participation rate of women grew significantly from the mid-1970s to 1986. The OECD labor force statistics defines participation as the ratio of the (female) labor force of all ages and the (female) population aged 15–64 including full- and part-time workers as well as those seeking employment. Table 5.1 shows that the Norwegian rate was lower than the French and West German rates until the early 1970s, but exceeded them after that (Brewster/ Rindfuss 2000). The sharpest increase took place in the 1970s, namely by more than 61% in Norway. It is the decade in which social policies started to modernize that country. In France and West Germany, the rise was not that steep during the whole time period but started from much higher initial values.

Table 5.1. Female labor force participation rates

	FRANCE	NORWAY	WEST GERMANY
1965		36.9	49.0
1970	48.2	38.8	48.1
1975	50.5	53.3	49.6
1980	54.3	63.2	50.0
1985	55.0	68.3	50.4
1990	56.6	71.2	55.8
1996	59.9	66.0	

Source: Brewster/ Rindfuss (2000): 276.

The labor market integration of women in socialist countries was traditionally very intense because of the high demand for labor. Moreover, the low wage levels re-

[34] Definition according to Eurostat 2012c: "The employment rate is calculated by dividing the number of persons aged 20–64 in employment by the total population of the same age group. The indicator is based on the *EU Labour Force Survey*. The survey covers the entire population living in private households and excludes those in collective households such as boarding houses, halls of residence and hospitals. The employed population consists of those persons who during the reference week did any work for pay or profit for at least one hour, or were not working but had jobs from which they were temporarily absent."

quired women's full-time economic activity (Robert/Blossfeld 1995, Haas et al. 2006). Combining employment and child-rearing was alleviated by job guarantees, low competition in the labor market, and the socialist ideology promoting fertility and female labor supply (Matysiak/Vignoli 2008).[35] In Hungary, the employment rate steadily rose after World War II: from 50% in 1960 to 60% in 1970 and to 70–75% in the 1980s (Robert/Blossfeld 1995). Female labor supply and work orientation of East German women are still high today (Kreyenfeld 2004). Summarizing the Eastern and Western part when quoting the proportion for Germany ignores different working cultures. This is especially observable when comparing labor force participation of married women because the East German rate exceeds the West German one by far in this subgroup (Fuchs/Weber 2004).[36] Before unification, rates differed much more strongly: the West German rate was much lower. While participation sank slightly in the Eastern part of the newly unified German Republic, it significantly rose in the Western part. Converging rates can hence be mainly ascribed to the changed behavior of West German women.

The low rate Hungarian women have been exhibiting since transformation diverges from the East German one. The rate of Hungarian men is also very low (Eurostat 2012c). While the male labor force participation rate amounted to 84.8% in Norway, to 80.1% in Germany, and to 75.5% in France in 2008, it totaled only 69% in Hungary. This points to a long-lasting economic crisis after the transformation (Barlai/Hartleb 2007). The labor market participation rate declined during the 1990s, which partly resulted from the redundancy of a part of the work force in the course of the transformation from a planned to a market economy (Aassve/Billari/Spéder 2006: 148). Consequently, the rate is much lower today than it was at the end of the 1980s. The economic crisis resulted in existential uncertainty which was accompanied by a reduction in the availability of public child care facilities (Matysiak/Vignoli 2008: 366). This interplay made it harder for women to combine employment and child-rearing and let both employment and fertility rates sink. Another factor that contributes to explaining the decreased activity rate is the growth of the university enrollment rate. During the socialist era, access to higher education was limited. The increase has been part of the post-transitional catching-up process. Between 1990 and 2002 the

[35] It was a situation that completely changed after the transformation (Haas et al. 2006). Economic insecurity increased and reconciliation became more difficult.

[36] Due to the diverging concept the report follows, no rates are reported.

enrollment rate in full-time education in the age-group 18–22 years rose from 11.9% to 39.5% (Aassve/Billari/Spéder 2006: 148).

A further explanation for the low employment rate of women is delivered by the high score on the masculinity dimension in Hofstede's system of cultural dimensions (Hofstede 1980). The masculinity dimension refers to the distribution of gender roles. In a masculine society gender roles are strictly separated, in a feminine culture (e.g. the Norwegian one), gender roles overlap. This presumption is supported by findings of the PPAS. According to this survey, Hungary is the only one of 14 mostly Eastern European countries involved in which the majority of respondents (61%) favors the model of a traditional distribution of gender roles – the man is responsible for the income and the woman cares for children and household (European Commission 2007: 52). While maternal employment is broadly accepted in France (Fagnani 2002), this is not very much the case in Hungary where more than half of the respondents have the opinion that a preschool child probably suffers from his or her mother's going to work (European Commission 2007: 51).[37]

The strong culture of masculinity is not only reflected by values but also by practiced behavior in Hungary. The difference between the employment rates of childless women and mothers of at least two minor children is extremely pronounced – the country ranks second with 28% compared to the OECD average of 13.4% (D'Addio/D'Ercole 2005: 35). In Norway, the difference totals 5%, in France 14%, and in Germany it is 21%.[38] Several reasons contribute to the high employment rate among mothers in Norway. Among others, individual taxation puts pressure on women to be economically active in an expensive country. Further reasons – such as the strong institutional support for working mothers accompanied by liberal societal attitudes towards them – have been mentioned above.

Participation rates cannot simply be compared with each other. First, in (West) Germany, the percentage of mothers among all women is lower. Consequently, the share of mothers with young children must be higher in the other countries. Secondly,

[37] Furthermore there is virtually no acceptance for the male homemaker model (European Commission 2007: 52). In the European Values Study 2008, the respective proportion was 55% for Hungarians. In contrast, the percentage of respondents aged 18–40 years was even much higher in West Germany: here 63% agree to the statement against to 36% in East Germany and 41% in France (Bujard et al. 2012).

[38] This statistic does not differentiate between East and West Germany. It can be assumed however that the difference is much smaller in the Eastern part.

the percentages of women in France, Norway, Hungary, and East Germany[39] employed full-time or in long part-time[40] are higher, (Schmeißer et al. 2012: 31, 46, 84, 160; Statistics Norway 2005; Haas et al. 2006)[41] while in West Germany many (married) women have worked short part-time and many jobs were not subject to social insurance contribution (Keller/Schulz/Seifert 2012). Furthermore, employment has frequently not corresponded to qualifications due to the lack of qualified part-time jobs (Del Boca/Locatelli 2006).

Whereas today female labor force participation rates and fertility seem to be positively correlated in OECD countries, the growing rates of economically active women were accompanied by a marked decline in fertility during the 1970s and the first half of the 1980s (see e.g. OECD 2007, Ahn/Mira 2002). The turnaround may be partly induced by social, family, and labor market policies – due to the creation of qualified and suitable part-time jobs that have been attuned to these social developments (Brewster/Rindfuss 2000). Apps and Rees show by means of comparative statics in an equilibrium model that policies caused this changed trend. They assume that "the reason lies in the combined effects of a country's tax system and system of child support" (Apps/Rees 2004: 760). Their results suggest that countries with individual rather than joint taxation and support for families through high availability of public child care rather than through direct child-related payments, are likely to have both higher female labor supply and more children. Kögel 2004 also deals with the occurrence of a positive association and analyzes it by means of panel data techniques applied to pooled cross-country and time series data (1960–2000) of OECD countries. He shows that in the time series dimension within countries, the (negative) sign did not change. However, the study finds "support for a falling magnitude and significance of the negative time series association after 1985" for non-Mediterranean countries (Kögel 2004: 46; the meta-analysis of Matysiak/Vignoli 2008 shows very similar results).

[39] But: apart from generally positive consequences of female labor market attachment a low wage level, the absence of a widow's pension, and limited possibilities to obtain alimony after divorce put economic pressure on women to work in the GDR (Frerich/Frey 1996: 396). West German women were entitled to a widow's pension (equivalent to 60% of the pension of the deceased spouse) and to alimony in case of divorce (Kreyenfeld 2004: 279, 281).

[40] "Long" part-time means between 20 and 35 hours of work per week while "short" part-time is less than 20 hours of work per week.

[41] In 2001 more than half of the employed women in Hungary worked more than 40 hours per week while only 9% worked less than 30 hours (Haas et al. 2006: 756).

Current labor force participation of women may be correlated either positively or negatively with fertility (while the correlation itself is undisputed), but the first has no causal impact on the latter as Schröder and Brüderl (2008) show on the basis of causality tests and the German *Family Survey*. Their analysis was prompted by the finding that employed women have a lower transition probability to a child. Women who are childless are usually employed (pp. 133–134). That means they are employed because they previously decided against children. This points to the biased time-serial cross-country correlations Kögel 2004 has already suggested. Rather than a causal effect, the suspicion of a self-selection effect could be confirmed by the authors. They assume that family orientations or long-term career orientations, attitudes, as well as the employment outlook, and thus – also – third variables, cause the association (Schröder/Brüderl 2008). By contrast, Bloom et al. 2007 confirm with the aid of a data panel of 97 countries over the period 1960–2000 that fertility negatively affects female labor supply. Their findings show that female labor force participation decreases on average by about 10–15% in the age group 25–39 years with each additional child, and about 5–10% in the age group 40–49 years. The results imply a reduction of about four years of paid work over a woman's lifetime per child.

Beyond the hitherto mentioned factors, participation in the labor market and the decision to have children are encouraged by an extensive public sector. Usually, it is connected with gender-segregated occupations which contributes to the Norwegian term "gender equality light" (see subsection 5.1.1). Working in the public sector reduces employment uncertainty: (most) jobs are protected and employees are mostly guaranteed to return to their previous workplace after a job break due to childbirth. Hence, it offers good opportunities for reconciling family and work (see also Adsera 2005 and Hobcraft/Kiernan 1995). Public sector employment accounted for around 31% of total employment in Norway and almost one fourth in France but only 15.5% in Germany in 1995 (Adsera 2005). A substantial part of employed women in Norway work in the public sector: 48% as opposed to 19% of men (Statistics Norway 2005).

6 Empirical Analysis of the Influence of Religiosity on Completed Fertility in Comparative Perspective

This chapter presents and interprets results of the comparative data analyses differentiated by country and gender based on the Generations and Gender Survey. Section 6.1 introduces the GGS data employed, describes the variables used and the statistical method. Thereafter, section 6.2 gives a descriptive overview about the relevant GGS data: completed fertility and parities (6.2.1) as well as religious indicators (6.2.2). Additionally, the suitability of the variables is discussed. Subsection 6.2.3 tries to find out whether the theoretical presuppositions made in chapter 4 apply. Subsection 6.2.4 investigates the question of whether religiosity influences individuals' behavior as postulated. Section 6.3 interprets and discusses the results of several Poisson (and negative binomial) regression estimations. First, the direct effects of religiosity are dealt with (6.3.1) followed by indirect effects and the influence of the covariates (6.3.2). In 6.3.3 the results of the estimations for Turkish Muslims are introduced.

6.1 Data, variables, and statistical methods

6.1.1 The Generations and Gender Survey (GGS)

The Generations and Gender Survey (GGS) is a panel survey of national samples representing the 18–79 year old resident population in each – at the moment 19 – participating country. At least three waves are planned.[1] The first wave was conducted in

[1] All information in this subsection relies on Netherlands Interdisciplinary Demographic Institute (NIDI)/United Nations Economic Commission for Europe (UNECE) 2011.

2005 in France and Germany, in 2004/2005 in Hungary, and in 2007/2008 in Norway. The survey is the core element of the Generations and Gender Programme (GGP), a cross-national, comparative, multidisciplinary, retrospective, and prospective study of the dynamics of family relationships in contemporary industrialized countries.[2] It draws on approaches and theories from a number of social science disciplines, such as demography, sociology, economics, and social psychology.

One person per household was interviewed face-to-face and computer-assisted (CAPI) or by paper and pencil (PAPI, in Hungary). The goal is to collect comparable data in several, mainly European, countries. To achieve this end, each participating country should follow the same survey design, questionnaire, and instructions. Each country needed to implement those in full, as well as four optional submodules on nationality and ethnicity, on previous partners, on intentions of breaking up, and on housing. They were also encouraged to include the optional submodules to facilitate comparative research on these topics (Vikat et al. 2007).

The GGS – whose forerunner was the Family and Fertility Survey (FFS) – deals with topics related to children, partners, parents, work and everyday life and was designed to improve the understanding of demographic and social developments and of the factors that influence these – in total, eleven distinguishable subject areas. A large part of the questionnaire is devoted to questions about the family situation at the time of the interview, family-related events experienced in the past, and the intentions of respondents to engage in vital events such as forming and dissolving a partnership, bearing children, retiring, and leaving the parental home. The selection of topics has the objective to identify factors that influence these processes and involve economic aspects, values, orientations, and attitudes, gender as well as intergenerational relationships, household composition and housing, residential mobility, kin and social networks and private transfers, education, health, and public transfers. By including all these topics, the GGS covers the important societal aspects of demographic choices in contemporary developed societies.[3]

[2] The GGP is coordinated by the Population Activities Unit (PAU) of the United Nations Economic Commission for Europe (UNECE) in Geneva. A consortium of leading European centers of population research was formed to develop the program, including the survey and its instruments. The consortium is composed – among many other centers, departments, and institutes – of the *Institut national d'études démographiques* (INED in France), the Max Planck Institute for Demographic Research (in Germany), the Hungarian Central Statistical Office, and Statistics Norway.

[3] See UNECE Population Activities Unit 2006, Vikat et al. 2007: 389–391.

In Germany, a supplemental survey of persons with Turkish citizenship was conducted in 2006. Migrants are continuously under-represented in large population surveys, which is a relatively common phenomenon that can be ascribed to lacking language and education skills. Numbers of observations are usually too low to analyze this group and even less to study different subgroups in detail (Ette et al. 2007: 8). The goal was hence to extend existing knowledge about demographic behavior of the largest migrant group living in Germany. The sample represents foreigners originating from Turkey. It is not representative of all Muslims living in Germany (although about two thirds of the Muslims living in Germany have a Turkish origin (Haug/ Müssig/Stichs 2009: 12)), nor of all individuals with Turkish roots (who may have become German nationals). If this is kept in mind, the data offer an outstanding opportunity to include Muslims into the analysis. Such an additional survey does not exist for France or Norway. The questionnaire of the additional sample is equivalent to the main one except for some migration-specific questions.[4] Not all interviewers were Turkish-speaking but the CAPI-interviews were accompanied by a translation assistance where needed. This procedure was devised so as not to exclude migrants with limited German (Ette et al. 2007: 12).

Of the Turkish migrants interviewed, 95% are Muslims. The remaining 5% have another or no religious affiliation and will be excluded from all analyses. Muslims in the main survey will be eliminated due to the high selectivity of the respondents. The Muslims from the supplemental sample are also selective because they are all Turkish citizens. However, this selectivity is more acceptable and the number of observations is much higher. In principle, it is not possible to simply merge the main and the supplemental survey. This procedure was not intended by the institute that collected the data and therefore it has not catered for this, for example by providing weights. However, one joint analysis will nevertheless be conducted (in subsection 6.3.3). Apart from this exception, Muslim-specific analyses will be realized. This procedure threatens comparability with the main survey in which a certain proportion of the respondents is unaffiliated and hence less religious on average.

[4] The additional information covers: Turkish and German language skills and writing literacy, first and second spoken language at home, desire to stay in Germany or to return to Turkey, visits to Turkey (Have you ever been to Turkey since you migrated to Germany? How much time have you spent in Turkey during the last two years?).

At the time of analysis only the first wave was available for all relevant countries.[5] Therefore all following results are cross-sectional. Country weights do not exist, so the data sets cannot be merged. Analyses will hence be carried out separately for country.[6] Table 6.1 contains whole as well as reduced sample sizes and mean age of respondents structured by region and gender. East and West Germany will be analyzed separately due to historical, political, and cultural reasons explained in the preceding chapters.[7] In total, twelve groups can be distinguished. Mean ages in the reduced sample do not greatly differ between gender or regions and lie between 56.6 and 59.0 years. On average, Turkish women are the youngest and Turkish men are the oldest group. Hence, the difference between these two is the only larger gender difference by region. As mean and median age correspond to each other in the majority of samples, the age distribution is almost normally distributed.

The special advantage of the GGS with respect to the work at hand is that it facilitates an international comparison of completed fertility patterns and fertility differences of several religious groups within diverging institutional, historical, political, and cultural settings. These data illustrate the interaction of religiosity with environmental factors when it comes to family decisions. The second advantage is the inclusion of partnership biographies with which the second parent of a respondent's children can be identified (except for non-resident children in Hungary and the second parent of an adopted child). The lack of some information – on religiosity and on the current partner as well as ex-partners – can be considered as disadvantages. Furthermore, it is not possible to analyze all five countries together due to the lack of country weights. Also problematic is that not all countries have implemented the full questionnaire, that is they have not strictly followed the GGS core questionnaire. Some variables are absent in one data set while this information has been collected in another national survey. Country specifications become problematic in cases where major variables, such as "frequency of attendance of religious services" are considered. Missing variables are referred to in the corresponding sections.[8]

---

[5] Except for Hungary where the second wave was already available.

[6] Hungarians and especially Norwegians would be oversampled without the use of any weights. The Norwegian data set is the largest, while the country itself has a much smaller population than France and Germany.

[7] West Berlin is counted as West Germany, East Berlin is counted as East Germany.

[8] See also `http://www.ggp-i.org/data/faq.html\#d3` (faq 3: Why is a variable from the GGS Core Questionnaire missing in a specific country survey?; visited on 14 Dec 2011).

Table 6.1. Global numbers of observation in the national GGS surveys

	FRANCE		HUNGARY		NORWAY		GERMANY					
							East		West		Tr. migs	
	Women	Men	Women	Men	Women	Men	Women	Men	Women	Men	Women	Men
Whole sample size (Nobs), 18–79 years	5,708	4,371	7,517	6,023	7,541	7,340	1,104	847	4,303	3,763	1,916	2,129
Mean age	45.9	45.2	48.0	45.2	46.2	45.4	48.1	45.6	47.1	45.8	39.7	40
Median age	45	44	48	45	45	44	48	45	46	44	37	37
Reduced sample size (Nobs), 45–74 years	2,640	2,122	3,837	2,821	3,542	3,484	552	444	1,856	1,790	463	501
Mean age	57.7	58.1	58.3	57.3	57.6	57.4	58.9	57.9	58.6	58.1	56.8	59.0
Median age	57	58	58	56	57	57	59	58	59	58	56	60

Tr. migs: Turkish migrants, Nobs: Numbers of observations. Reduced samples without respondents affiliated to denominations excluded from empirical analysis due to low numbers of observations (see subsection 6.2.2).

6.1.2 The dependent variable: completed fertility

The Generations and Gender Survey collects information on all children the respondents have and discriminates between biological, adopted, step, and foster children. Resident children are recorded in the scope of the household grid:

> To begin, I would like to ask you about all persons who live in this household. Who are they? To help me keep track of your answers, please tell me their first names and how they are related to you.

Possible answers with respect to offspring are: "Biological child with current partner or spouse", "biological child with former partner or spouse", "stepchild", "adopted child" (not in Norway[9]), and "foster child" (the latter two were not collected in Hungary as separate categories).[10] Furthermore, information on all non-resident children is collected:

> We already talked about those children who currently live in your household. In addition to them, have you given birth to/ fathered any other children or have you ever adopted any other children?

(for respondents with resident children; excluding step-children) respectively

> Have you given birth to/ fathered any children or have you ever adopted any children?

(for respondents without resident children; excluding step-children); if the answer is "yes", information on the type of the children are collected. Possible answers are: "Biological child" (later these children are attached to corresponding partners), "adopted child" (not available in Norway), and "foster child" (the latter were are not recorded in Hungary). In the following, the number of children will be restricted to biological and adopted offspring; step and foster children will be excluded. Step-children in times of higher divorce rates usually have a second biological parent and foster children are frequently "temporary" children.

It is assumed that fertility is completed by the age of 45 years. In official statistics, for example in Germany (according to the Statistisches Bundesamt (Federal Statistical

---

[9] It is of course possible to adopt a child in Norway, even though this information was not collected (Statistics Norway 2012a).

[10] A pregnancy or expected fatherhood at the time of the interview is treated as resident, biological child with the current partner. According to GGS data, only a maximum of two children can be expected at once.

office)) or Norway (according to Statistics Norway) fertility is deemed to be completed when a woman has reached her 50th birthday. The number of births in the age range 45–50 is rather small, so a younger age is fixed in order not to lose too many observations. On average the husband is (about two years) older than his wife. Nevertheless, the same age boundaries are set for men and women in the empirical analyses. The uncertainty associated with these measures will be neglected.

Fertility and partnership histories in the German GGS have proven to partly deviate (see Naderi/Dorbritz/Ruckdeschel 2009[11] and Kreyenfeld/Hornung/Kubisch 2010 for details). Childlessness and singleness among West German women born before 1955 are too high when comparing GGS data with the *Microcensus* (a 1% sample), the *Socio-Economic Panel* (GSOEP), or population statistics. For female cohorts born after 1959 numbers of children are somewhat too high.[12] The data for birth cohorts 1955–1959 are reliable. However, the biases seem not to systematically correlate with religious affiliation and religiosity. Therefore, the data of the German GGS will be applied. Nevertheless have these issues to be taken into account when interpreting the regression results. Finally, data problems of the French, Hungarian or Norwegian data are not known.

6.1.3 The main explanatory variables: religious affiliation and religiosity

The GGS offers some variables referring to religion and religiosity. They have not been collected completely equally in France, Hungary, Norway, and Germany. Not all available variables can be ascribed to one of the dimensions of the multi-dimensional religiosity concept. Table 6.2 gives an overview of the indicators:

Table 6.2. Variables in the GGS with religious reference

	FRANCE	HUNGARY	NORWAY	GERMANY
Religious affiliation (country-specific list)	X	X	X	X
Frequency of attending religious services	X		X	X
Attitudes towards religious ceremonies – baptism, wedding, funeral	X	X	X	X
Religious faith as a value for children		X	X	X

[11] Of special interest is figure 1 on p. 15 where the percentage of childless women in the GGS and *Microcensus* are compared with each other.

[12] Naderi/Dorbritz/Ruckdeschel 2009 reports high accordance with parities 1–4 (p. 15, figure 2). They also show that the data are representative of the population (p. 17).

Religious affiliation means self-defined (France and Hungary) or official (Norway and Germany) affiliation to a religious group and has been collected with the aid of a country-specific list:

Which religious denomination do you adhere to, if any?

In France, the categories are Roman Catholic, Orthodox, Protestant, Muslim, Jewish, Buddhist, Hindu, other, and none. The numbers of observations of the following categories are sufficiently high enough to be used in the empirical analyses: *Roman Catholic*, *Protestant*, *Muslim*, and *without religious affiliation*. All other affiliations will be excluded in descriptive and multivariate analyses. In Hungary, the categories available were: Roman Catholic, Greek Catholic, Calvinist, Lutheran, Faith Church, Unitarian, Greek Orthodox, Jewish, Buddhist, Hindu, other affiliation, and none. This large variety of affiliations is reduced to: *Roman Catholic*, *Greek Catholic*, *Calvinist*, *Lutheran*, and *without religious affiliation*. All other affiliations will be disregarded and dropped from the data set. In Norway, the country-specific list consists of the *Lutheran* state church (the Church of Norway), *other Christian affiliation* (Christianity outside the Church of Norway), *non-Christian affiliation* as well as *without religious affiliation*. In Germany, only the categories *Christian*, Muslim, other, and *without religious affiliation* can be differentiated. Protestants and Catholics cannot be distinguished from each other. As the supplemental survey covers Muslims, they are excluded from the main survey. A comparison of Muslims from the main survey with those from the supplemental survey documents the high selectivity of the few Muslims in the main survey concerning several indicators, e.g. fertility. "Other" (non-Christian) affiliations will also not be considered in the analyses.

In the terminology of Riesebrodt, a denomination – with which one can declare to be affiliated – is not a religion, but a religious tradition. Therefore, the definition of religion and the meaning of denominations do not completely correspond to each other. An individual without religious affiliation – affiliation here and in the following refers to the individual trait – does not adhere to one of the officially recognized religious denominations. This need not mean that this person is irreligious.

The frequency of attending religious services is an indicator for the dimension of ritual. The categories in France, Norway, and Germany differ from each other. In Hungary, this information was not collected. While in France the exact frequency of attendances per year was asked, in Germany the variable was categorized as follows: daily, more than once per week, once per week, more than once per month, once per month, more than once per year, once per year, rarely, and never and in Norway it was daily, weekly but not daily, monthly but not weekly, a few times a year, less often, and never. The categories and frequencies are summarized as follows in the descriptive analyses: *(more than) once per week/ weekly (at least 52 times a year), more than once per month/ several times a month (24–48 times a year), once per month (12–20 times a year), 7–10 times a year, more than once per year/ few times a year (4–6 times a year), Once per year/ less often (1–3 times a year, rarely*, and *never*. In regression analyses the categories have to be dichotomized for methodical reasons with *frequent attendance of religious services*, which means that a person attends worship at least once per month or 12 times a year. A frequent attendee is assumed to be more religious than a person who rarely or never attends (*rare attendance*).[13]

Using the current frequency of attending religious services is not entirely unproblematic. This applies especially to East Germany and Hungary because most relevant demographic events occurred during the socialist period and the frequency was presumably different then.[14] A certain percentage of respondents has reached an age where physical restrictions can occur that prevent them from attending church. Rather, they watch masses on TV (see also Stark/Glock 1968: 86–89) or changed their forms of expression, e.g. they increase their frequency of prayers or they read religious literature. Increasing age usually affects religiosity, because people start to deal with the finiteness of life. In contrast to the cohort effect, this age effect cannot be considered in a cross-sectional regression estimation.

The GGS contains indicators that reflect attitudes associated to religious traditions and can be subsumed under the title "attitudes towards religious ceremonies at turning points in life":

> I am going to read out some statements about religious ceremonies and I would like you to tell me to what extent do you agree or disagree with each one.

They comprise

(i) baptism: It is important for an infant to be registered in the appropriate religious ceremony,

[13] It is difficult to definitively state the exact frequency of attendances. From US studies it is known that respondents often overestimate frequencies (see e.g. Hadaway/Marler/Chaves 1998).

[14] It can however be expected that religious people whose religiosity survived 40 years of socialism increased attendance frequency after the collapse of the system.

(ii) wedding: It is important for people who marry in registry offices to have a religious wedding too, and
(iii) funeral: It is important for a funeral to include a religious ceremony.

The scale of possible answers is equal in all three cases: 1 means "strongly agree", 5 means "strongly disagree". The developers of the questionnaire intended to explain fertility patterns and developments by changed attitudes, norms, and values by integrating these subjective variables:

> The link between values and demographic behavior is one of the central explanatory threads in explaining the demographic trends in the Western countries since the mid-1960s, for which Lesthaeghe and van de Kaa (...) coined the term Second Demographic Transition (Vikat et al. 2007: 418).

It is also their theoretical concept behind potential effects of (religious) values on demographic behavior.[15] The GGS collects an extensive set of attitudes and values, and "religiosity and secularization" are one dimension of it. Attitudes or values do not measure a core dimension of religiosity (see subsection 3.1.2), but as they have a religious reference they will be considered exploratively in the empirical analyses.

As the attitudes towards religious practices at turning points in life are highly inter-correlated with each other (see tables A.1 and A.2 in the appendix for the distribution of the original variables measuring attitudes and for a correlation matrix), an additive "values index" will be constructed.[16] After having recoded the initial values (1=0, ..., 5=4) and added them up, the index ranges from 0 which means "strong disagreement with religious ceremonies" to 12 expressing "strong agreement with religious ceremonies".

Baptism is a Christian practice which is reflected in the answer behavior of Muslims for that ceremony: they either did not respond to the question, answered "not applicable" or ascribed less importance to that kind of religious rite. To not adulterate the index values, the agreement value for baptism will be replaced by, i.e. imputed from the mean of the sum of the agreement values of the both other rites.

[15] "The central role of this dimension in explaining demographic behavior is emphasized in several approaches that aim to explain demographic change, including that of the Second Demographic Transition" (Vikat et al. 2007: 418, see also Surkyn/Lesthaeghe 2004).

[16] Alternatively, a dimension analysis that bundles and explains the common variance of these three variables in the form of an artificial factor could be calculated. However, the values of an index are easier to interpret and it is therefore preferred. As a trial, a principal component analysis was computed. The correlation was strong in magnitude, so that these two options can be treated almost interchangeably.

The fourth variable with religious reference collects the respondents' attitude towards the importance of religious faith as a "quality" or virtue[17] a child can acquire:

> Here is a list of qualities that children can acquire. Which, if any, do you consider to be especially important? Please choose up to three and mention them in the order of importance.

The pre-specified qualities – beside religious faith – respondents could opt for were: "good manners", "independence", "hard work", "feeling of responsibility", "imagination", "tolerance and respect for other people", "thrift, saving money, and things", "determination, perseverance", "unselfishness" as well as "obedience". In the empirical analysis no distinction will be made between the position at which a respondent stated religious faith as an important quality for children. The main point is that it was mentioned. In Norway, the number of important traits that could be stated was neither limited to three as in the other countries nor did the qualities have to be ranked. To believe that "religious faith" is a significant area for children to be "educated" in during childhood is also not an official indicator that measures religiosity according to the multi-dimensional concept. Not everybody who is of the opinion that to hand down religious faith to children is meaningful, has actually done so. Moreover, it is dependent on having children. But presumably, a larger share of parents who do think that it is an important quality passed it down.

In general, it may be criticized that the variables used reflect current statuses, attitudes, characteristics, and practices. Nevertheless, it is hardly imaginable that people start to attend church frequently with rising age – despite the above mentioned age effect. The other way round is indeed more noticeable. People who may have been socialized religiously but over (a long) time stopped attending church or do so much more rarely than during their fertile phase are characterized as non-practicing even though they do not belong to this category when it comes to their incorporated values. Other people may disagree with religious ceremonies at an early age but changed their attitudes after having concluded their fertility period.

6.1.4 The covariates

Several determinants of birth behavior cannot be used in the empirical analysis because they refer to current events, traits, and situations whereas fertility was partly

[17] The term "child quality" has been directly taken from the English questionnaire.

completed years before. Time-constant traits are unproblematic. If the assumption of time constancy is insecure but probable, such as in the case of religious affiliation, it will be made. In general, the probability of validity rises inversely to age. Due to the differences between men and women listed in subsection 5.2.1, parallel analyses for men and women will be conducted. This separation – together with the country-specific one – eliminates a part of the variance in the data.

One important covariate is the *birth cohort* as proxy for situations and developments during the fertile phase. The birth years *1930–1942* are summarized as the old cohort, the birth years *1939–1952* build the middle cohort, and persons who were born between *1949 and 1962* form the young cohort. The cohorts overlap slightly across countries but not within a country, because the reference parameter for the groups was the age of the respondents and not their stated year of birth. Data were also collected in different years. The youngest respondent is 45 years old. That is an age at which the probability to bear a(nother) child or to become father is very low. Due to varying years of data collection, the youngest birth cohort also varies by country. The oldest respondent was born in 1930 to measure exclusively post-war fertility. The downward limitation furthermore avoids an increasing survival selectivity of cohorts born earlier. The majority of the oldest cohort group married and had children during the golden age of marriage and the family (as reported in chapter 2).

Two criteria were used to generate the cohort groups. The middle cohort group should by and large have completed fertility before unification or transformation so that the impact of the temporal collapse of fertility can be read from cohort fertility of the youngest East German and Hungarian cohort group, especially the better educated members of those groups. The use of cohorts prevents misinterpreting the influence of religiosity as in truth merely a cohort effect because older cohorts were both more religious and more fertile. Furthermore, it partly accounts for the fact that no longitudinal data are available. In addition, some interaction dummies between religious affiliation, religiosity, and birth cohort will be used: *birth cohort * frequency of attendance of religious services * (un-)affiliated.*[18] This procedure takes account of changed behavior over the course of time differentiated by religiosity indicators.

[18] The single dummies are called *birth cohort 1930–1942 * frequent attendance, birth cohort 1930–1942 * rare attendance * affiliated, birth cohort 1930–1942 * unaffiliated, birth cohort 1939–1952 * frequent attendance, birth cohort 1939–1952 * rare attendance * affiliated, birth cohort 1939–1952 * unaffiliated, birth cohort 1949–1962 * frequent attendance, birth cohort 1949–1962 * rare attendance * affiliated*, and *birth cohort 1949–1962 * unaffiliated.*

The family of origin can be ascribed a significant influence on fertility behavior. A set of characteristics fall under this umbrella term, such as migration history, socioeconomic traits of mother and father, growing up with both parents or having divorced parents, the number of siblings, etc. Also the desired number of children could be attached to this cluster because the foundations for tastes, attitudes, preferences, and values are already shaped during childhood. Two characteristics are considered here: "migration background"[19] as well as the "number of siblings". The number of siblings is simply measured by the sum of brothers and sisters the respondent has. The number of siblings indirectly measures passed down family orientations. Having (more) siblings is associated with having positive attitudes towards children and family in general. Hitherto, research results have shown significant positive effects of a higher number of siblings on family size or the probability to form a family at all (e.g. Berinde 1999, Adsera 2004, Tölke 2004, White/Bernardi 2008).

An individual has a migration background if she or he is foreign, either with (first generation migrant) or without own migration experience (at least second generation migrant). Furthermore, a person with national citizenship is counted as a migrant if she or he has experienced migration (first generation migrant), or if the person did not migrate from another country herself or himself but at least one parent did so, or at least one parent is or was foreign (second or third generation migrant). All Turkish migrants in the supplemental survey are foreigners with direct migration experience.

Much information on migration background is available in the German and French data sets, but not in the Hungarian and Norwegian ones. In addition to this information, the answer categories of equivalent variables are country-specific. These facts necessitate a country-specific measurement of migration background. In the Hungarian data the only information given is "ethnic group", that means self-defined ethnicity, while the French or Norwegian data do not contain this information. This informational scarcity might be traced back to the fact that Hungary is not a (typical) destination for migrants, unlike France, Norway, and Germany. A respondent in Hungary can count herself among one of the following ethnic groups: Gypsy, Hungarian of Gypsy origin, Greek, Croatian, Polish, German, Hungarian of German origin, Armenian, Romanian, Ruthenian, Serbian, Slovak, Hungarian of Slovak origin, Slovenian, Ukrainian, Hungarian, Other. This large number of different ethnicities will be grouped. In addition to

[19] A migration background can also be "in-law", that means the partner has a migration history while the respondent might be autochthonal. This could have an effect on fertility because migration background is a meaningful cultural factor.

the autochthonal population (Hungarian), the following clustered categories remain: *Gypsy/ Hungarian of Gypsy origin*, and *East European/ German/ Other* (including Hungarians of German origin).

In the Norwegian questionnaire, the respondents were asked whether they were born in Norway and the answer option was just binary (yes/no). The second piece of information collected was current citizenship. Possible answers were not categorized in advance. As a great variety of nations is represented, each with low numbers of observations, the information that will be used in the analyses remains dichotomous: *migration background* means that someone was not born in Norway and/ or holds another citizenship than the Norwegian one. A majority of foreigners stems from other Scandinavian countries sharing a similar culture.

Respondents interviewed in France or Germany are assumed to have a migration background if one or more points of the following itemization apply:

1. the persons were not born in the country of interview,
2. they belong to another ethnic group (not available for France; categories in Germany: "German", "EU before 2003", "Additional EU country after 2004", "Russian", "Other EU country", "Turkish/ Kurdish", "Other"),
3. they currently have another citizenship (categories in France: "French by birth, including by restoration of nationality", "French by naturalization", "marriage, declaration or acquisition at age 18", "Foreign", "Stateless", "Both French by birth, including by restoration of nationality, and foreign", and "Both French by naturalization, marriage, declaration or acquisition at age 18, and foreign"; categories in Germany: "German", "Russian", "Turkish", "other", "German and other" "EU15 (2003)", and "Other country of Europe") or they do have the national citizenship but not from birth,
4. one or both parents of the respondent were not born in the country of interview,
5. one or both parents of the respondent belong to another ethnic group (not available in France; categories in Germany as above),
6. one or both parents of the respondents currently have another citizenship (categories as above) or they have the national citizenship but not from birth (the latter is neither available for mother nor father in France; categories in Germany as above).

In the French GGS possible backgrounds are *(North)African* and "European or other" (called *migration background* in the regression tables). About one half of the North

Africans are Roman Catholics who most probably are *Pieds-noirs*, basically autochthonal French citizens, even if they and their parents were born in North Africa. Around the year of Algeria's independence (1962) they migrated to France. They have French citizenship from birth. Hence, they will be counted among the persons "with migration background" but not among the North Africans. In Germany, the category *migration background* means European, Russian or other.[20] Less than ten Turkish migrants were left in the German GGS after Muslims had been excluded.[21]

The GGS collects educational attainment and professional qualification according to the International Standard Classification of Education (ISCED). ISCED was designed

> to serve as an instrument suitable for assembling, compiling and presenting comparable indicators and statistics of education both within individual countries and internationally. It presents standard concepts, definitions and classifications. ISCED covers all organized and sustained learning opportunities for children, youth and adults including those with special needs education, irrespective of the institution or entity providing them or the form in which they are delivered (United Nations Educational, Scientific and Cultural Organization (UNESCO) 2006: 7).

The basic concept and definitions of ISCED have therefore been developed to be universally valid and invariant to the particular circumstances of a national education system. After having updated and revised the taxonomy, the present classification is known as ISCED 1997 and primarily covers two cross-classification variables: levels and fields of education.[22] Possible values are: 0: preprimary education, 1: primary level, 2: lower secondary level, 3: upper secondary level, 4: post secondary non-tertiary education, 5: first stage of tertiary education, and 6: second stage of tertiary education. The following levels include labor market relevant training: 2C, 3C, 4B, 5A, and 5B. Some country specifications exist concerning the non-collection

---

[20] No information on deceased parents is available in the German data set. Respondents whose parents are already deceased are treated as nationals.

[21] For migration history, it would have been desirable to separate East and West Germans based on the place where they were born or socialized. In this work, East and West Germans are defined as such on the basis of where they lived of the time of the interview. This ignores the fact that especially the well-qualified women left the Eastern region, moved to the West, and are hence also migrants with a divergent cultural background affecting a variety of matters.

[22] For further information see United Nations Educational, Scientific and Cultural Organization (UNESCO) 2006.

of levels: Level 4 was not collected in France, level 6 was not collected in Hungary, and level 0 was not available in Germany. Therefore migrants from countries without compulsory education (or those who did not actually attend school) probably had to sort themselves into the category "other education" or level 1 while in France, Hungary, and Norway migrants could select the correct category. To make educational attainment more comparable between the countries, the original ISCED levels are summarized to three categories: *low educational attainment (isced 0–2)*,[23] *medium educational attainment (isced 3–4)*, and *high educational attainment (isced 5–6)*. In the model estimations of the Turkish migrants, medium and high education are pooled. Educational attainment is available for the respondent and the current partner, but not for ex- or already deceased partners. Income is not considered due to the advanced age of many respondents. Retirement pay is usually lower than income from employment. Periods of employment can also not be used in the analyses.[24]

Marital status is constructed from GGS data and is composed of a variety of variables. In the GGS "partnership" is defined as cohabitation especially when information on previous partnerships are collected. Only when it comes to the current partner, and no partner lives in respondent's household, is the question posed of whether a "relationship to somebody without cohabitation" exists: "Are you currently having an intimate (couple) relationship with someone you're not living with? This may also be your spouse if he/she does not live together with you. Our survey not only covers heterosexual relationships, but also same-sex relationships. If you have a partner of the same sex, please answer the following questions as well."

The respondents' marital status will be described with one of the following categories: *never married* with the subcategory *single* (never had partnership), *married for the first time* (including PACS), *divorced*, *widowed* (once or twice; never divorced), *remarried* (including PACS; second time – previous marriage divorced; 3rd/ 4th time – at least one previous marriage divorced). In Norway respondents were not asked whether a marriage ended in divorced, but merely who started the legal process of divorce. All marriages that broke up will be treated as divorced except for the few cases where the respondent explicitly states that the partners "moved apart".

23 Some respondents in Germany – the majority of them Turkish migrants – stated that they are "still a pupil" (N=18), "still in training" (N=4) or "other education" (N=145). Those respondents are assigned to the category "low education".

24 Social status – e.g. measured by the qualification of the (male) partner – must also be ignored as it is only available if there is currently a partner. Moreover, many missings exist.

Being single only means that the respondent never cohabited with a partner. But, she or he may have had living apart together relationships. This cannot be ascertained with the data. In the multivariate analysis, respondents who have been divorced at least twice count among the "remarried" category because they had more than one institutionalized relationship. A stable marriage is an ex-post indicator for a divorce risk that ex-ante was anticipated as low and due to which spouses did not restrict their marital investments.

Fertility not only varies across countries or individual characteristics but also within countries across different sizes of settlements. Generally, in rural regions family life is more traditional. In urban areas, especially large cities, birth rates are lower (Kulu/Boyle/Andersson 2009: 916 cite a variety of studies also for France, Norway, and Germany confirming this result, see also p. 936). Among other things, rents are higher than in the suburbs and rural areas. Many young parents prefer – conditional on their economic resources – another surrounding for their young family and want to buy or build an own house with garden so that they move out of the cities if they were living there before. The size of the city hence only causally influences fertility under certain conditions, namely insofar as selective movements can be ruled out. The following variables take account of the size of the municipality of residence. Using this information presupposes that there is not much movement between rural and urban areas after the children were born and have grown up. Data collection was country-specific, making comparisons difficult but accounting for differing population sizes and densities.

In France the categories are: *rural* (less than 5,000 inhabitants), urban (more than 5,000 inhabitants), and *town*. In Norway, four categories were collected: *centrality level 0: completely rural*, *centrality level 1*, *centrality level 2*, and *centrality level 3: urban.*[25] In Germany, the categories are much clearer and have been (partly) aggregated as follows: *up to 19,999 inhabitants*, *peripheral area from 50–100,000/ central area from 20–100,000 inhabitants*, *peripheral area from 100,000/ central area from 100–500,000 inhabitants*, *more than 500,000 inhabitants*. In Hungary, regional information will be represented by subdividing the respondents into four categories:

[25] Exact explanations for these categories do not seem to exist.

capital (Budapest), *city*, *town*, and *village*.[26] The distribution of the covariates is displayed in tables A.8, A.9, and A.10 in the appendix.

6.1.5 Statistical method: Poisson regression

Poisson is the central statistical tool used in this study. Its main features are explained in this section. The exposition follows Greene 2012: 842–850. Poisson regression models are employed if the dependent variable only attains non-negative integers. Hence, the Poisson distribution is a discrete probability distribution that inter alia can be used to model the number of events within a given interval of time. If these events occur with a constant rate, it has only one parameter, λ, that is generally chosen to be the mean value. The model specifies that each value of the dependent variable is drawn from a Poisson population. It can be used to explain the non-linear relationship between religiosity (and further variables) and fertility in cross-sectional data.

The basic Poisson model is expressed by

$$\Pr(Y = y) = \frac{e^{-\lambda}\lambda^{y}}{y!}, \quad y = 0, 1, 2, \ldots \tag{6.1}$$

where λ represents the Poisson parameter and y is the single count. With the aid of this basic model the theoretical probabilities for each count (0, 1, ... children) can be calculated on condition that λ is estimated from the empirical distribution. The results of both the empirical and the theoretical distribution can be found in table 6.4 in subsection 6.2.1. λ can be made a function of covariates. The most commonly link function is the logarithm. One sets

$$\ln \lambda_i = x_i'\beta. \tag{6.2}$$

where x denotes a set of explanatory variables, i.e. religiosity and the covariates (birth cohort, educational attainment, marital status, number of siblings, migration background or ethnic group, size of settlement) and β is a set of regression coefficients

[26] "City" means settlements that have special "county-level" rights. They include county seats and a few other big cities (50,000 or more inhabitants) that are regional centers and have special rights and responsibilities. "Towns" are all the other urban settlements, usually middle-sized or smaller ones. "Villages" are the smaller, rural settlements. These information have been provided by Livia Murinkó who is research fellow at the HCSO Demographic Research Institute in Budapest.

expressing the quantitative linear relationship between $\ln \lambda_i$ and x_i. The parameters are estimated by maximum likelihood techniques. The log-likelihood function is

$$\ell(\beta) := \ln L(\beta) := \sum_{i=1}^{n} \left[-\lambda_i + y_i x_i' \beta - \ln y_i! \right]. \tag{6.3}$$

One possible measure of fit is based on the ratio of the log likelihoods of the estimated model and the empty model and is defined as $1 - \ell(\text{model})/\ell(\text{null})$. This is McFadden's pseudo R^2. It will generally be reported in preference to likelihood values. Principally, McFaddden's pseudo R^2 does not share all the properties of the R^2 of ordinary least squares regression. Therefore, McFadden's pseudo R^2, which is only one out of a variety of pseudo R^2 statistics, should only be interpreted with some caution.[27]

A further measure of fit reported will be (the value of) the likelihood-ratio test (LR χ^2). It globally tests if at least one β coefficient is significantly different from zero. The degrees of freedom are defined by the number of explanatory variables. The LR test statistic is calculated as $-2 * [\ell(\text{null}) - \ell(\text{model})]$. $\Pr > \chi^2$ indicates the asymptotic probability of observing a more extreme value of LR χ^2 than the one obtained if in fact the explanatory variables have no impact on the dependent variable (this means that all regression coefficients must together be equal to zero). If the probability is below one of the common significance levels ($p < 0.05$, $p < 0.01$, $p < 0.001$), the null hypothesis that all coefficients are equal to zero is rejected.[28]

The Poisson model implies equi-dispersion, i.e. $\mathbb{E}(Y) = \text{var}(Y) = \lambda$. As will (also) be shown in subsection 6.2.1, the distribution in most groups complies with this model implication – the presupposition of equi-dispersion is not violated – so that the basic method can be applied. Sometimes, however, data are over-dispersed: the variance is larger than the mean – or under-dispersed, i.e. the variance is smaller than the mean (Winkelmann 1994: 25–26).

In the case of over-dispersion, negative binomial regression models will be estimated. To check for over-dispersion, a goodness-of-fit test of the model estimation is performed. The test is distributed χ^2 with 1 degree of freedom. If the test is significant ($\Pr > \chi^2 \rightarrow p < 0.05$), the estimated Poisson regression model may be inappropriate.

---

[27] Also see the STATA website: `http://www.ats.ucla.edu/stat/stata/output/stata_poisson_output.htm` (18 Jun 2013).

[28] Also see the STATA website: `http://www.ats.ucla.edu/stat/stata/output/stata_poisson_output.htm` (18 Jun 2013).

The negative binomial model arises from a natural formulation of cross-section heterogeneity. By introducing an individual, unobserved effect into the conditional mean, the Poisson model is generalized:

$$\ln \mu_i := x_i^{'}\beta + \varepsilon_i = \ln \lambda_i + \ln u_i \tag{6.4}$$

where the disturbance ε_i reflects either the common specification error or the usual cross-sectional heterogeneity. In this case, the distribution of y_i conditioned on x_i and u_i which is ε_i remains Poisson with conditional mean and variance μ_i:

$$f(y_i \,|\, x_i, u_i) = \frac{e^{-\lambda_i u_i}(\lambda_i u_i)^{y_i}}{y_i!}. \tag{6.5}$$

If u is a random variable with a fixed gamma distribution, a negative binomial distribution results (Greene 2012: 847). The negative binomial distribution is over-dispersed in comparison to the Poisson distribution,

$$var(Y) = 1/p\mathbb{E}(Y) > \mathbb{E}(Y).$$

An alternative to count data models are event data models but they demand high standards of the data as they not only model the number of counts but also their spacing and event times. The data used in the following are somewhat deficient or required information is simply missing. Data collection in the countries was not strictly homogeneously conducted. Therefore it seems to be prudent to concentrate only on the number of events and to ignore more detailed information even if it is present.

For France, Norway, and Germany GGS supplies a weighting factor that is constructed on the basis of socio-demographic information such as level of education, income, size of household, etc. that should lead to the adjustment of the sample distributions to the distributions of the respective population.[29] Descriptive analyses will be calculated using weighting adjustments. Regression estimations will not be weighted. Analyses are conducted with Stata 10.0. Figures are constructed with R 2.15.1.

[29] Concerning the weighing procedure the consortium made no guidelines. No standards exist. Information on sampling and weighing procedures can be found on the website of the GGP (`www.ggp-i.org/`). For Hungary, there is also a weighting factor. However, information seem to be only available in Hungarian.

6.2 Descriptive analysis

The present section contains the first empirical results: 6.2.1 describes fertility, 6.2.2 deals with religious affiliation and religiosity. In subsection 6.2.3 assumptions advanced in chapter 4 are tested against reality. Finally, subsection 6.2.4 shows whether religiosity has an effect on completed fertility among respondents born between 1930 and 1962.

6.2.1 Fertility

The values for completed fertility in the following tables are structured by country and gender. Fertility has declined over the course of time as already shown. Therefore, birth cohort serves as an additional differentiation factor in table 6.3 displaying the average number of children people have in France, Hungary, Norway, and Germany. The table also documents that the completion age for men and women can be set equal.

Table 6.3. Completed fertility by country, gender, and cohort

		FRANCE			HUNGARY			NORWAY			GERMANY								
											East			West			Turkish migrants		
Age group / birth cohort		Total	Women	Men	Total	Women	Men	Total	Women	Men	Total	Women	Men	Total	Women	Men	Total	Women	Men
1	45–54 (1949–1962)	2.03	2.11	1.94	1.83	1.90	1.74	2.06	2.08	2.04	1.77	1.76	1.78	1.52	1.63	1.41	2.33	2.42	2.22
2	55–64 (1939–1952)	2.16	2.12	2.19	1.84	1.84	1.84	2.12	2.11	2.12	1.61	1.75	1.47	1.54	1.60	1.47	2.18	2.17	2.20
3	65–74 (1930–1942)	2.50	2.61	2.36	1.76	1.75	1.78	2.38	2.41	2.35	1.95	2.01	1.89	1.78	1.84	1.71	1.96	2.25	1.80
1–3	45–74 (1930–1962)	2.20	2.25	2.14	1.81	1.84	1.78	2.14	2.15	2.12	1.78	1.84	1.71	1.61	1.69	1.52	2.19	2.28	2.10

Weighted data. Numbers of observations: table A.8 in the appendix.

The bottom row shows average fertility for all relevant birth cohorts together. It is highest among Turkish migrants who are restricted to Muslims (95% of original sample) and the French followed by Norwegians with 2.2 respectively 2.14 children per person. Differences are marginal. East Germans and Hungarians with 1.8 children per person on average basically not do differ. West Germans are least fertile. Men report fewer children than women (see details in section 5.2.1). Fertility differences are more pronounced between the oldest cohort group and the medium one than between the medium and the youngest cohort (the Hungarian and migrant data exhibit diverging distributions). Presumably this gap, which is largest in France, is – among others – associated with the post-war golden age of marriage and the family, a period within which the oldest cohort group had its fertile period while the both other cohorts largely had it afterward.

Cohort differences by gender are similar to the total group. Hungary is an exception: in the descriptive perspective, gender and cohort show little variance. The oldest cohort has least children (women and men are taken together), which reflects the diverging course of the fertility rate presented above. Fertility of Turkish migrants (also) increases in the opposite direction. Older migrants are less fertile, which could be a migration effect. The gender difference reinforces this assumption because it is the men who have fewer children. Many migrants who were recruited as workers during the time of Germany's economic miracle due to a scarcity of domestic labor force, moved to Germany early in their lives when they had not yet had children. Later, not all of them caught up on their postponed fertility. While the workforce mainly consisted of men, processes of family reunion taking place later contributed to raising the female share in the migrant population (Nauck 1993). These developments explain the fertility differences by gender in the oldest cohort and moreover, why 28.6% of the men but only 17.4% of the women belong to the oldest cohort (see table A.8 in appendix). In later cohorts, fertility converged due to the more strongly balanced proportions of women and men in those cohorts and the ban on recruitment abroad by the government in 1973.

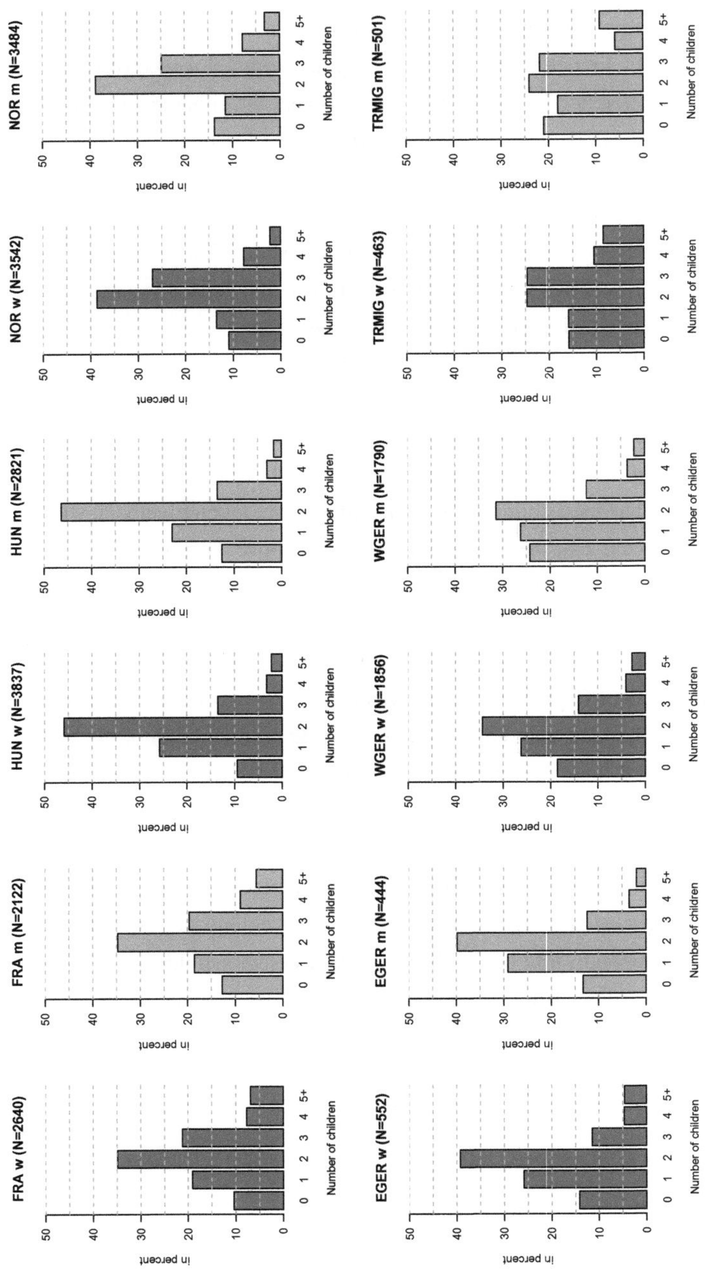

Fig. 6.1. Parity distribution by country and gender

The parity distributions largely accord with the values introduced in section 2.1. Childlessness is lowest among Hungarian women (9.5%) followed by French (10.4%) and Norwegian women (10.9%) (see figure 6.1[30]). Only West Germans and Turkish migrants show levels of childlessness above 15%. The proportion of childless individuals in East Germany is a bit higher than expected. The share of men without children exceeds the share of women except for East Germany. In the further course of this work it becomes obvious that the behavior of East German women contradicts a variety of assumptions. To have a small family with only one child is most popular among Germans, especially East German men. Almost one third of them father an only child. On the other side of the distribution, Turkish migrants most often have a large family with four or more children (women: 19%, men: 15.1%). The French follow with 14.5%. While having so many children is uncommon among Norwegians, they rank second behind Turkish migrants when all families with at least three children are summarized (migrants: 43.6% respectively 36.9%; Norwegians: 37% respectively 35.9%; French: 35.7% respectively 34%). In Hungary and Germany, large families are less widespread. The shares among men amount to less than 19%, and to about 20% among women. Finally, there seems to be a two-child norm, especially in Hungary with 46% of all respondents. The incidence is not that prevalent in any other country, but is also very pronounced among East Germans and Norwegians.

Table 6.4 compares the empirical with the theoretical Poisson distribution for each group. The single distributions are reflected by their mean and variance (λ). The very small variance with respect to the Hungarians clearly expresses the two-child dominance with low shares at the edges of the distribution. A similar explanation holds for the Norwegian data where the variance is also small. That means the Hungarian and Norwegian data are under-dispersed because the variance is smaller than the mean (the same applies to the data of East German men). Equi-dispersion is guaranteed by the data of women and men in France and West Germany as well as women in East Germany. It is only the data of the male Turkish migrants that are over-dispersed: the variance is larger than the mean. Parities are more equally distributed than in all other groups. The edges accumulate higher shares than expected by the theoretical distribution. Therefore, in section 6.3.3 negative binomial models are estimated and for the reason of comparability for both female and male migrants.

30 Only values above 4 are summarized in this figure.

Table 6.4. Comparison of empirical and theoretical distributions

	FRANCE				HUNGARY				NORWAY				GERMANY East				GERMANY West				GERMANY Turkish migrants			
	Women		Men		Women		Men		Women		Men		Women		Men		Women		Men		Women		Men	
	E	P	E	P	E	P	E	P	E	P	E	P	E	P	E	P	E	P	E	P	E	P	E	P
0	10.4	10.6	12.7	11.7	9.5	16.0	12.5	16.8	10.9	11.6	13.8	12.0	14.2	15.8	13.3	18.0	18.6	18.6	24.3	21.8	15.9	10.0	21.0	12.2
1	19.1	23.8	18.5	25.1	25.8	29.3	23.0	29.9	13.5	25.0	11.5	25.4	25.9	29.2	29.1	30.9	26.2	31.3	26.2	33.2	15.9	23.1	18.1	25.6
2	34.9	26.7	34.8	26.9	45.9	26.9	46.4	26.7	38.7	26.9	38.8	27.0	39.2	26.9	39.8	26.5	34.3	26.3	31.3	25.3	24.6	26.5	24.0	27.0
3	21.1	20.0	19.6	19.2	13.5	16.4	13.5	15.9	27.0	19.3	25.0	19.0	11.4	16.7	12.3	15.1	14.1	14.8	12.3	12.9	24.6	20.3	21.8	19.0
4	7.7	11.2	8.9	10.3	3.2	7.5	3.0	7.1	7.8	10.4	7.8	10.1	4.7	7.6	3.5	6.5	4.1	6.2	3.7	4.9	10.5	11.7	5.9	10.0
5+	6.9	7.7	5.5	6.8	2.2	3.9	1.6	3.6	2.2	6.8	3.1	6.5	4.6	3.8	2.0	3.0	2.8	2.8	2.2	1.9	8.5	8.4	9.1	6.2
Nobs	2,640		2,122		3,837		2,821		3,542		3,484		552		444		1,856		1,790		463		501	
Mean (Variance)	2.2 (2.3)		2.1 (2.1)		1.8 (1.2)		1.8 (1.3)		2.2 (1.5)		2.1 (1.6)		1.8 (1.8)		1.7 (1.3)		1.7 (1.6)		1.5 (1.5)		2.3 (2.5)		2.1 (3.2)	

Age group 45–74 years, birth cohorts 1930–1962. In %; weighted data. E: Empirical distribution, P: Theoretical Poisson distribution, Nobs: Numbers of observations.

The excess-zero problem which usually emerges in association with fertility (and usually leads to the application of zero-inflated models) does not apply here because only completed fertility is considered. Due to low childlessness in the majority of the groups, the application of a hurdle model that divides the decision about children in two parts (1. Children "yes" or "no", 2. in case of "yes": how many?) does not answer the question posed. The estimation of "ordinary" Poisson models serves the purpose and the efficiency is high enough (merely in case of the migrants will negative binomial models be estimated). The only issue that has to be handled is the excess-two problem. But an alternative model would not deliver better answers to solve that striking characteristic in most of the distributions.

6.2.2 Religiosity

Religious affiliation

The percentage of religiously affiliated individuals, the frequency of church attendance as well as involvement in church life, etc. has declined during the last 40 years in many European countries (secularization processes at the individual level). These developments affect mainly Christianity while the religiosity of Muslims – mostly migrants – is higher on average. It has confused some of the autochthonal citizens in the countries of immigration (see also Sengers/Sunier 2010). More than a few feel "threatened" by the Muslims' self-confidence and their requests for mosques. Muslims massively contributed to religion's jump back onto the public agenda (see also Casanova 2007: 346–348, Banchoff 2007: 6–8, Reuter 2009: 39–40, Just 2011: 189–190). Suddenly many Europeans have started to reconsider their secular or Christian cultures, core values, and the foundation of the constitutions on Christian principles. Nevertheless, this process has not been reflected by re-growing individual religiosity of Christians. Table 6.5 contains the distributions of religious affiliation in France, Hungary, Norway, and Germany.

Affiliation rates significantly differ between the five countries. In France, religious affiliation is – due to the separation of state and church – not recorded by official authorities. All data on the population's denominational composition rely on (survey) estimates or originate from the religious groups themselves. Statements on affiliation rates vary considerably. While the rate of affiliates in the GGS exceeds 85%, in the 1998 International Social Survey Programme (ISSP) little more than half of the French respondents reported that they were affiliated (53%). In the European Social Survey

(ESS) of 2008 this statement applied to 40%, while the remainder reported being unaffiliated.[31] These remarkable variations are presumably not due to biases during the recruitment process. All three surveys demand a great deal of the selection process for respondents so that this probability should be rather small. The survey method, i.e. the way the question is posed (ISSP: Which religious denomination do you adhere to? ESS: Do you consider yourself as belonging to any particular religion or denomination? GGS: Which religious denomination do you adhere to, if any?) is very similar in each survey and hence can hardly generate variation. The main problem, however, may be found in the very high proportion (compared to the other countries) of contacted persons who refused to take part in the ISSP survey. The share of unit non-responses of all contacted persons added up to 89% (East Germany: 34%, West Germany: 40%, Hungary: 48%; Zentralarchiv für empirische Sozialforschung 2001: 42, 44, 50). While in West Germany "only" half of the non-responses were refusals, in France almost all non-responses were refusals. This fact reinforces the problem.

80% of French respondents are Roman Catholics, women somewhat more frequently than men. The proportion of Muslims exceeds the proportion of (Reformed) Protestants.[32] Accordingly, Islam is the second most widespread religious tradition in France. One cannot read in table 6.5 that 0.8% of the French population are Jews.[33] Jewish respondents are part of the pooled category "other". Their percentage in the GGS is 0.8% (women) respectively 0.4% (men).

With about 83%, most affiliated Norwegians are members of the (Lutheran state) Church of Norway. Compared to population, the proportion is only slightly elevated. The category "Christianity outside the Church of Norway" is composed of members of several evangelical free churches, the Catholic Church as well as further Christian groups (Statistics Norway 2012h, table 3). Muslims account for only a small proportion of non-Christians. 6% of female non-Christians are Muslims and 17% of the

[31] This information is based on the author's own calculations with ISSP (available at `www.gesis.org`) and ESS data (available at `www.europeansocialsurvey.org/`).

[32] The Reformed Protestants (also called Huguenots), were killed or expelled in one of the eight religious wars in the second half of the 16th century so that since 1685 the number of Protestants has been rather small (see Hinrichs/Haupt 2008: 144–206).

[33] According to the World Jewish Congress and the American Jewish Yearbook 2006 500,000 Jews live in France (Institute for Jewish Community Research 2006). In the 1950s and 1960s, the Ashkenazi community of veteran French Jews and immigrants from Eastern Europe underwent a major demographic transformation with the arrival of 300,000 Jews from North Africa, mainly from Morocco, Tunisia, and Egypt. As a result, the Sephardi Jews now comprise 60% of the French Jewish community.

males (included in category "other"). In the population, the share of Christians outside the Church of Norway is somewhat higher than the share of non-Christians. This is not reflected in the data. Only a small share of Norwegians is unaffiliated. Official statistics recognize what they call "life stance communities" and count them among other religious denominations.

The majority of Hungarians is Catholic, most of them are Roman Catholic (60%) but also a small minority of Greek Catholics lives in the country (3%).[34] Greek Catholics can be mainly found in a small delimitable region in the Eastern part of the country.[35] The difference with regard to France consists in the existence of another meaningful religious group, the Reformed Protestants who follow the teachings and ideas of Calvin or Zwingli. Every fifth respondent in Hungary characterizes herself or himself as Reformed Protestant. Beside Reformed Christians, Lutherans live in Hungary albeit with a much smaller share of 4%. As mentioned in 3.2.4, the proportion of Hungarians affiliated to Orthodox Christianity is extremely low, which is due to shifts in the national borders in the last century. One tenth do not adhere to any of the organized religious denominations. The country can traditionally be characterized as religiously pluralist and this has been the case since the 16th century (see Tomka 1999: 29–30).

[34] The national Greek Catholic churches (Albanian, Bulgarian, Croatian, Greek, Hungarian, Italo-Greek, Macedonian, Melkite, Romanian, Russian, Ruthenian, Slovak, and Ukrainian) denote a set of Byzantine-rite churches that are unified with Rome. The Byzantine rite came into existence in the Byzantine Empire and belongs to the liturgies of the Eastern churches.

[35] The website http://commons.wikimedia.org/wiki/File:Vall\%C3\%A1sos_\%C3\%A9s_nem_h\%C3\%ADv\%C5\%91_k\%C3\%B6z\%C3\%B6ss\%C3\%A9gek_Magyarorsz\%C3\%A1gon.png (10 May 2012) displays a very informative figure showing the regional distribution of religious affiliates in Hungary based on the 2001 Census data. The name of the creator of the figure is "Beroesz".

Table 6.5. Religious affiliation by country and gender

	FRANCE		HUNGARY		NORWAY		GERMANY					
							East		West		Tr. migs	
	Women	Men	Women	Men	Women	Men	Women	Men	Women	Men	Women	Men
Christian	84.0	80.0	89.1	84.5	87.7	86.5	32.5	27.9	89.0	81.3	(0.7)	(0.4)
Roman Catholic	81.9	78.2	61.1	59.1								
Greek Catholic			2.8	2.9								
Reformed Protestant (Calvinist)	1.8	1.7	20.9	18.4								
Lutheran			4.0	3.9								
Church of Norway					83.1	82.6						
Christianity outside the Church of Norway					4.6	3.9						
Other Christian affiliation	(0.3)	(0.1)	(0.4)	(0.2)								
Muslim	2.1	4.0					(0.0)	(0.3)	(0.7)	(2.1)	95.6	94.1
Other	(1.1)	(1.5)	(1.2)	(1.4)	5.2	5.2	(0.8)	(0.5)	(1.6)	(1.1)	(1.6)	(2.3)
Without affiliation	4.7	6.2	8.6	12.0	6.1	7.6	65.5	71.2	8.5	15.1	(1.3)	(2.2)
No response/ refusal	8.4	8.0	(1.2)	(2.0)	(1.0)	(0.9)	(1.2)	(0.3)	(0.2)	(0.5)	(0.8)	(1.0)
Numbers of observations	2,679	2,157	3,945	2,927	3,571	3,508	560	449	1,907	1,854	485	540

Age group 45–74 years, birth cohorts 1930–1962. In %; weighted data. Tr. migs: Turkish migrants. The list of denominations is country-specific. Respondents with an affiliation whose share is in brackets are excluded from all other tables and analyses due to their small proportion. The numbers of observations are hence higher here. French respondents who did not respond are merely excluded from analyses in which information on affiliation is needed.

Although the variations between the different data sets are smaller, they are also discernible in the case of Hungary. In the 1998 ISSP 49% stated that they were Roman Catholic, 16% were Protestants (either Reformed or Lutheran), and 30% did not adhere to any denomination. In the 2008 ESS the share of affiliated was even smaller (Roman Catholics: 39%, Protestants: 16.6%).[36] The share of respondents without any affiliation amounted to 40%. The parallels between France and Hungary in relation to the surveys are obvious. The proportion of unaffiliated individuals is lowest in the GGS and highest in the ESS. The question on religious affiliation fortunately arose in the Census 2001 so that official data can be used for comparison as opposed to France. The majority of the population avows itself to the Catholic Church (55%), Roman and Greek Catholics are taken together. 16% are Reformed Protestants, and 3% are Lutherans. One fourth declared themselves to be unaffiliated or did not specify an affiliation. Summarized, this means that the proportions of Catholics and Protestants are slightly elevated in the GGS – but still closer to the "real" value than in the ISSP and particularly the ESS – while unaffiliated respondents are under-represented.

The proportion of affiliated individuals in Hungary has grown since the breakdown of the socialist system. According to the analysis of Pickel 2011 that is based on data from the project "Church and religion in an enlarged Europe 2006" (C&R), the shares were 65% in 1991, 67% in 2000, and 78% in 2006 (p. 175). Hungary in this context is representative for most of the other post-socialist societies where rates of affiliation have also re-grown after 1990. The majority of Catholics live in the wealthier and more modern West,[37] while the Reformed Protestants are to be found in the East.[38] Predominantly older industries and agriculture are located in the East, which means that many regions are economically weak there while the West has strongly modernized after the transformation. This regional distribution delivers clues about the social profiles of religious groups. With respect to Lutherans and

[36] Values relating to ISSP and ESS are based on the author's own calculations.

[37] See the very informative figure on the website http://commons.wikimedia.org/wiki/File:Vall\%C3\%A1sos_\%C3\%A9s_nem_h\%C3\%ADv\%C5\%91_k\%C3\%B6z\%C3\%B6ss\%C3\%A9gek_Magyarorsz\%C3\%A1gon.png (10 May 2012).

[38] Great regional urban-rural disparities exist in centralist Hungary following on from the planned economy and transformation of the economic system (Barlai/Hartleb 2007). The Budapest region, where 17% of the whole population lives, the Balaton region, and some other urban agglomerations (mainly in the North-west) have benefited from the transformation, from the market economy and foreign investments, while areas shaped by agriculture and heavy industry in the East and North-east, have enormous difficulties keeping up with international competition. Unemployment has significantly risen there.

Reformed Protestants, socioeconomic differences do exist. Lutherans have a higher education and are younger on average (while theological differences are rather small; Tomka 2006: 46).

Less than one third of the East Germans belong to one of the Christian churches, which is the lowest share of all countries included (see table 6.5). The large majority of remaining affiliates are members of the Protestant Church, a few are Roman Catholics who are spread over East Germany in diaspora regions. This part of Germany has had a Protestant cultural tradition since the Reformation although in the years following World War II, the proportion of Catholics grew significantly due to the return of millions of expellees (Knauft 1980: 13–14). In 1950, the proportion of Catholics was 11%. At the end of the 1980s only 4% still adhered to the Catholic Church. 80% were Lutherans in 1950 and 26% forty years later.[39] Hardly any Muslims live here. The percentage of individuals without membership multiplied tenfold in the years in-between. Today, the rate of affiliated individuals within East Germany varies greatly by region. In the Northern part, it is much lower than in many regions of the Southern part. In rural areas it is much higher than in urban areas (Storch 2003: 233, 241). The latter indeed is a common finding for most countries, but the general level distinguishes East Germany from those.

Church member losses did not occur continuously in the years between 1950 and 1990 (Storch 2003: 237). At the end of the 1950s, the number of church leavers reached a peak. Afterward it fell but still remained at a high level. It was not before the middle of the 1970s that the number of exits strongly decreased. The quantity of church entries was numerically negligible by contrast. Whereas during the first years of the existence of the GDR the losses could be traced back to church exits, later another factor gained importance: the relation between baptisms and funerals changed. The number of funerals steadily increased while the number of baptisms diminished. Even many church members did not have their children baptized.

Consequently, individuals without religious affiliation can be leavers or never baptized individuals. In West Germany the latter reason has not played a prominent role until recently. Baptisms are still common but the number of leavers is slowly increasing. In 1950, 96% of the population belonged to one of the two churches, and, according to the GGS, in 2005 the proportion still amounted to 87% (according to official statistics: 83% are affiliated; Statistisches Bundesamt 2008: 380). The

[39] Knauft's information rests on church sources and statistical yearbooks of the GDR and has hence to be treated with care.

relation between Catholics and Protestants is relatively balanced with a small edge in favor of Catholics because the number of Protestant church leavers was somewhat higher in recent years.[40] Before the 1980s, the number of Protestant church members exceeded the number of Catholics (Pollack 2000: 19). A small share of 1.8% of West Germans adheres to the Orthodox Church. Somewhat less than two thirds of the whole population living in Germany are members of a Christian church (data: Evangelische Kirche in Deutschland 2008).

The proportion of Muslims in France (based on extrapolation) accounts for 5–7% of the total population (Banchoff 2007: 6), and in Germany for 4.6–5.2%. Of the latter, 45% are German citizens with a migration background. The majority has a foreign citizenship (Haug/Müssig/Stichs 2009: 11). Three fourths of the Turkish Muslims are Sunnis, 19% are Turkish or Kurdish Alevis, 2.3% Shiites, and 4.2% are followers of another tradition (Haug/Müssig/Stichs 2009: 137).[41] Alevis do not recognize all five pillars of Islam (Sökefeld 2008: 33, Tan 1999: 66–69). For example, they are not obliged to participate in Friday worship and can be characterized in total as a quite secular group. Discussions – also among Alevis themselves – deal with the question of if they are Muslims at all. This debate is mainly relevant for Germany – but not for France – because Alevis mainly originate from Turkey.

Hungary and the GDR did not experience mass immigration – neither of Muslims nor in general. Some workers from other Socialist countries such as Vietnam were temporarily permitted to work there. After World War II the government of the Federal Republic of Germany recruited guest workers from countries neighboring the Mediterranean Sea (Herbert 1986: 198, Goldberg/Halm/Şen 2004: 4, Beauftragte der Bundesregierung für Migration, Flüchtlinge und Integration 2007: 50). Most of those workers originated from Christian countries such as Italy and Greece, but a large number of workers were also recruited from Turkey and a small group of workers came from the Maghreb. After having fulfilled the recruitment contracts, a high proportion of workers did not move back to their countries of origin as had been expected by the government but stayed – and brought their families to live with them. By shifting their main place of residence from Turkey to West Germany, migration turned them

[40] See also section 3.2 where this point is presented in more detail.

[41] Within Sunni Islam four legal schools are established: Hanafi, Maliki, Shafi'i, and Hanbali. Maghrebi Sunnis follow the Maliki school whereas Sunnis who immigrated from Turkey follow the Hanafi school (see Glasenapp 2005: 397–398). Differences between the schools are not considerable (Breuer 2008: 8).

from temporary to permanent residents (Bundesministerium des Innern 2008: 15). These developments resulted in a fast increase of both the number of foreigners and of Muslims. Later, the civil war in Yugoslavia further increased the number of Muslims by the inflow of refugees. These reasons lead to the fact that wherever Muslims stem from they do not belong to the autochthonal population: either they are still foreigners belonging to the first, second, or third generation, or they are Germans with a migration background. Immigration of Muslims to France has a somewhat longer history due to the colonial past and recruitment already after World War I (see e.g. Fetzer/Soper 2006: 63–69, Hervieu-Léger 2007: 204). The recruitment of guest workers was similarly arranged as to in Germany. The recruitment processes differed concerning the countries of origin the workers were recruited from. The Maghrebi countries were one of the main recruitment regions because of their former colonial status (Wihtol de Wenden 2007: 140).[42]

Religious affiliation can at most be understood as a base category of religiosity and seems to have few consequences with respect to the religious self-concept of and what an individual believes. Affiliation is a rather passive indicator that moreover is frequently associated with national identity or traditions without expressing religiosity. In countries were belonging is still a norm, social desirability effects have to be taken into account. These issues require the consideration of further indicators. But one matter has to be pointed out: beside the huge country differences the observation that more women than men are religiously affiliated is obvious.

Frequency of attendance of religious services

Table 6.6 contains data on the frequency of attendance of religious services in France, Norway, and Germany. In spite of a significantly higher affiliation rate, more French respondents – especially men – never attend church than East Germans. In contrast, more French respondents (women: 16.8%, men: 9.4%) attend church frequently, that means 12 times a year or more often, than people in East Germany (women: 10.3%, men: 7.9%). The differences between East and West Germans are observable. In the Western part of Germany, respondents are by far more active with considerable gender differences (women: 32.1%, men: 23%). Also only a minority never attends. Only a small share of Norwegians – by far the smallest share in comparison – attends

[42] In contrast to the Turkish migrants in Germany, the majority of Maghrebi migrants in France possesses French citizenship because they were born in France.

religious services at least once a month (women: 8.2%, men: 6.1%). Less people never attend than in France or East Germany. Turkish migrants, all of them Muslims, offer a completely different picture, i.e. they attend mosque with a much higher frequency. Half of the women and two thirds of the men take part in congregational prayer once a month or more frequently. It is observable that in general more women attend frequently than men (see also the theoretical reasoning for this gender-specific behavior among Christians by Azzi/Ehrenberg 1975) while Muslims diverge from this pattern. Participation in Friday prayer is often not regarded as mandatory for women contrary to men. This implies they more rarely take part in collective forms of practice and pray more often at home instead (Haug/Müssig/Stichs 2009: 149, 159–161, Wunn 2008: 63). These women cannot be characterized as less religious than men on the basis of a single indicator. Alevi women and men jointly take part in collective prayer.

The shares presented have up to now not controlled for affiliation rates. Therefore, the lower part of table 6.6 discriminates between affiliated and unaffiliated individuals. It bundles the attendance categories so that only two remain. Basically, hardly any of the unaffiliated attend religious services at least once a month. Rather, intense attendees are a subgroup of the affiliated. In Norway and France it is a small subgroup. In Germany it is a visible minority. However, in East Germany it is a minor group within a small minority which explains the high percentage, referred to the whole population, that rarely or never attends in that region. The affiliated in West Germany are slightly more active. While most affiliated in East Germany are Protestants, in the Western part of the Republic there is parity (about one half is Protestant while the other half is Catholic). Data usually show that Catholics still attend church more often (see subsection 3.2.4). In France, it is the minority of Protestants (24.8%) whose activity rate is more pronounced than that of the Roman Catholics (13.5%). Muslims living in France attend collective prayer less often (26.3%) than those living in Germany. This corresponds to the remaining population and shows that several other factors – beside affiliation – influence religious practice.

Table 6.6. Frequency of attending religious services by country and gender

		FRANCE		NORWAY		GERMANY					
						East		West		Tr. migs	
Frequency		Women	Men	Women	Men	Women	Men	Women	Men	Women	Men
(More than) once per week/ weekly/ daily (at least 52 times a year)		9.7	5.5	3.5	3.2	4.2	3.0	12.9	10.9	33.5	43.2
More than once per month/ some times a month (24–48 times a year)		2.3	1.8	4.7	2.9	2.8	2.3	11.4	5.7	11.0	15.3
Once per month (12–20 times a year)		4.8	2.1			3.3	1.6	7.8	5.3	5.5	7.1
7–10 times a year		1.4	1.4								
More than once per year/ few times a year (4–6 times a year)		5.0	3.9	12.7	9.7	8.2	9.7	25.4	24.3	10.7	9.5
Once per year/ less often (1–3 times a year)		10.4	10.0	21.8	20.0	9.5	7.7	7.6	10.3	5.4	2.3
Rarely						8.4	10.8	19.7	20.3	13.3	6.8
Never		66.4	75.4	57.3	64.3	63.6	64.9	15.3	23.3	20.6	15.8
Numbers of observations		2,624	2,111	3,542	3,484	552	444	1,856	1,790	463	501
At least once per month	affiliated	17.8	10.3	8.6	6.5	31.0	22.5	34.8	25.6	50.0	65.7
	unaffiliated	0.7	0.9	2.9	0.9	0.0	0.8	3.6	1.4		
Less than once per month	affiliated	82.3	89.7	91.5	93.5	69.0	77.5	65.2	74.4	50.0	34.3
	unaffiliated	99.3	99.1	97.1	99.1	100.0	99.2	96.4	98.6		

How often do you attend religious services (apart from weddings, funerals, baptisms, and the like)? Age group 45–74, birth cohorts 1930–1962. In %; weighted data. Tr. migs: Turkish migrants. Information not collected in Hungary.

Attitudes towards religious *rites de passage* and importance of religious faith as child quality

Table 6.7 presents the results of the index explained in subsection 6.1.3. In the regional perspective, the support for religious ceremonies at turning points in life is highest in Hungary (taken together the values 10–12) followed by France.[43] They are lowest in East Germany where almost no one regards them as very important.[44] While church attendance rates in Norway are substantially lower than in West Germany, agreement with religious rites is higher. Women's attitudes are more approving than men's, except for East Germany and the Turkish migrants (referred to the mean). As there are also many people in France who disagree with rites at turning points in life, the second highest mean is realized in West Germany where only a small proportion of respondents disapproves of rites. The lowest mean by far is realized by East Germans which coincides with the lowest proportion of affiliated individuals. While religious rites traditionally accompany turning points in life in Hungary, France, Norway, and West Germany, this tradition almost ceased to exist in East Germany. It is therefore understandable that someone does not regard a rite as important if he or she grew up without it.

[43] See also Chélini-Pont 2007: 82–83: According to the Catholic newspaper *La Croix* in June 2003, 60% of the French population as a whole still went to church in connection with births, 50% for marriages, and 80% for funerals. However, the large majority of French Catholics does not know, understand or accept the Christian belief. Catholic specificities have disappeared. Catholics are hardly distinguishable from the rest of the French population. In a poll carried out in 2003, two thirds felt that the adoption of the PACS did not endanger the family as an institution, and almost three fourths said that homosexuality is an acceptable way of living one's sexuality. Also a large majority sees sexuality and procreation on the one hand and religion on the other hand as two separate spheres. Chélini-Pont 2007: 84 reports that the traditionally close relationship between behavior and faith has now been lost by French Catholics. In his view the importance attributed by Catholic's doctrine to sin in the regulation of human behavior has almost vanished.

[44] The number of executed religious rites has continuously been on the decline in the last decades (Grosser 2009: 58): e.g. in France 80% of newborns were still baptized in 1975 while it was only 46.5% in 2004.

Table 6.7. Attitudes towards religious ceremonies at turning points in life (*rites de passage*) by country, gender, and religious affiliation

	FRANCE		HUNGARY		NORWAY		GERMANY					
							East		West		Tr. migs	
Index values	Women	Men	Women	Men	Women	Men	Women	Men	Women	Men	Women	Men
0–3	17.0	18.2	11.5	14.9	9.4	10.0	49.3	45.0	8.4	12.2	5.7	4.4
4–6	13.0	14.8	13.9	16.6	12.0	11.4	22.5	27.6	15.2	16.2	11.0	9.2
7–8	14.2	14.5	9.8	10.5	9.9	10.2	6.9	9.0	16.9	16.4	2.9	6.4
9	7.1	8.5	6.1	7.1	11.1	11.2	10.8	9.6	25.2	24.8	25.7	26.1
10	8.4	8.7	8.6	6.8	7.8	6.7	2.8	1.4	6.9	6.6	9.6	8.7
11	7.2	7.5	3.8	3.7	4.0	4.1	2.3	1.3	4.3	4.4		
12	31.9	26.2	44.6	38.2	25.1	20.2	3.0	3.7	22.0	17.8	41.7	41.7
No response/ not applicable	1.3	1.6	1.7	2.2	20.8	26.4	2.5	3.6	1.1	1.7	3.5	3.5
Nobs (excl. "no response")	2,607	2,092	3,775	2,762	2,854	2,605	538	429	1,838	1,758	446	482
Mean	8.1	7.8	9.0	8.4	8.5	8.2	4.3	4.4	8.4	7.9	9.6	9.7
→ by religious affiliation:												
With religious affiliation	8.4	8.2	9.3	8.9	8.8	8.5	7.4	8.0	8.8	8.6	9.6	9.7
Christian	8.4	8.1	9.3	8.9	9.1	8.8	7.4	8.0	8.8	8.6		
Roman Catholic	8.3	8.1	9.5	9.1								
Greek Catholic			10.2	9.7								
Reformed Protestant (Calvinist)	8.5	8.0	8.8	8.4								
Lutheran (Hungary)/ Church of Norway			8.7	8.8	9.1	8.8						
Christianity outside the Church of Norway					9.7	9.4						
Muslim	10.3	8.8									9.6	9.7
Other					3.9	3.6						
Without religious affiliation	2.9	3.4	4.8	4.2	3.9	4.1	2.7	2.9	4.2	4.1		
No response	8.1	7.2										

Age group 45–74; birth cohorts 1930–1962. In %; weighted data. Tr. migs: Turkish migrants.

With regard to the initial variables (see table A.1 in the appendix), it can be reported that agreement with a religious funeral is highest in all countries while the lowest importance is ascribed to a religious wedding. Norwegians have the highest non-response rate. East German men most often have no opinion or do not care about religious rites ("neither agree nor disagree"). These individuals can be referred to as indifferent. The share in all groups is most pronounced regarding a church wedding. In general, Hungarians most often "strongly agree". The French are most often polarized. The highest proportions in the category "agree" are found among West Germans. They seem to consider religious rites more as traditions that belong to turning points in life but not as expressions of religiosity. This fine difference may exist between the two categories "strongly agree" and "agree".

Religious traditions have been shown to decrease in importance in everyday life but are still relevant at turning points.[45] This comprises the possibility that also non-religious people approve of religious ceremonies. Tomka substantiates this presumption with data from the Hungarian population: not all devout persons, i.e. those strongly believing in god, insist upon such rites and the other way round: also a majority of people with a fluctuating or undecided world view and even a minority of atheists affirm religious rites (Tomka 1999: 112).[46] To check this finding, the lower part of table 6.7 as well as the tables A.3 and A.4 in the appendix discriminate between different religious affiliations. This is also to control for the varying percentages of affiliated individuals across countries. It delivers evidence that unaffiliated individuals agree less with the statements. The unaffiliated, independent of gender and country, exhibit strongly downwards deviating values compared to the affiliated. One can however also observe that not all of the unaffiliated hold the opinion that religious ceremonies are unimportant. This especially applies to Hungarians without any affiliation (see the summarized distribution of index values in table A.3). The East German population distribution is mainly due to the very pronounced proportion of unaffiliated individuals. But: in the country with the most pronounced approval of the rites, the unaffiliated also agree more strongly than those in the remainder. The indicators must hence be partly confounded with traditional and national values.

---

[45] Nevertheless, there is a remarkable cohort effect. The lower part of table A.5 clearly shows that the importance, expressed by the lowering mean of the index values, has sunk with rising cohort.

[46] Especially the rural population regards religious ceremonies as important.

Referring to the single religious groups, agreement is highest among Greek Catholics in Hungary followed by Muslims in Germany and France. Ignoring the gender-specific difference of Muslims in France, Muslims in France and Germany approve very similarly of religious ceremonies. Roman Catholics in Hungary agree more than those in France. In Hungary alone, the index means of the Catholics express higher affirmation than those of the Protestants. Protestants in Hungary deem the rites more important than Catholics in France. Lutherans and the Reformed hardly differ from each other. In Norway, Christians who do not adhere to the state church regard them as more significant than the Lutherans do. Apart from this, both groups have a high level of agreement. The Norwegian Protestants agree more than Protestants in Hungary or France. The attitudes towards religious rites differ between Christians in both Germanies: agreement is much lower in East than in West Germany. This is especially true with respect to the East German female Christians who consider the ceremonies less important than men do.

Table 6.8 presents the results of the respondents' attitude towards the importance of religious faith as child quality.[47] Only a small minority in each group considers it significant. The list of competing qualities is hard, however. They refer to basic human characteristics (such as "good manners", "feeling of responsibility", and "tolerance and respect for other people"). Not mentioning religious faith does not mean that socializing a child religiously is dispensable but only that it is not among the three most important qualities a child should possess according to the people's opinion. One third of the Turkish migrants counts religious faith among the three most important child qualities. Also an observable minority of the Norwegians do so. They were however not required to limit the number of qualities they could state. Comparability is hence not ensured. The percentage of non-responses among Norwegians equals the non-responses in table 6.7. Hardly any East Germans rate religious faith highly. In that region, it is the most rarely mentioned child quality out of all eleven possible qualities (this also applies to Hungarian men). The uneven distribution of this indicator in East Germany enforces its exclusion from multivariate analyses.

The lower part of the table again discriminates the summarized percentages by religious affiliation. Christians outside the Church of Norway most often regard religious faith as an important child quality (women: 67.1%; men: 59.8%). Among members of the Church of Norway it is about every fifth person. Referring to re-

[47] The term "quality" has been directly taken from the English questionnaire.

spondents who had to rank the qualities, Muslims strongly deviate from persons who adhere to another denomination. One third of them support a religious socialization. Not too surprisingly, almost nobody without an affiliation give larger weight to it. Referring to affiliated individuals, more West German than East German or French respondents support a religious socialization. The largest gender difference can be observed among Greek Catholics: almost twice as many women as men regard a religious socialization as important. Roman Catholics ascribe more importance to this trait than Protestants in Hungary do, but both groups realize lower values than the pooled group of Christians in West Germany.

Table 6.8. Importance of religious faith as child quality by country and gender

	HUNGARY		NORWAY		GERMANY					
					East		West		Tr. migs	
	Women	Men	Women	Men	Women	Men	Women	Men	Women	Men
Most important quality	1.1	0.6			0.3	0.1	1.2	1.2	14.0	12.5
Second most important quality	1.2	0.9			0.2	0.8	2.0	2.2	9.8	9.3
Third most important quality	2.7	1.8			1.4	0.9	3.9	4.7	10.2	11.2
Applies (sum)	5.0	3.3	16.9	14.3	1.9	1.9	7.1	8.1	34.0	33.0
Does not apply	94.7	95.8	62.2	59.0	97.7	97.7	92.2	91.2	64.4	64.8
No response/ not applicable	0.3	0.9	21.0	26.7	0.4	0.4	0.6	0.7	1.6	2.2
Nobs (exkl. "no response")	3,826	2,798	2,846	2,595	550	442	1,848	1,777	457	492
→ Applies (sum) by religious affiliation:										
With religious affiliation	5.4	3.7	22.4	20.5	4.9	6.6	7.7	9.5	34.6	33.6
Christian	5.4	3.7	22.8	20.7	4.9	6.6	7.7	9.5		
Roman Catholic	5.5	3.9								
Greek Catholic	12.3	6.7								
Reformed (Calvinist)/ Lutheran	4.5	3.0								
Church of Norway			20.3	19.1						
Christianity outside the Church of Norway			67.1	59.8						
Muslim									34.6	33.6
Other			16.4	17.2						
Without religious affiliation	0.7	0.3	5.8	7.7	0.5	0.0	1.2	1.2		

Age group 45–74, birth cohorts 1930–1962. In %; weighted data. Tr. migs: Turkish migrants, Nobs: numbers of observations. Information not collected in France; no ranking in Norway.

In table 6.9 the indicators are related to each other to check whether they measure the same thing or something different. The correlation of attendance with the value index is weaker in Norway, and stronger in East Germany, but in no case very strong. In all groups, intense attendees of religious services consider religious ceremonies very important and furthermore more important than rare attendees. Frequent attendees regard religious faith as much more important than rare attendees do. The values and differences strongly vary across groups. The most extreme case are the Norwegians. In Germany, remarkable gender differences are visible. Men who often take part in religious services attach much more importance to religious faith. The correlation of religious faith with the index expressing agreement with religious rites is – except for Norwegians – rather low. Female Muslims who rarely go to mosque realize higher values concerning religious faith than male Muslims. This may again indicate that they have to fall back on alternative forms of expressing their religiosity. The last row shows that attitudes towards rites and the attitude towards the importance of religious faith as child quality do not correlate very closely and hence represent two different aspects.

Denz (2000) clustered European countries on the basis of several indicators that are associated with church and Christianity. According to his typology, Norway and France are a "little churchly", have an unchristian to atheistic foundation, and are rather irreligious. East Germany is "unchurchly", has the same basic structure as France, and is a "very irreligious country". West Germany is "formally churchly", "little Christian", and "irreligious". Finally, Hungary is "churchy" and "religious" but "little Christian". Summarized, this means that none of the countries considered is "highly churchly", "highly Christian", and "very religious" (Denz 2000: 73–74).

Table 6.9. Associations between the variables

	FRANCE		HUNGARY		NORWAY		GERMANY					
							East		West		Tr. migs	
	Women	Men	Women	Men	Women	Men	Women	Men	Women	Men	Women	Men
Correlation of attendance with index (Pearson's *r*)	0.32	0.23			0.23	0.22	0.44	0.44	0.39	0.32	0.30	0.33
Intense attendance: mean index	11.0	10.7			10.9	10.9	8.9	9.9	10.1	9.8	10.4	10.3
Rare attendance: mean index	7.5	7.5			8.2	8.0	3.7	4.0	7.6	7.4	8.7	8.5
Intense attendance: percentage religious faith					79.5	83.5	9.9	22.8	17.4	27.1	50.9	46.6
Rare attendance: percentage religious faith					11.3	9.9	1.0	0.3	2.2	2.9	17.2	6.9
Correlation of religious faith with index (Pearson's *r*)			0.14	0.13	0.36	0.34	0.16	0.26	0.20	0.23	0.11	0.22

Age group 45–74, birth cohorts 1930–1962. In %; weighted data. Tr. migs: Turkish migrants.

6.2.3 Testing the theoretical presuppositions

This subsection will answer the question if divorce is more uncommon among religiously affiliated and religious couples than among unaffiliated and nonreligious persons as assumed in chapter 4. There it was argued that anticipating a low divorce risk raises the willingness of spouses to invest in their marriage. The "risk" must be measured by the ex-post indicator "stable marriage" comprising all persons who ever married but never experienced a divorce. Furthermore, it will be checked if marital stability, independent of its association with religiosity, has an effect on completed fertility. As characteristics of ex-partners cannot be re-constructed and the current partner in several cases is not the father of the children, the consideration of traits of the respondent must be sufficient. It cannot be controlled whether possible (ex-)partner(s) exhibited features that elevate the divorce probability. Before particularizing the general hypothesis formulated in chapter 4, the marital status of the respondents will be described.

Table A.10 in the appendix presents the marital status of the respondents including those who never married in the upper part and without them in the lower part. To keep track of different partnership biographies, cohabitations are not included. The majority of respondents is still married for the first time. Gender differences are considerable: the proportion of married men is noticeably higher. The largest gender difference is reported for Turkish migrants and for Hungarians. The latter exhibit the lowest proportions of persons married for the first time. Observably more women are widowed, which is also a cross-border phenomenon and correlated with their higher life expectancy. The difference is highest in Hungary where the gender gap in life expectancy is most pronounced. Respondents who were once widowed and once divorced are allocated to the "divorced"-category. The percentage of remarried individuals is higher among men. Most of the remarried experienced at least one divorce. The proportion of single respondents is highest by far in Germany (for details on that topic see subsection 6.1.2). Most respondents who never married have lived at least temporarily in a partnership and cannot be classified as lifelong singles. Being "separated" is rare because it is rather a temporary status.

The lower part of table A.10 shows that being married for the first time is now more than before the dominant type of living among persons who ever married. The status is least widespread in Hungary, followed by Norway, and in either case especially among women. The share of widowed women remains pronounced in

Hungary. Still more men are remarried. Norwegian women, followed by Hungarian women, are most often divorced. Turkish migrants exhibit the lowest proportions of ever divorced persons, followed by West Germans. The huge differences concerning divorce between West and East Germans plotted in subsection 2.2.2 cannot be attested by GGS data. While before only a very general hypothesis has been formulated, it is specified here in greater detail:

H_{1a} The religiously affiliated have more stable marriages than the religiously unaffiliated.

H_{1b} Catholics have more stable marriages than Protestants. The analysis is restricted to France, Hungary, and Norway. In the latter country, Lutherans and Christians outside of the Church of Norway are compared with each other. The latter group also comprises adherents of evangelical free churches and is only partly composed of Catholics.

H_{1c} Attending religious services frequently positively influences marital stability.[48]

H_{1d} A high acceptance of religious rites at turning points in life has a positive effect on marital stability.

H_{1e} People who regard religious faith as an important child quality have more stable marriages than persons who do not.

Table 6.10 presents descriptive results (without respondents who never married). The upper part shows the percentage of married for the first time (respectively widowed) structured by religious affiliation. It can be documented that the proportion of stable marriages among affiliates is clearly higher than the proportion among the unaffiliated. The most noticeable cleavage can be observed in West Germany. While merely 58.8% (women) respectively 64.4% (men) of the unaffiliated are still married for the first time, the percentage points are 26% respectively 23% higher among the affiliated. The difference is least pronounced among East Germans followed by Hungarians. Moreover, no differences exist between affiliates in West and East Germany. There are slight but continuous gender differences across countries independent of being affiliated or unaffiliated. In Norway, stability rates by gender differ strongest especially with respect to the unaffiliated. Where Catholics and Protestants can be distinguished, results indicate that the former do not have more stable marriages than

[48] A further differentiation between Catholics and Protestants could only be realized in Hungary where both groups are sufficiently large but where the frequency of church attendance was not collected.

the latter. The proportions of stable marriages are similar across Christian denominations within the same country (not tabulated here). Altogether, Turkish migrants – who are all Muslims – as well as Christian West German men live most often in stable marriages. Stability rates are not pronounced among French Muslims to the same extent. Additionally, the rates are lower than among Christians in France.

People who frequently attend religious services can be characterized as subgroup of the affiliated. They have even more stable marriages (except for East German men).[49] Call/Heaton 1997 use several religiosity indicators to prove evidence for the effect on marital stability. They attest the indicator "church attendance" the greatest effect. Turkish migrants score the highest proportions, followed by West Germans and the French. Rare attenders can be subdivided into affiliated and unaffiliated persons. There are reasons to assume that they differ enough from each other. Affiliates may be religious and express their religiosity in another form than measurable here whereas this cannot be expected from unaffiliated individuals. The data document that it is also worthwhile to discriminate these three groups with respect to marital stability – except for East Germany where frequent attenders do not have more stable marriages than rare attending affiliates. The difference between rarely attending affiliates and rarely attending unaffiliated persons is again most considerable in West Germany, followed by the French. In West Germany, it is of greater importance to be religiously affiliated at all. Also in the group of the Turkish migrants, frequent attendance raises the probability to be still married for the first time. Altogether, marriages of unaffiliated Norwegian women are least stable. Almost every second marriage broke up.

[49] It has been mentioned that the influence of worship on marital stability is notably lower if only one spouse attends religious services regularly compared with a couple in which both are frequent attenders. These two groups cannot be distinguished. As there is a small minority whose marriages broke up, it would have been desirable to be able to do it.

Table 6.10. Association between religiosity and marital stability

	FRANCE		HUNGARY		NORWAY		GERMANY					
							East		West		Tr. migs	
	Women	Men	Women	Men	Women	Men	Women	Men	Women	Men	Women	Men
Religious affiliation												
With religious affiliation	79.4	80.6	74.7	76.2	68.7	73.8	84.3	87.7	84.5	87.0	87.5	92.3
Without religious affiliation	60.4	65.3	64.5	66.7	52.5	62.4	78.4	79.5	58.8	64.4	–	–
Frequency of attending religious services												
At least once per month	91.9	88.6	–	–	83.0	86.8	85.0	84.1	90.5	93.2	93.7	94.7
Less than once per month	75.8	78.6	–	–	66.4	72.0	79.8	81.8	78.3	80.9	80.8	87.8
Less than once per month (affiliated)	75.7	79.6	–	–	67.3	72.8	84.0	88.9	80.9	84.7	80.8	87.8
Less than once per month (unaffiliated)	60.4	64.9	–	–	51.4	62.1	78.4	79.4	60.6	64.1	–	–
Index of attitudes towards religious ceremonies												
Values 10–12	82.6	84.3	78.5	78.3	73.7	78.8	79.7	84.2	89.3	91.4	89.2	94.8
Values 0–9	74.6	76.1	67.9	72.8	64.7	70.3	80.4	82.5	78.6	80.6	85.3	88.9
Religious faith												
Mentioned as important child quality	–	–	78.1	80.8	74.2	82.6	–	–	91.9	86.3	90.4	94.8
Not mentioned as important child quality	–	–	73.7	74.8	67.5	71.7	–	–	81.6	83.4	85.8	90.8

Age group 45–74; birth cohorts 1930–1962. In %; weighted data. Tr. migs: Turkish migrants. The stated proportions reflect respondents who are still married for the first time (without respondents who never married).

A high approval of religious ceremonies at turning points in life is also associated with higher marital stability, except for East Germans, but the difference is not very pronounced. The correlation strength across countries and gender is even quite weak. The differences concerning the importance of religious faith as important child quality are also far from being impressive. It is only noticeable among Norwegian men and West Germans. While hypotheses H_{1a} and H_{1c} can be accepted, this is not the case for the remainder. Group differentiation is not great enough. Grouping affiliated and attenders into three groups reflects differences in marital stability strongest.

As seen so far, French Muslims have less stable marriages and exhibit lower participation rates with regard to attendance of religious services than Turkish Muslims in Germany. This "collides" with their higher fertility. However, these are only aggregated group results. Evidence at the individual level will be tested later. Another example are Hungarians if they are compared with East Germans. Fertility is higher in the former country, while marital stability is higher in the latter one. While both fertility and marital instability are low in West Germany, both are noticeably higher in France and especially Norway. To illustrate the associations directly, in table 6.11 fertility is calculated dependent on different statuses.

Women and men married for the first time do not have most children. This means that marital stability does not seem to promote fertility which does not correspond to the presuppositions nor to other study results (Thomson et al. 2012, Coppola/Di Cesare 2008, Meggiolaro/Ongaro 2010). Anticipating a divorce risk need not equal actual marital disruption. Many spouses might have restricted their investments and increased their labor supply but remain married (South/Bose/Trent 2004). Insofar, the non-visibility of the marital stability effect might be a measurement problem. Other spouses did not anticipate divorce, invested into the marriage, and have been deserted by their partner, a risk that has risen after *de facto* unilateral divorce was legalized (Kneip/Bauer 2009). Only Norwegian women corroborate the assumption. Both married for the first time as well as widowed (and never divorced) women have most children in Norway. If union stability is already measured by the marriage itself – because unmarried unions are more unstable – the hypothesis holds. Women and especially men who never married have fewest children (also if only individuals are considered who cohabited at least once). Women and men behave rather reluctantly in investing in a relationship they do not assume to be stable.[50] Therefore, the hypothesis

[50] The frequency of cohabitation has gained importance only in the youngest cohort so that lower fertility could also be the outcome of a cohort effect. But only a small share of the

could be divided in two parts. Then the first part would be true, while the second part does not hold.

Among men, the result is obvious: the remarried father most children. This result supports findings by Klein 2003 and Billari 2005 (see section 4.4). In general, women and men in West Germany who are separated or divorced more than once have most children. Separated persons are also most fertile in France. The number of observations is not too high but it seems as if parents avoid a divorce after marital breakdown because they have several children resulting in a vice versa argumentation. A comparison cannot be done among the Turkish migrants because group sizes are too low. Marital status does not provoke much variance regarding family size among Hungarian women. However, women who experienced a divorce are less fertile than all other women who married at least once, independent of the current status.

While religious affiliation and frequent attendance of religious services raise marital stability, no clear evidence can be provided concerning the influence of marital stability on completed fertility. In section 6.3 it will be tested whether interaction effects between religiosity, marital stability, and fertility can be discovered if regarded jointly.

lower fertility is a cohort effect. If the perspective is restricted to the youngest cohort, their fertility is still lowest in comparison with the remaining statuses.

Table 6.11. Association between marital stability and completed fertility

	FRANCE		HUNGARY		NORWAY		GERMANY					
							East		West		Tr. migs	
	Women	Men	Women	Men	Women	Men	Women	Men	Women	Men	Women	Men
Married (1st time)	2.35	2.28	1.93	1.89	2.36	2.33	1.76	1.74	1.75	1.63	2.32	2.10
Separated (never divorced)	(2.96)	(2.76)	1.89	(1.93)					(2.03)	(2.07)		
Divorced once	2.21	2.28	1.74	1.81	2.08	2.13	1.98	1.86	1.86	1.54	(2.20)	
Divorced more than once	(2.10)		1.87	2.09	1.92	1.93			(1.99)	(2.28)		
Remarried	2.17	2.77	1.99	2.15	2.19	2.50	(2.70)	(2.25)	1.71	1.84		
Widowed	2.68	2.10	1.88	1.79	2.29	1.85	1.65	(1.94)	1.67	1.63	(2.06)	
Never married (but not lifelong single)	1.28	1.06	1.38	0.61	1.17	1.07	(1.36)	(0.93)	0.96	0.90		

Age group 45–74; birth cohorts 1930–1962. In %; weighted data. Tr. migs: Turkish migrants. Empty cells indicate low numbers of observations (<20). Observations between N=20 and N=29 are in brackets.

6.2.4 Religiosity's impact on fertility

This subsection descriptively investigates if religiosity positively influences fertility as postulated in chapter 4. As in the preceding section, firstly hypotheses are specified in greater detail:

H_{2a} Religiously affiliated persons have more children than religiously unaffiliated persons. It is assumed that the decisive "parting line" runs between the affiliated and the unaffiliated.

H_{2b} Catholics have more children than Protestants (1). The analysis is restricted to France, Hungary, and Norway.[51] Muslims have more children than Christians (2).

H_{2c} Attending religious services frequently positively influences completed fertility.[52]

H_{2d} A high approval of religious rites at turning points in life has a positive effect on completed fertility.

H_{2e} People who regard religious faith as important child quality have more children than persons who do not.

Table 6.12 shows that persons without religious affiliation have fewer children than the affiliated: the differences range from 0.18 (East German men and Hungarian women) to 0.41 (Norwegian women) children on average. The only exceptions are East German women and Hungarian men. In these two groups unaffiliated individuals are slightly more fertile. Consequently, the differences are smallest in the two former socialist countries. Fertility gaps between affiliated and unaffiliated persons are compared restricted to the country where the respondents live because the unaffiliated in one country (France) have more children than the affiliated in another country (Germany, Hungary). Unaffiliated East Germans have more children than affiliated West Germans. This is due to the large number of further factors causing variance not only across individuals but also across countries.

---

51 In the latter country, Lutherans and Christians outside of the Church of Norway are compared with each other. That group also comprises evangelical free churches and is only partly composed of Catholics.

52 A further differentiation between Catholics and Protestants could only be realized in Hungary where both groups are sufficiently large but where the frequency of church attendance was not collected.

Table 6.12. Completed number of children (cohort fertility) by country, gender, and religious affiliation

	FRANCE		HUNGARY		NORWAY		GERMANY					
							East		West		Tr. migs	
	Women	Men	Women	Men	Women	Men	Women	Men	Women	Men	Women	Men
With religious affiliation	2.24	2.17	1.85	1.77	2.18	2.15	1.77	1.84	1.72	1.57	2.28	2.10
Christian	2.21	2.08	1.85	1.77	2.17	2.14	1.77	1.84	1.72	1.57		
Roman Catholic	2.21	2.08	1.86	1.75								
Greek Catholic			2.10	2.06								
Reformed Protestant (Calvinist)	2.32	2.07	1.81	1.84								
Lutheran			1.87	1.64								
The Church of Norway					2.17	2.13						
Christianity outside the Church of Norway					2.18	2.29						
Muslim	3.61	3.88									2.28	2.10
Other					2.41	2.34						
Without religious affiliation	2.00	1.87	1.67	1.84	1.77	1.81	1.87	1.66	1.43	1.27		
No response/ refusal	2.42	2.07										
Nobs	2,624	2,111	3,837	2,821	3,542	3,484	552	444	1,856	1,790	463	501

Age group 45–74; birth cohorts 1930–1962. In %; weighted data. Tr. migs: Turkish migrants, Nobs: numbers of observations.

Table 6.13. Completed number of children (cohort fertility) by country, gender, and frequency of worship

	FRANCE		NORWAY		GERMANY					
					East		West		Tr. migs	
	Women	Men	Women	Men	Women	Men	Women	Men	Women	Men
(More than) once per week (52–1820 times a year)	2.68	3.20	2.55	2.87			1.84	1.98	2.42	2.29
More than once per month (24–48 times a year)	2.11	2.26	2.56	2.70			1.71	1.83	2.24	1.57
Once per month (12–20 times a year)	2.49	2.14			1.62	2.14	1.71	1.34	1.95	2.77
7–10 times a year	2.31	2.13								
More than once per year (4–6 times a year)	2.31	2.20	2.21	2.36	1.72	1.60	1.72	1.57	2.56	2.04
Once per year/ less often (1–3 times a year)	2.25	2.21	2.23	2.19	1.67	2.02	1.68	1.36	1.96	1.97
Rarely					1.55	1.90	1.55	1.41		
Never	2.16	2.05	2.06	2.01	1.95	1.62	1.68	1.41	2.31	1.90
Dichotomized										
Frequent attendance of religious services	2.55	2.78	2.56	2.79	1.62	2.14	1.76	1.78	2.33	2.18
Rare attendance of religious services	2.18	2.08	2.12	2.08	1.86	1.68	1.66	1.45	2.23	1.96
Less than once per month (affiliated)	2.17	2.10	2.14	2.11	1.84	1.78	1.69	1.50	2.23	1.96
Less than once per month (unaffiliated)	2.02	1.87	1.78	1.80	1.87	1.65	1.43	1.27		
Nobs	2,624	2,111	3,542	3,484	552	444	1,856	1,790	463	501

Age group 45–74; birth cohorts 1930–1962. In %; weighted data. Tr. migs: Turkish migrants, Nobs: numbers of observations.

The most fertile persons by far are Muslims in France. Male Muslims have on average two children more than unaffiliated men. Muslims in Germany have considerably fewer children. Possible reasons are the different countries of origin which are also partly associated with different traditions within Islam that the Muslims follow, the history of migration, the generally higher fertility level in France because of several factors, etc. Neither in France nor Hungary do Roman Catholics have larger family sizes than Reformed Protestants. But the small locally restricted confessional group of Greek Catholics has the most fertile adherents in Hungary. This means that Roman and Greek Catholics significantly differ from each other in their demographic behavior. Possible reasons have already been discussed. Male Lutherans have slightly fewer children than their Reformed peers. In Norway, male members of Christian denominations outside the Church of Norway outnumber members of the state church with respect to achieved fertility. "Others" (non-Christians) are most fertile. Referring to all groups, West German men without religious affiliation have fewest children. While hypothesis H_{2a} holds, this is only partly the case for hypothesis H_{2b}. Catholics do not have more children. A further check, including holding a variety of variables constant, follows in the next section.

Table 6.13 shows the average number of children of rare and frequent attenders of religious services. Frequent worshipers achieve a noticeably higher fertility. Moreover, the gender differences are remarkable. It is striking that attending church frequently is stronger visible in men's reproductive behavior (while the percentage of religious individuals is higher among women). They have on average 0.7 more children in Norway and France, 0.46 in East Germany, and 0.33 in West Germany. Among the more homogeneous group of Muslims, the difference amounts to 0.22 children. The respective difference between frequent and rare female attenders sums to 0.44 in Norway, 0.37 in France, and 0.1 among West Germans and Muslims. The only exception are – again – East German women. Among them, frequent church attendees have 0.24 children less. Frequently attending Norwegian and French men have the highest fertility of all, with almost 2.8 children on average. Apart from their lower fertility compared with men, frequent attenders among Norwegian and French women are also equal with respect to the number of children they have. The share of frequent attenders is larger among the French, however.

Rare attenders can again be subdivided into affiliated and unaffiliated persons. This makes sense in view of the fact the religiosity can be differently expressed, as mentioned previously. As was the case for marital stability, these two categories also exhibit differences with respect to completed fertility. The gap is however much smaller. The "frequent attendance" effect exceeds the "affiliation" effect (especially among Norwegian and French men) but the former does not fully explain the difference between the affiliated and the unaffiliated. The exception are again East German women whose fertility difference is counter-intuitive. The "affiliation effect" is greater among West German women – there is hardly any additional "attendance effect" – and almost equals the frequent attendance effect among West German men. For the sake of completeness, completed fertility is also listed for the single frequency categories. The association between the number of children and the frequency of church attendance is not strictly linear for either women or men. Hypothesis H_{2c} holds in the descriptive perspective apart from the exception mentioned: women in Germany.

The higher fertility among frequent attenders of religious services can be traced to diverging parity distributions (see table A.7 in the appendix). Frequent attenders have higher incidence rates of large families. This is especially observable in France and Norway. For example, almost 59% of Norwegian men have at least three children if they frequently attend religious services but only 35% have so many children if they are rare attending affiliates. The rate decreases to 26% among unaffiliated individuals (rates for Norwegian women: 53.6%, 36%, 26.4%). French women (49.3%) and men (54%) also have larger families more often if they are frequent attenders. However, rare attending affiliated and unaffiliated individuals hardly differ: almost one third of these in France have at least three children.

The upper part of table 6.14 shows the average number of children respondents have conditional on their value on the measure of the importance they ascribe to religious rites at turning points in life. The correlation coefficients indicate that no strong positive, linear associations between the number of children and the strength of approval exist. Weak correlations are detectable among the French, West German men and Norwegians. East German women who regard the celebration of religious ceremonies as important have least children in that region. In Hungary, numbers of children are equal for all index values. There is no variance. Hungarians who did not respond have fewest children on average.

Whether respondents who consider religious faith to be an important child quality (lower part of table 6.14) have a larger family depends on country and gender. Whereas in Hungary neither men nor women can be differentiated with respect to fertility by this indicator,[53] it is the case for West German men. The difference totals 0.6 children followed by Norwegian men and female Turkish migrants (differences total 0.3 children each). In the remaining groups the difference is smaller. Male Turkish migrants have fewer children if they attach value to a child's religious socialization. Hypotheses H_{2d} and H_{2e} are only true in a few cases which can be understood as an indication that in surveys asking for forms of expression is preferable to asking about attitudes.

[53] Only Hungarians of the opinion that religious faith is the most important child quality have more children on average.

Table 6.14. Completed number of children (cohort fertility) by country, gender, and values of index of attitudes towards religious ceremonies or importance of religious faith as child quality

	FRANCE		HUNGARY		NORWAY		GERMANY					
							East		West		Tr. migs	
	Women	Men	Women	Men	Women	Men	Women	Men	Women	Men	Women	Men
Index values												
0–3	2.03	1.90	1.74	1.82	1.96	1.96	1.95	1.71	1.58	1.53	2.35	1.55
4–6	1.90	2.05	1.80	1.78	2.00	2.02	1.80	1.77	1.65	1.27	2.34	2.11
7–8	2.31	2.08	1.77	1.76	2.14	2.06	1.69	1.77	1.70	1.32	2.04	2.08
9	2.14	2.08	1.84	1.73	2.11	2.13	1.81	1.85	1.65	1.62	2.30	2.17
10	2.17	2.07	1.86	1.77	2.17	2.13			1.63	1.54		
11	2.54	2.14	1.81	1.76	2.28	2.18			1.81	1.50	2.04	2.47
12	2.48	2.43	1.89	1.81	2.23	2.30	1.54	1.74	1.80	1.84	2.32	2.01
No response			1.49	1.42	2.24	2.11						
Nobs (without “no response”)	2,607	2,092	3,775	2,762	2,854	2,605	538	429	1,838	1,758	446	482
Mentioned as important child quality			1.83	1.74	2.27	2.39			1.89	2.08	2.46	1.95
Not mentioned as important child quality			1.84	1.79	2.11	2.08			1.68	1.48	2.17	2.22
No response					2.20	2.08						
Nobs (without “no response”)			3,826	2,798	2,846	2,595			1,848	1,777	457	492

Age group 45–74; birth cohorts 1930–1962. In %; weighted data. Tr. migs: Turkish migrants, Nobs: numbers of observations. Index: In further analyses the values will not be summarized as they are here. Missing values are due to low numbers of observations.

6.3 Regression analysis

Section 6.3 deals with the results of the regression model estimations separated by gender and country to find evidence for the assumptions made with respect to the effects of religiosity on completed fertility. Using Poisson regression, completed fertility is regressed on a vector of religiosity variables and covariates. Due to the dependent variable – completed fertility – estimations are mainly restricted to time-constant traits and characteristics. Cross-sectional cross-country analyses are tainted with the problem that they do not account for unobserved country heterogeneity. The explanatory variables of central interest are listed in table 6.15.

Table 6.15. Model estimations by country

	FRA	NOR	HUN	GERMANY			
				E	W	Tr.m	GER(r)
Model I: religious affiliation (binary)	X	X	X	X	X		
Model II: religious affiliation (differentiated)	X	X	X				X
Model III: frequency of attending religious services	X	X		X	X	X	
Model IV: attitudes towards religious ceremonies at turning points in life	X	X	X	X	X	X	
Model V: importance of religious faith as child quality		X	X		X	X	

FRA: France, HUN: Hungary, NOR: Norway; E: East, W: West, Tr.m: Turkish migrants, GER(r): Germany restricted to Germans and Turkish migrants from the supplemental survey (without non-Turkish migrants).

The first central variable is religious affiliation as a binary indicator; secondly, religious affiliation in a different form that specifies affiliations; thirdly, frequency of attendance of religious services (later subdivided by affiliation and birth cohort); fourthly, the values index concerning attitudes towards religious ceremonies at turning points in life; and fifthly, religious faith as child quality. Only the Norwegian data set contains all variables with religious reference. That means that not all religious indicators can be used simultaneously. Respondents with missing values on core variables are excluded from the analysis. This is of special importance. A significant proportion of Norwegian respondents did not answer the question of how strongly they approve or disapprove of religious ceremonies. The number of observations is hence much lower in the respective model. Missing variables and values also prevents building an index that integrates all variables. To nevertheless construct an index would result in country-specific index values that could not be compared with each other.

Subsection 6.3.1 discusses the direct effects of religious affiliation and religiosity on fertility. Subsection 6.3.2 elaborates on the effects of the covariates and indirect effects of religiosity and subsection 6.3.3 focuses on the Turkish migrants living in Germany and asks if their higher fertility is caused by religiosity or the lower level of modernization of their country of origin. The arrangement of the tables containing regression results differs from the tables with descriptive results. While it seemed reasonable in the latter case to put women and men of one country together due to the general fertility level in that country, a gender-specific arrangement of the tables makes more sense when comparing the effects of religiosity and several covariates on fertility.

6.3.1 The effects of religiosity on completed fertility

Religious affiliation

In table 6.16 and 6.17 first multivariate results are displayed. Controlling for several covariates, religious affiliation significantly affects the fertility of Norwegians as well as of West German men. It has already been shown descriptively that the fertility gap is largest in these three groups. In the other countries, the tendency is in accordance with the hypothesis but not strong enough to be significant when controlling for a variety of covariates. The sign in the group of East German women has – contrary to Hungarian men – taken the expected (positive) direction. Hypothesis H_{2a} cannot be evaluated before associations between religious affiliation and the covariates have been tested.

Several reasons come into consideration to explain why religious affiliation does not significantly affect fertility. Religious affiliation is a rough indicator to measure fertility differences because it is only the basic category of religiosity. Besides, it solely informs about the direct effect of religiosity so that not the whole effect is captured. An additional reason is that the group of religious individuals within the group of affiliates is not great enough to provoke an effect for the whole group. The frame may be very supportive and in this way superimpose any religiosity effect.

In Norway, the religious within the group of affiliated is small – albeit a highly fertile group – but a significant effect can nevertheless be identified. Therefore, it must be asked if the argumentation also works the other way round. As already mentioned, every Norwegian citizen is a member of the state church from birth on. Citizens who are not members of the Church of Norway seem hence to explicitly reject it. These persons can be characterized as a selective group, apparently also with respect to fertility. For example, unaffiliated Norwegian women have observably fewer children than unaffiliated French women on average (shown in table 6.12). The significant effect of religious affiliation can hence be explained with the unaffiliated on the one hand and the small religious group – the frequent attenders in this context[54] – within the large group of affiliates on the other hand.

[54] In this work, frequent attenders are defined as "the religious" because it is measurable. It does not exclude that rare attenders are not also religious. But this has already been made rather clear in chapter 3.

Table 6.16. Results of model I: Effects of religious affiliation on completed fertility (women)

	FRA	NOR	HUN	EGER	WGER
Affiliated	0.010	0.117*	0.002	0.014	0.104
(Base category: unaffiliated)					
Birth cohort 1949–1962	−0.238***	−0.083**	0.143***	−0.114	−0.146**
Birth cohort 1939–1952	−0.235***	−0.105**	0.103***	−0.139	−0.191***
(Base category: birth cohort 1930–1942)					
Low educ. attainment (isced 0–2)	0.139***	0.077**	0.112***	0.108	0.082
High educ. attainmen (isced 5–6)	0.043	0.000	0.048	0.002	0.094*
(Base category: medium educational attainment (isced 3–4))					
Lifelong single	−0.583***	−1.313***	−1.796***	−0.080	−0.107
Never married but not lifelong single	−0.566***	−0.691***	−0.449***	−0.312	−0.526***
Remarried/ divorced more than once	0.037	−0.092**	0.044	0.262*	0.161*
Divorced once	0.008	−0.105**	−0.079*	0.118	0.048
(Base category: married for the 1st time/ widowed but never divorced)					
Number of brothers and sisters	0.027***	0.023***	0.027***	0.029	0.048***
Migration background	0.023	−0.071		−0.089	0.015
FRA: (North) African	0.292***				
(Base category: no migration background)					
Ethnic group: Gypsy/ Hungarian of Gypsy origin			0.573***		
Ethnic group: East European/ German/ other			−0.141		
(Base category: ethnic group: Hungarian)					
FRA: rural	0.199***				
FRA: urban	0.147***				
(Base category: FRA: town)					
NOR: centrality level 0: completely rural		0.159***			
NOR: centrality level 1		0.138***			
NOR: centrality level 2		0.076*			
(Base category: NOR: centrality level 3: urban)					
HUN: village			0.210***		
HUN: town			0.170***		
HUN: city			0.099*		
(Base category: HUN: capital)					
GER: up to 19,999 inhabitants				−0.009	0.180**
GER: peripheral area from 50–100,000/ central area from 20–100,000 inh.				−0.060	0.195***
GER: peripheral area from 100,000/ central area from 100–500,000 inh.				0.069	0.139**
(Base category: GER: more than 500,000 inhabitants)					
Constant	0.661***	0.690***	0.269***	0.597***	0.290***
Numbers of observations	2639	3526	3825	545	1807
Wald chi^2	410.710	433.794	410.234	25.130	122.788
Pr > χ^2	0.0000	0.0000	0.0000	0.0333	0.0000
McFadden's pseudo R^2	0.045	0.038	0.036	0.014	0.022

Estimations are based on Poisson regression. Significance levels: * $p < 0.05$, ** $p < 0.01$, *** $p < 0.001$; FRA: France, NOR: Norway, HUN: Hungary, EGER: East Germany, WGER: West Germany, GER: Germany.

Table 6.17. Results of model I: Effects of religious affiliation on completed fertility (men)

	FRA	NOR	HUN	EGER	WGER
Affiliated	0.083	0.108*	−0.069	0.083	0.111*
(Base category: unaffiliated)					
Birth cohort 1949–1962	−0.173***	−0.053	0.103**	−0.007	−0.179***
Birth cohort 1939–1952	−0.103**	−0.091**	0.088*	−0.108	−0.174***
(Base category: birth cohort 1930–1942)					
Low educ. attainment (isced 0–2)	0.032	0.008	0.133***	−0.293	0.018
High educ. attainment (isced 5–6)	0.034	−0.011	0.080*	−0.145	0.165***
(Base category: medium educational attainment (isced 3–4))					
Lifelong single	−1.574***	−1.466***	−3.887***	−0.471**	−0.710***
Never married but not lifelong single	−0.818***	−0.752***	−1.170***	−0.713**	−0.644***
Remarried/ divorced more than once	0.207***	0.042	0.131**	0.347**	0.283***
Divorced once	0.029	−0.068	−0.036	0.026	−0.028
(Base category: married for the 1st time/ widowed)					
Number of brothers and sisters	0.034***	0.021***	0.012	0.006	0.040***
Migration background	0.019	0.048		0.154	0.165**
FRA: (North) African	0.384***				
(Base category: no migration background)					
Ethnic group: Gypsy/ Hungarian of Gypsy origin			0.313***		
Ethnic group: East European/ German/ other			0.027		
(Base category: ethnic group: Hungarian)					
FRA: rural	0.167**				
FRA: urban	0.158***				
(Base category: FRA: town)					
NOR: centrality level 0: completely rural		0.111***			
NOR: centrality level 1		0.132***			
NOR: centrality level 2		0.061			
(Base category: NOR: centrality level 3: urban)					
HUN: village			0.219***		
HUN: town			0.162**		
HUN: city			0.130*		
(Base category: HUN: capital)					
GER: up to 19,999 inhabitants				−0.045	0.231***
GER: peripheral area from 50–100,000/ central area from 20–100,000 inh.				−0.017	0.108
GER: peripheral area from 100,000/ central area from 100–500,000 inh.				−0.097	0.111*
(Base category: GER: more than 500,000 inhabitants)					
Constant	0.520***	0.694***	0.385***	0.604***	0.217**
Numbers of observations	2122	3462	2810	443	1753
Wald chi^2	610.325	516.909	481.952	37.704	216.900
Pr > χ^2	0.0000	0.0000	0.0000	0.0006	0.0000
McFadden's pseudo R^2	0.083	0.045	0.057	0.028	0.040

Estimations are based on Poisson regression. Significance levels: * $p < 0.05$, ** $p < 0.01$, *** $p < 0.001$; FRA: France, NOR: Norway, HUN: Hungary, EGER: East Germany, WGER: West Germany, GER: Germany.

Except for the German data, the binary indicator "religious affiliation" can be subdivided into alternative affiliations. In the French model, Roman Catholics are the main group. There are too few Reformed Protestants in the French models for them to be included. To do so would result in large confidence intervals strongly restricting the coefficients' validity. The number of observations of the Muslims is also low. To be able to nevertheless include them, the number is augmented by individuals from the Maghreb and the rest of Africa. On the whole, these two groups overlap.[55] Fertility of the two initial groups is comparable and moreover similarly elevated. While the other French model estimations involve two items of information on migration background, namely (North) African and other migration background, model II merely involves one integrative indicator for migration history.

The Muslim effect in the model estimations for men is stronger than for women. This can be explained by the higher fertility of the male Muslims and the simultaneously lower fertility of the unaffiliated men, both compared to women. However, the fertility difference between unaffiliated and Muslim women amounting to 1.6 children is also extreme. The sign of the coefficient for male Catholics exhibits the expected tendency but is not significantly different from zero. The sign for Roman Catholic women in France is unexpectedly negative. But the puzzle's answer can be found in cohort effects. The difference between Roman Catholic and unaffiliated French women is largely restricted to the oldest cohort but negligible in the medium and young cohort, though positive. To control for cohort "eliminates" a large part of the positive effect of being Catholic. Slight interactions with further covariates turn the neutral effect to a negative one. Apart from the negative sign, the coefficient almost equals zero.

Among Hungarians, no significant effects can be attested although the fertility of Greek Catholic women exceeds fertility of unaffiliated women by 0.43 children on average. Among men, Roman Catholics, Lutherans, and Calvinists have fewer children than the unaffiliated, the sign of the coefficients is hence negative. Only Greek Catholics have a higher fertility. Their attendance rate remains unknown, but they regard religious faith as child quality as important much more often than affiliates

[55] Every seventh respondent who gave no response or refused the answer (see table 6.5) originates from the Maghreb. They do not need to be Muslims but can also be (Sephardi) Jews who immigrated in the 1950s and 1960s mainly from Morocco, Tunisia, and Egypt (Institute for Jewish Community Research 2006). That means, for one analysis they count among the mixed category.

of other denominations and also appreciate religious ceremonies at turning points in life more highly. It may hence be concluded that they are more religious. High fertility rates among diaspora groups are not uncommon (Adsera 2004, Adsera 2006). Besides, they are a local minority. It can therefore be assumed that, on the one hand, they exhibit high intra-marriage rates (their marital stability rate is in fact much higher than that of the Roman Catholics) and are part of a close network structure on the other hand. Finally, it is remarkable that although the coefficient indicating Greek Catholics is not significant, their higher fertility differs strikingly in an ex-socialist country where religious affiliation otherwise generates little variance with respect to fertility.

In contrast, Norwegians, no matter which denomination they are affiliated to, have significantly more children. The effect of adherents who are not members of the state church – other Christians and non-Christian affiliates comprising Muslims – is thereby stronger. The special position of the unaffiliated in Norway has already been referred to. Additionally, 40% of the other Christians are frequent church attenders and 64.2% regard religious faith as an important child quality so that the proportion of religious adherents within the group is very large. This explanation does not work with respect to non-Christians. Their rate of frequent attenders is low (7.8%) as is the rate of respondents who consider religious faith as important. The strength of the effects does not vary by gender. Hence, all affiliated Norwegians contribute to the effect of religious affiliation on fertility. About 27% of other Christians and the non-Christians have a migration background which is controlled for. The respective percentage concerning Lutherans is 2.7%. To conclude, multivariate analyses show that hypothesis H_{2b} can be accepted apart from French Roman Catholics. An integrative regression for Germany will be presented in an extra subsection later in this chapter.

Table 6.18. Results of model II: Effects of different religious affiliations on completed fertility

	Women			Men		
	FRA	NOR	HUN	FRA	NOR	HUN
Roman Catholic	−0.011		0.005	0.045		−0.076
Greek Catholic			0.076			0.015
Lutheran		0.102*	0.038		0.097*	−0.105
Calvinist			−0.023			−0.050
Other Christian affiliation		0.154**			0.150**	
Non-Christian affiliation		0.214**			0.187**	
Muslim (and/or from North Africa)	0.323***			0.451***		
(Base category: unaffiliated)						
Birth cohort 1949–1962	−0.241***	−0.087**	0.141***	−0.182***	−0.054	0.101**
Birth cohort 1939–1952	−0.234***	−0.107***	0.103***	−0.119**	−0.091**	0.087*
(Base category: birth cohort 1930–1942)						
Low educ. attainment (isced 0–2)	0.117***	0.077**	0.111***	0.021	0.008	0.130***
High educ. attainment (isced 5–6)	0.055	−0.008	0.049	0.031	−0.014	0.081*
(Base category: medium educational attainment (isced 3–4))						
Lifelong single	−0.671***	−1.311***	−1.797***	−1.466***	−1.464***	−3.884***
Never married but not lifelong single	−0.534***	−0.690***	−0.452***	−0.869***	−0.754***	−1.166***
Remarried/ divorced more than once	0.026	−0.094**	0.045	0.189***	0.039	0.129**
Divorced once	−0.002	−0.107**	−0.078*	0.013	−0.070	−0.034
(Base category: married for the 1st time/ widowed)						
Number of brothers and sisters	0.026***	0.023***	0.027***	0.035***	0.021***	0.011
Migration background	0.014	−0.097		0.005	0.023	
(Base category: no migration background)						
Ethnic group: Gypsy/ Hungarian of Gypsy origin			0.574***			0.312***
Ethnic group: East European/ German/ other			−0.150			0.036
(Base category: ethnic group: Hungarian)						
FRA: rural	0.207***			0.158**		
FRA: urban	0.152***			0.149**		
(Base category: FRA: town)						
NOR: centrality level 0: completely rural		0.162***			0.115***	
NOR: centrality level 1		0.141***			0.136***	
NOR: centrality level 2		0.078*			0.064	
(Base category: NOR: centrality level 3: urban)						
HUN: village			0.211***			0.216***
HUN: town			0.171***			0.160**
HUN: city			0.099*			0.130*
(Base category: HUN: capital)						
Constant	0.689***	0.701***	0.269***	0.577***	0.700***	0.389***
Numbers of observations	2395	3526	3825	1936	3462	2810
Wald chi^2	374.489	439.168	412.848	547.485	520.137	483.916
Pr > χ^2	0.0000	0.0000	0.0000	0.0000	0.0000	0.0000
McFadden's pseudo R^2	0.045	0.038	0.036	0.081	0.045	0.057

Estimations are based on Poisson regression. Significance levels: * $p < 0.05$, ** $p < 0.01$, *** $p < 0.001$; FRA: France, NOR: Norway, HUN: Hungary.

Frequency of attendance of religious services

The effects of attendance frequency of religious services on achieved fertility are tested in several ways and presented in the following tables. Tables 6.19 and 6.20 show the "simple" direct effect of frequent attendance compared to rare attendance for both genders. As was already the case in the descriptive analyses, it can be observed that effects in the model estimations for men are much stronger across countries than for women and mostly highly significant. For East German women the effect is negative which is a recurring finding. The coefficient for West German women exhibits a very low value near zero due to the fact that the larger difference regarding realized fertility exists between affiliated and unaffiliated persons and not between frequent and (affiliated) rare attenders. Altogether, the effect is largest for Norwegian and French men. Moreover, the effect of this religiosity indicator is much more noticeable than of affiliation alone which was expected. Frequent attenders are a subgroup of the affiliated (unaffiliated persons who often worship are exceptions) but rare attenders (also comprising people who never attend) are not a homogeneous group. They comprise almost all unaffiliated as well as affiliated persons who may either be irreligious or express religiosity in another form. Hence, it seems advisable to subdivide rare attenders into affiliated and unaffiliated persons. This has already been done descriptively and the results recommend this procedure. Furthermore, rare attending affiliates regard both religious ceremonies at turning points in life as well as religious faith as child quality across all countries as much more important than (rare or never attending) unaffiliated individuals do.

Tables 6.21 and 6.22 present the results of the further subdivision. Effects, that is the demographic differences between affiliated and unaffiliated individuals who utmost rarely attend, are stable and consistently positive but they are not strong enough to be significant. Among Norwegian women the fertility gap between rare attending affiliated and unaffiliated persons is almost as high as the gap between frequent and rare attenders in general (as displayed in table 6.13). But the effect is only significant at the 10% level. The effect for frequent attendance becomes even more visible in most groups which is due to the stronger contrasting reference category. For women and men from East Germany, no effect can be documented. With respect to West German women there was only a small fertility gap between rare and frequent attenders. To separate the affiliates from all rare attenders has hence apparently been promising. Though the coefficients remain insignificant, they grow observably. Compared to the "simple" estimation, the value multiplied many times in the differentiated estimation. To conclude, hypothesis H_{2c} holds in most cases.

Table 6.19. Results of model IIIa: Effects of frequency of worship on completed fertility (women)

	FRA	NOR	EGER	WGER
Frequent attendance of religious services	0.105**	0.144***	−0.023	0.009
(Base category: rare attendance of religious services)				
Birth cohort 1949–1962	−0.213***	−0.081**	−0.118	−0.148**
Birth cohort 1939–1952	−0.220***	−0.103**	−0.141	−0.194***
(Base category: birth cohort 1930–1942)				
Low educ. attainment (isced 0–2)	0.142***	0.080**	0.109	0.084
High educ. attainment (isced 5–6)	0.040	−0.021	0.001	0.088
(Base category: medium educational attainment (isced 3–4))				
Lifelong single	−0.612***	−1.317***	−0.080	−0.105
Never married but not lifelong single	−0.560***	−0.685***	−0.314	−0.535***
Remarried/ divorced more than once	0.047	−0.087*	0.257*	0.149*
Divorced once	0.028	−0.100**	0.120	0.041
(Base category: married for the 1st time/ widowed)				
Number of brothers and sisters	0.027***	0.022***	0.029	0.048***
Migration background	0.016	−0.083	−0.090	0.015
FRA: (North) African	0.285***			
(Base category: no migration background)				
FRA: rural	0.204***			
FRA: urban	0.162***			
(Base category: FRA: town)				
NOR: centrality level 0: completely rural		0.161***		
NOR: centrality level 1		0.144***		
NOR: centrality level 2		0.076*		
(Base category: NOR: centrality level 3: urban)				
GER: up to 19,999 inhabitants			−0.006	0.189**
GER: peripheral area from 50–100,000/ central area from 20–100,000 inh.			−0.060	0.205***
GER: peripheral area from 100,000/ central area from 100–500,000 inh.			0.067	0.147**
(Base category: GER: more than 500,000 inhabitants)				
Constant	0.626***	0.790***	0.607***	0.378***
Nobs	2624	3526	545	1807
Wald chi^2	420.181	442.197	25.130	120.256
$\Pr > \chi^2$	0.0000	0.0000	0.0333	0.0000
McFadden's pseudo R^2	0.046	0.038	0.014	0.021

Estimations are based on Poisson regression. Significance levels: * $p < 0.05$, ** $p < 0.01$, *** $p < 0.001$; FRA: France, NOR: Norway, EGER: East Germany, WGER: West Germany, GER: Germany.

Table 6.20. Results of model IIIa: Effects of frequency of worship on completed fertility (men)

	FRA	NOR	EGER	WGER
Frequent attendance of religious services	0.203***	0.230***	0.192	0.118**
(Base category: rare attendance of religious services)				
Birth cohort 1949–1962	−0.157***	−0.047	−0.018	−0.172***
Birth cohort 1939–1952	−0.093*	−0.085**	−0.105	−0.167***
(Base category: birth cohort 1930–1942)				
Low educ. attainment (isced 0–2)	0.025	0.013	−0.276	0.012
High educ. attainment (isced 5–6)	0.024	−0.027	−0.152	0.150***
(Base category: medium educational attainment (isced 3–4))				
Lifelong single	−1.564***	−1.466***	−0.484**	−0.706***
Never married but not lifelong single	−0.809***	−0.747***	−0.716**	−0.642***
Remarried/ divorced more than once	0.211***	0.047	0.338**	0.272***
Divorced once	0.038	−0.058	0.027	−0.025
(Base category: married for the 1st time/ widowed)				
Number of brothers and sisters	0.033***	0.019***	0.004	0.038***
Migration background	0.017	0.023	0.151	0.154**
FRA: (North) African	0.348***			
(Base category: no migration background)				
FRA: rural	0.168**			
FRA: urban	0.157***			
(Base category: FRA: town)				
NOR: centrality level 0: completely rural		0.118***		
NOR: centrality level 1		0.140***		
NOR: centrality level 2		0.060		
(Base category: NOR: centrality level 3: urban)				
GER: up to 19,999 inhabitants			−0.039	0.233***
GER: peripheral area from 50–100,000/ central area from 20–100,000 inh.			−0.026	0.113
GER: peripheral area from 100,000/ central area from 100–500,000 inh.			−0.104	0.113*
(Base category: GER: more than 500,000 inhabitants)				
Constant	0.579***	0.779***	0.630***	0.286***
Numbers of observations	2111	3462	443	1753
Wald chi^2	616.821	538.194	38.529	219.379
Pr $> \chi^2$	0.0000	0.0000	0.0004	0.0000
McFadden's pseudo R^2	0.084	0.047	0.029	0.041

Estimations are based on Poisson regression. Significance levels: * $p < 0.05$, ** $p < 0.01$, *** $p < 0.001$; FRA: France, NOR: Norway, EGER: East Germany, WGER: West Germany, GER: Germany.

Table 6.21. Results of model IIIb: Effects of frequency of worship on completed fertility (women)

	FRA	NOR	EGER	WGER
Frequent attendance of religious services	0.106**	0.233***	−0.015	0.101
Rare attendance * affiliated	0.027	0.095	0.026	0.102
(Base category: unaffiliated)				
Birth cohort 1949–1962	−0.214***	−0.079*	−0.115	−0.147**
Birth cohort 1939–1952	−0.220***	−0.102**	−0.139	−0.192***
(Base category: birth cohort 1930–1942)				
Low educ. attainment (isced 0–2)	0.142***	0.080**	0.106	0.082
High educ. attainment (isced 5–6)	0.039	−0.013	0.002	0.094*
(Base category: medium educational attainment (isced 3–4))				
Lifelong single	−0.612***	−1.316***	−0.080	−0.107*
Never married but not lifelong single	−0.561***	−0.681***	−0.311	−0.527***
Remarried/ divorced more than once	0.046	−0.084*	0.261*	0.160*
Divorced once	0.028	−0.097**	0.119	0.048
(Base category: married for the 1st time/ widowed)				
Number of brothers and sisters	0.027***	0.022***	0.029	0.048***
Migration background	0.016	−0.078	−0.087	0.015
FRA: (North) African	0.284***			
(Base category: no migration background)				
FRA: rural	0.204***			
FRA: urban	0.162***			
(Base category: FRA: town)				
NOR: centrality level 0: completely rural		0.159***		
NOR: centrality level 1		0.141***		
NOR: centrality level 2		0.074*		
(Base category: NOR: centrality level 3: urban)				
GER: up to 19,999 inhabitants			−0.007	0.181**
GER: peripheral area from 50–100,000/ central area from 20–100,000 inh.			−0.061	0.196***
GER: peripheral area from 100,000/ central area from 100–500,000 inh.			0.068	0.139**
(Base category: GER: more than 500,000 inhabitants)				
Constant	0.625***	0.697***	0.597***	0.292***
Numbers of observations	2624	3526	545	1807
Wald chi^2	420.371	445.575	25.234	122.651
$Pr > \chi^2$	0.0000	0.0000	0.0469	0.0000
McFadden's pseudo R^2	0.046	0.039	0.014	0.022

Estimations are based on Poisson regression. Significance levels: * $p < 0.05$, ** $p < 0.01$, *** $p < 0.001$; FRA: France, NOR: Norway, EGER: East Germany, WGER: West Germany, GER: Germany.

Table 6.22. Results of model IIIb: Effects of frequency of worship on completed fertility (men)

	FRA	NOR	EGER	WGER
Frequent attendance of religious services	0.264***	0.314***	0.207	0.188**
Rare attendance * affiliated	0.064	0.091	0.060	0.085
(Base category: unaffiliated)				
Birth cohort 1949–1962	−0.155***	−0.044	−0.016	−0.170***
Birth cohort 1939–1952	−0.093*	−0.085**	−0.111	−0.163***
(Base category: birth cohort 1930–1942)				
Low educ. attainment (isced 0–2)	0.025	0.013	−0.287	0.011
High educ. attainment (isced 5–6)	0.024	−0.022	−0.150	0.156***
(Base category: medium educational attainment (isced 3–4))				
Lifelong single	−1.561***	−1.463***	−0.478**	−0.705***
Never married but not lifelong single	−0.807***	−0.740***	−0.705**	−0.633***
Remarried/ divorced more than once	0.212***	0.050	0.346**	0.288***
Divorced once	0.041	−0.057	0.029	−0.016
(Base category: married for the 1st time/ widowed)				
Number of brothers and sisters	0.033***	0.019***	0.004	0.038***
Migration background	0.017	0.032	0.149	0.156**
FRA: (North) African	0.349***			
(Base category: no migration background)				
FRA: rural	0.167**			
FRA: urban	0.158***			
(Base category: FRA: town)				
NOR: centrality level 0: completely rural		0.115***		
NOR: centrality level 1		0.138***		
NOR: centrality level 2		0.057		
(Base category: NOR: centrality level 3: urban)				
GER: up to 19,999 inhabitants			−0.046	0.222**
GER: peripheral area from 50–100,000/ central area from 20–100,000 inh.			−0.029	0.101
GER: peripheral area from 100,000/ central area from 100–500,000 inh.			−0.101	0.106*
(Base category: GER: more than 500,000 inhabitants)				
Constant	0.517***	0.691***	0.615***	0.218**
Numbers of observations	2111	3462	443	1753
Wald chi^2	617.823	541.919	38.935	221.593
Pr > χ^2	0.0000	0.0000	0.0007	0.0000
McFadden's pseudo R^2	0.084	0.047	0.029	0.041

Estimations are based on Poisson regression. Significance levels: * $p < 0.05$, ** $p < 0.01$, *** $p < 0.001$; FRA: France, NOR: Norway, EGER: East Germany, WGER: West Germany, GER: Germany.

Attitudes towards religious *rites de passage* and importance of religious faith as child quality

The attitudes towards the importance of religious ceremonies and religious faith as child quality are exploratively involved because these indicators are not part of the religiosity measurement model (see tables 6.23, 6.24, and 6.25). Considering religious rites at turning points in life, a significant influence on achieved fertility can be attested for French women as well as French, Norwegian and West German men while no significant effect for people from the former socialist countries can be documented. The coefficients for East German women and Hungarian men even exhibit a negative sign. In the group of French women there is, as already shown, no linear effect of the index values on the number of children they have. But women who regard religious ceremonies as very important have as many children (about 2.5) as frequent church attenders. Three quarters of the frequent attenders realize high index values (above 10). But the minority of those with high index values attends church frequently. Insofar, it is not the same group of individuals. The significant impact found in France may be explained by country-specific factors. The incidence of religious ceremonies strongly decreased in importance and it is no longer self-evident that they still accompany funerals and especially weddings (Grosser 2009: 58) so that evaluating them as important is also reflected in fertility. The significant influence among men can be presumably traced back to the parallelism of traditional attitudes and traditional behavior. Men who have traditional attitudes also behave traditionally with all the consequences discussed in chapter 4 leading to a higher fertility.

Norwegian women who are convinced that religious faith is an important child quality have significantly more children. West German women with the same conviction also have a higher fertility but the impact is insignificant. Men who find that religious faith is important have more children than men who disagree or do not rank religious faith among the three most important child qualities. The effect is highly significant among Norwegian and West German men. The latter group who have the opinion that children should be socialized religiously have even more children – namely 2.1 – than men who attend church once a week (2.0) at a population mean of 1.5 children. Referred to Norwegian men, the margin amounts to 0.31 children. Among West German men it is hence twice as high (0.6). Hungarians do not differ in their demographic behavior according to their attitudes; the negative coefficient which is almost equal to zero has been evoked by the covariates.

The percentage of religious men is smaller compared to women, but men who are religious more often have larger families than non-religious men. This statement is however principally restricted to societies without a socialist past. Two related reasons come into consideration to explain this phenomenon. A religious man has a higher probability to marry a religious woman (due to the higher percentage of religious women) which again has the well-known consequences. The second reason is that he – while not claiming a larger part of the commodities produced jointly – uses his, compared to his wife's, improved bargaining position (she has given up employment) to request another child. If his desired number of children exceeds hers, his desire prevails over his wife's. Berinde finds that religious activity does not influence the transition risk to a third birth in Sweden (see details in 3.3). She ascribes the absent effect to the highly secular surrounding that enables women to reconcile family and occupation (Berinde 1999: 355, 366). While her conclusion cannot be transferred to Norway according to the results of this study, it may be valid with respect to Hungary and East Germany. Berinde neglects however that it is not only the frame that decides on fertility decisions but also preferences or utilities ascribed to children. Even if the former influences the latter (which can be assumed), it does not completely determine it. Finally, hypotheses H_{2d} and H_{2e} hold for men who live in a country without a socialist past. For women, they only hold in one group each.

Table 6.23. Results of model IV: Effects of attitudes towards religious ceremonies on completed fertility (women)

	FRA	NOR	HUN	EGER	WGER
Religious ceremonies important (index)	0.009*	0.005	0.000	−0.011	0.001
Birth cohort 1949–1962	−0.218***	−0.079*	0.142***	−0.147	−0.149**
Birth cohort 1939–1952	−0.223***	−0.115**	0.104***	−0.151	−0.197***
(Base category: birth cohort 1930–1942)					
Low educ. attainment (isced 0–2)	0.141***	0.072*	0.113***	0.142	0.088
High educ. attainment (isced 5–6)	0.067	0.009	0.046	−0.018	0.088
(Base category: medium educational attainment (isced 3–4))					
Lifelong single	−0.588***	−1.496***	−1.778***	−0.085	−0.110
Never married but not lifelong single	−0.555***	−0.689***	−0.450***	−0.259	−0.512***
Remarried/ divorced more than once	0.046	−0.084*	0.045	0.267*	0.158*
Divorced once	0.017	−0.115**	−0.070	0.126	0.043
(Base category: married for the 1st time/ widowed)					
Number of brothers and sisters	0.027***	0.025***	0.027***	0.025	0.048***
Migration background	0.018	−0.112		−0.059	0.016
FRA: (North) African	0.282***				
(Base category: no migration background)					
Ethnic group: Gypsy/ Hungarian of Gypsy origin			0.572***		
Ethnic group: East European/ German/ other			−0.158		
(Base category: ethnic group: Hungarian)					
FRA: rural	0.193***				
FRA: urban	0.144***				
(Base category: FRA: town)					
NOR: centrality level 0: completely rural		0.160***			
NOR: centrality level 1		0.134***			
NOR: centrality level 2		0.088*			
(Base category: NOR: centrality level 3: urban)					
HUN: village			0.205***		
HUN: town			0.165***		
HUN: city			0.092*		
(Base category: HUN: capital)					
GER: up to 19,999 inhabitants				0.029	0.194**
GER: peripheral area from 50–100,000/ central area from 20–100,000 inh.				−0.035	0.212***
GER: peripheral area from 100,000/ central area from 100–500,000 inh.				0.077	0.154***
(Base category: GER: more than 500,000 inhabitants)					
Constant	0.584***	0.742***	0.280***	0.653***	0.369***
Numbers of observations	2607	2843	3763	533	1789
Wald chi^2	413.903	357.080	399.337	26.913	117.697
Pr > χ^2	0.0000	0.0000	0.0000	0.0198	0.0000
McFadden's pseudo R^2	0.045	0.039	0.035	0.016	0.021

Estimations are based on Poisson regression. Significance levels: * $p < 0.05$, ** $p < 0.01$, *** $p < 0.001$; FRA: France, NOR: Norway, HUN: Hungary, EGER: East Germany, WGER: West Germany, GER: Germany.

Table 6.24. Results of model IV: Effects of attitudes towards religious ceremonies on completed fertility (men)

	FRA	NOR	HUN	EGER	WGER
Religious ceremonies important (index)	0.010*	0.008*	−0.002	0.010	0.014*
Birth cohort 1949–1962	−0.164***	−0.063	0.103**	0.009	−0.173***
Birth cohort 1939–1952	−0.101**	−0.089*	0.087**	−0.089	−0.173***
(Base category: birth cohort 1930–1942)					
Low educ. attainment (isced 0–2)	0.021	0.000	0.138***	−0.235	0.027
High educ. attainment (isced 5–6)	0.041	0.012	0.078	−0.162*	0.166***
(Base category: medium educational attainment (isced 3–4))					
Lifelong single	−1.550***	−1.541***	−3.860***	−0.463**	−0.698***
Never married but not lifelong single	−0.798***	−0.763***	−1.144***	−0.740**	−0.631***
Remarried/ divorced more than once	0.210***	0.045	0.133**	0.410***	0.295***
Divorced once	0.023	−0.089	−0.031	0.030	−0.027
(Base category: married for the 1st time/ widowed)					
Number of brothers and sisters	0.034***	0.023***	0.011	0.012	0.038***
Migration background	0.016	−0.001		0.151	0.159**
FRA: (North) African	0.381***				
(Base category: no migration background)					
Ethnic group: Gypsy/ Hungarian of Gypsy origin			0.308***		
Ethnic group: East European/ German/ other			0.027		
(Base category: ethnic group: Hungarian)					
FRA: rural	0.170**				
FRA: urban	0.159***				
(Base category: FRA: town)					
NOR: centrality level 0: completely rural		0.115**			
NOR: centrality level 1		0.105*			
NOR: centrality level 2		0.077*			
(Base category: NOR: centrality level 3: urban)					
HUN: village			0.198***		
HUN: town			0.140**		
HUN: city			0.110*		
(Base category: HUN: capital)					
GER: up to 19,999 inhabitants				−0.001	0.227***
GER: peripheral area from 50–100,000/ central area from 20–100,000 inh				0.001	0.117
GER: peripheral area from 100,000/ central area from 100–500,000 inh.				−0.094	0.111*
(Base category: GER: more than 500,000 inhabitants)					
Constant	0.521***	0.715***	0.366***	0.565***	0.195*
Numbers of observations	2092	2591	2751	428	1725
Wald chi^2	591.424	373.470	462.372	39.986	214.029
$Pr > \chi^2$	0.0000	0.0000	0.0000	0.0003	0.0000
McFadden's pseudo R^2	0.081	0.043	0.055	0.031	0.040

Estimations are based on Poisson regression. Significance levels: * $p < 0.05$, ** $p < 0.01$, *** $p < 0.001$; FRA: France, NOR: Norway, HUN: Hungary, EGER: East Germany, WGER: West Germany, GER: Germany.

Table 6.25. Results of model V: Effects of importance of religious faith as child quality on completed fertility

	Women			Men		
	NOR	HUN	WGER	NOR	HUN	WGER
Religious faith important	0.076*	−0.007	0.064	0.118***	−0.001	0.217***
(Base category: Religious faith not mentioned as one of the three most important traits)						
Birth cohort 1949–1962	−0.083*	0.145***	−0.152**	−0.063	0.112**	−0.177***
Birth cohort 1939–1952	−0.112**	0.101***	−0.191***	−0.085*	0.085*	−0.169***
(Base category: birth cohort 1930–1942)						
Low educ. attainment (isced 0–2)	0.081*	0.114***	0.087	0.000	0.132***	0.014
High educ. attainment (isced 5–6)	−0.001	0.047	0.090	0.002	0.084*	0.157***
(Base category: medium educational attainment (isced 3–4))						
Lifelong single	−1.505***	−1.782***	−0.104	−1.483***	−3.825***	−0.687***
Never married but not lifelong single	−0.690***	−0.447***	−0.510***	−0.756***	−1.320***	−0.645***
Remarried/ divorced more than once	−0.088*	0.044	0.150*	0.048	0.134***	0.266***
Divorced once	−0.112**	−0.080*	0.042	−0.079	−0.036	−0.054
(Base category: married for the 1st time/ widowed)						
Number of brothers and sisters	0.025***	0.027***	0.048***	0.024***	0.012	0.038***
Migration background	−0.117		0.023	−0.031		0.163**
(Base category: no migration background)						
Ethnic group: Gypsy/ Hungarian of Gypsy origin		0.546***			0.270**	
Ethnic group: East European/ German/ other		−0.141			0.022	
(Base category: ethnic group: Hungarian)						
NOR: centr. level 0: completely rural	0.158***			0.125**		
NOR: centrality level 1	0.137***			0.099*		
NOR: centrality level 2	0.088*			0.081*		
(Base category: NOR: centrality level 3: urban)						
HUN: village		0.208***			0.212***	
HUN: town		0.170***			0.158**	
HUN: city		0.099*			0.131*	
(Base category: HUN: capital)						
GER: up to 19,999 inhabitants			0.191**			0.253***
GER: peripheral area from 50–100,000/ central area from 20–100,000 inh.			0.212***			0.126*
GER: peripheral area from 100,000/ central area from 100–500,000 inh.			0.145**			0.123*
(Base category: GER: more than 500,000 inhabitants)						
Constant	0.777***	0.271***	0.380***	0.760***	0.326***	0.285***
Numbers of observations	2835	3814	1799	2581	2787	1740
Wald chi^2	361.755	398.991	116.229	367.907	463.000	223.233
Pr > χ^2	0.0000	0.0000	0.0000	0.0000	0.0000	0.0000
McFadden's pseudo R^2	0.039	0.035	0.021	0.043	0.055	0.042

Estimations are based on Poisson regression. Significance levels: * $p < 0.05$, ** $p < 0.01$, *** $p < 0.001$; NOR: Norway, HUN: Hungary, WGER: West Germany, GER: Germany.

6.3.2 The effects of the covariates on completed fertility

This subsection deals with the indirect impact religiosity can exert. Each subsection starts with a short description of the covariates and their group-specific distributions followed by a discussion of the coefficients and their effects. All statements refer to tables 6.16 to 6.26.

Birth cohort

Roughly one third of the respondents belong to each birth cohort group (see table A.8 in the appendix for the distribution of most covariates). The oldest group is somewhat smaller and comprises about one fourth of the respondents.

In general, the cohort effects are strong. Individuals of the oldest cohort[56] who had their fertile period during the golden age of marriage and the family have born more children than subsequent birth cohorts (exceptions will be mentioned later) and this is represented by the coefficients. But there is – apart from French men – no linear effect. Hence, it is reasonable to not use birth cohort as a continuous variable but to group the birth cohorts. The grouped birth cohorts 1939–1952 and 1949–1962 do not greatly differ from each other when it comes to achieved fertility. In some groups the coefficient for the middle cohort is – after having controlled for several covariates – even more strongly negative than for the youngest cohort. This applies to the Norwegians, East Germans and to West German women. Apart from East Germany, where men in the middle cohort have only 1.47 children but men in the young cohort have 1.78 children, a lower fertility of the middle cohort cannot be inferred from descriptive analysis (see table 6.3).[57] Cohort effects in the East German estimations exhibit the expected tendency, but remain insignificant. In Norway, cohort effects are significant – except for the youngest male cohort – but less strong than in France and West Germany. While the level of fertility in Norway and France does not differ very much in the middle and younger cohorts of either country, it was observably higher in France in the older cohort which explains the difference in the strength of the effects.

Hungarians' fertility does not show the common negative cohort effects. Rather, the effects are positive: weakly positive in the middle cohort and strongly positive in

[56] Remember: The cohorts only overlap across countries not within them.

[57] An education effect can be excluded. Principally, this cannot be a transformation effect. Men in the middle cohort were already too old at that time.

the youngest cohort in the model estimations of men, and both highly significant in the model estimations of women. Chapter 2 has already shown that the Hungarian fertility rate does not correspond to the typical demographic pattern documented for Western and Northern Europe. However, only slight positive cohort effects can be inferred from the descriptive data. The stronger effects are set up by the control for educational attainment. The variables interact with each other when it comes to realized fertility. Moreover, cohort effects among highly-educated women are more strongly visible between the oldest and the middle cohort while there is hardly any difference between the middle and the young cohort group. The small group of highly-educated women in the older cohort has only 1.37 children. Among low and medium educated women the effect is positive and linear. Cohort effects among men also vary by educational attainment. While the youngest cohort group of low-educated men has fewer children than both older cohort groups, it is the other way round with respect to highly-educated men. Furthermore, cohort effects among men are restricted to the unaffiliated while within the group of affiliates there are none.

Tables 6.26 and 6.27 present model estimations that take account of the claim made in the theoretical approach with respect to behavioral changes. Usually, studies that research the effects of religiosity on fertility do not consider that behavioral changes – decreasing fertility over the course of time – have taken place. They only argue why religious individuals have more children than non-religious people. But this argumentation is incomplete. Therefore, the model estimations test whether fertility has not only fallen among the unaffiliated but also among the affiliated. Several reasons support this assumption. The binding power of religious norms has weakened. Moreover, general conditions have changed, e.g. with respect to the price of time. The divorce risk has risen due to an increase of heterogamous marriages as explained in chapter 4. However, individuals with a functionally autonomous religious motivational system should be an exception. Functional autonomy means that motivational impulses assert themselves independent of external circumstances.[58] In addition, their probability of intra-marriage is higher. It can however not be assumed that those individuals can be fully identified on the basis of the few indicators available in the GGS.

The test is effected by generating interaction terms between affiliation, attendance of religious services, and birth cohort. The base category is unaffiliated respondents

[58] See further explanations in section 3.1.2.

belonging to the youngest cohort. In comparison, all coefficients should be significantly different from zero. The effects for the affiliated (rare attenders) and the (affiliated) frequent attenders should be stronger, and additionally they should be the stronger the earlier the people were born. For Spain, Adsera found that in younger birth cohorts affiliated and unaffiliated persons no longer differ in their reproductive behavior (Adsera 2004, Adsera 2006 and section 3.3). It is now necessary to include religious practice in order to discriminate between them while in older birth cohorts "affiliation" alone was a sufficient indicator. This means that all coefficients should be significantly different from zero except for the one indicating rare attending affiliates belonging to the youngest cohort group.

It would have been preferable to estimate separate models for each cohort. However, in several groups, the number of observations is too low to attain reliable results. In some cases, the group of unaffiliated persons is very small, in other cases, the group of religious people is too small. Alternatively, tables A.5 and A.6 in the appendix show descriptive results. First, religiosity has decreased over time. Younger people are less active participants than older ones. The only exception is East German men because their religious activity rate has always been low. No linear cohort effects by religiosity category can be measured. In general however, fertility has fallen over the cohorts but, as assumed, the decrease was weakest among religious people. Religious French men of the youngest cohort are even more fertile than of the older cohorts. In the descriptive perspective, demographic behavior in the group of younger French people does not differ between the affiliated and the unaffiliated while fertility of the religious people is much higher. This clearly confirms Adsera's results for Spain.

Now, the estimation results are interpreted. Some cells are empty due to the reasons just mentioned. In the French and Norwegian model estimations unaffiliated respondents of the older and middle cohort are summarized. Frequent attenders cannot be subdivided by cohort in the East German data, they are pooled. The result is that statistically significant effects in the model estimations of women are mainly restricted to the older cohort. The effects are much stronger for frequent attenders in that cohort so that not only a cohort effect but also an additional religiosity effect can be documented. For Norwegian women an additional religiosity effect can be confirmed independent of the birth cohort. In total, the effects are weaker than expected. This may be due to relatively small group sizes: French women who often attend and belong to the youngest cohort are also much more fertile (2.61) than their unaffiliated peers but the group size is small.

The results in the male groups differ slightly. Religiosity effects are measurable in almost all cohorts but also decrease with cohort (except for East German men). Hence, they are strongest in the oldest cohort. Because of the extremely low fertility of unaffiliated, younger men in West Germany (they only have 0.95 children on average, see also table A.6), all effects are significantly different from zero. Finally, fertility differences between affiliated and unaffiliated individuals in the older and middle cohort can be interpreted as disproof of the suggestion that the higher religiosity of earlier birth cohorts merely reflects an age-related return to faith (see also Norris/ Inglehart 2006, Voas/Crockett 2005).

Adsera's finding for Spain can by and large be confirmed for the countries relevant in this work. In the youngest cohort, affiliated and unaffiliated respondents do not significantly differ from each other any more (except for West German men) while frequent attenders still have a higher fertility although the difference is not statistically significant across all groups (sometimes the small group size is responsible for the lack of significance). The coefficients are however continuously much larger than for religious affiliation alone. Within the oldest cohort, both frequent attenders and also "pure" affiliates have a higher fertility than unaffiliated individuals.

Table 6.26. Results of model IIIc: Effects of cohort*religiosity on completed fertility (women)

	FRA	NOR	EGER	WGER
Birth cohort 1930–1942 * frequent attendance	0.254**	0.333***		0.266*
Birth cohort 1930–1942 * rare attendance (* affiliated)	0.188*	0.167*	0.275*	0.250*
Birth cohort 1930–1942 * unaffiliated			0.004	−0.023
Birth cohort 1939–1952 * frequent attendance	0.025	0.213*	0.014	0.007
Birth cohort 1939–1952 * rare attendance (* affiliated)	−0.032	0.062	−0.169	0.063
Birth cohort 1939–1952 * unaffiliated	0.065	−0.015	0.035	0.052
Birth cohort 1949–1962 * frequent attendance	0.192	0.200*		0.115
Birth cohort 1949–1962 * rare attendance (* affiliated)	−0.051	0.091	−0.058	0.099
(Base category: birth cohort 1949–1962 * unaffiliated)				
Low educ. attainment (isced 0–2)	0.146***	0.081**	0.105	0.085
High educ. attainment (isced 5–6)	0.034	−0.013	0.002	0.092
(Base category: medium educational attainment (isced 3–4))				
Lifelong single	−0.608***	−1.315***	−0.064	−0.111*
Never married but not lifelong single	−0.558***	−0.683***	−0.313	−0.525***
Remarried/ divorced more than once	0.044	−0.084*	0.271*	0.152*
Divorced once	0.027	−0.097**	0.109	0.048
(Base category: married for the 1st time/ widowed but never divorced)				
Number of brothers and sisters	0.026***	0.022***	0.030	0.048***
Migration background	0.016	−0.077	−0.091	0.014
FRA: (North) African	0.287***			
(Base category: no migration background)				
FRA: rural	0.205***			
FRA: urban	0.162***			
(Base category: FRA: town)				
NOR: centrality level 0: completely rural		0.158***		
NOR: centrality level 1		0.140***		
NOR: centrality level 2		0.073*		
(Base category: NOR: centrality level 3: urban)				
GER: up to 19,999 inhabitants			0.004	0.177**
GER: peripheral area from 50–100,000/ central area from 20–100,000 inh.			−0.060	0.192***
GER: peripheral area from 100,000/ central area from 100–500,000 inh.			0.072	0.138**
(Base category: GER: more than 500,000 inhabitants)				
Constant	0.447***	0.625***	0.486***	0.148
Numbers of observations	2624	3526	545	1807
Wald chi^2	423.235	446.780	30.941	125.618
Pr > χ^2	0.0000	0.0000	0.0203	0.0000
McFadden's pseudo R^2	0.046	0.0039	0.018	0.022

Estimations are based on Poisson regression. Significance levels: * $p < 0.05$, ** $p < 0.01$, *** $p < 0.001$; FRA: France, NOR: Norway, EGER: East Germany, WGER: West Germany, GER: Germany.

Table 6.27. Results of model IIIc: Effects of cohort*religiosity on completed fertility (men)

	FRA	NOR	EGER	WGER
Birth cohort 1930–1942 * frequent attendance	0.386***	0.389***		0.528***
Birth cohort 1930–1942 * rare attendance (* affiliated)	0.181	0.114	0.072	0.415***
Birth cohort 1930–1942 * unaffiliated			0.008	0.378**
Birth cohort 1939–1952 * frequent attendance	0.280*	0.304***	0.172	0.295*
Birth cohort 1939–1952 * rare attendance (* affiliated)	0.097	0.034	−0.059	0.251*
Birth cohort 1939–1952 * unaffiliated	0.037	−0.049	−0.105	0.277*
Birth cohort 1949–1962 * frequent attendance	0.238	0.192*		0.418***
Birth cohort 1949–1962 * rare attendance (* affiliated)	0.024	0.083	0.083	0.273**
(Base category: Birth cohort 1949–1962 * unaffiliated)				
Low educ. attainment (isced 0–2)	0.026	0.013	−0.285	0.010
High educ. attainment (isced 5–6)	0.025	−0.023	−0.154	0.151***
(Base category: medium educational attainment (isced 3–4))				
Lifelong single	−1.560***	−1.464***	−0.483**	−0.701***
Never married but not lifelong single	−0.807***	−0.743***	−0.707**	−0.617***
Remarried/ divorced more than once	0.212***	0.049	0.346**	0.284***
Divorced once	0.041	−0.058	0.026	−0.012
(Base category: married for the 1st time/ widowed)				
Number of brothers and sisters	0.033***	0.019***	0.004	0.040***
Migration background	0.017	0.032	0.154	0.153**
FRA: (North) African	0.350***			
(Base category: no migration background)				
FRA: rural	0.166**			
FRA: urban	0.158***			
(Base category: FRA: town)				
NOR: centrality level 0: completely rural		0.116***		
NOR: centrality level 1		0.137***		
NOR: centrality level 2		0.059		
(Base category: NOR: centrality level 3: urban)				
GER: up to 19,999 inhabitants			−0.046	0.218**
GER: peripheral area from 50–100,000/ central area from 20–100,000 inh.			−0.028	0.100
GER: peripheral area from 100,000/ central area from 100–500,000 inh.			−0.100	0.105*
(Base category: GER: more than 500,000 inhabitants)				
Constant	0.397***	0.661***	0.606***	−0.122
Numbers of observations	2111	3462	443	1753
Wald chi^2	617.151	544.523	39.206	228.592
Pr > χ^2	0.0000	0.0000	0.0017	0.0000
McFadden's pseudo R^2	0.084	0.047	0.029	0.042

Estimations are based on Poisson regression. Significance levels: * $p < 0.05$, ** $p < 0.01$, *** $p < 0.001$; FRA: France, NOR: Norway, EGER: East Germany, WGER: West Germany, GER: Germany.

The family of origin

Table A.8 presents the number of brothers and sisters the respondents have. All respondents and supposedly the majority of siblings were born before the second demographic transition occurred and the Wall was constructed, the breakdown of religiosity in the GDR began, and socialist ideology could have affected fertility decisions. The numbers of siblings East and West German respondents have does not differ much, but it is much lower in Germany than in Hungary and Norway. French respondents have most brothers and sisters. Their mothers had on average more than four children. This seems to be high, but childless women naturally remain ignored in this perspective. The population mean must hence be lower. One fifth of all respondents are only children in Germany, but less than one tenth in France. More than one half of the French respondents have at least three brothers and sisters. This only applies to one fourth of East German and one third of West German respondents. Hungary and Norway are in-between but closer to France than to Germany with more than 41%.

The number of siblings strongly positively influences realized fertility of women and men. Except for the French, the association is closer among women. Among Hungarian men and East Germans the influence is not significant. If the argument that religiosity positively affects fertility is pursued, it is self-evident to assume that respondents from large families have (had) religious parents. On the basis of the available indicators, only weak associations between the religiosity indicators and the number of siblings can be established. In Hungary, unaffiliated persons have fewest siblings and Greek Catholics have most, which largely corresponds to denomination-specific fertility levels. However, contrary to expectations, unaffiliated people in France have slightly more siblings than Roman Catholics, and in Germany – neither in the East nor in the West – no difference between affiliated and unaffiliated respondents is measurable. For Eastern Germany, this finding is not surprising. Most unaffiliated people in the data set were still baptized but left the Church during the SED-regime. People who attend church frequently indeed have observably more siblings than rare attenders of religious services[59] and gender-specific differences exist. While the impact of siblings on fertility is stronger among women, men differ more strongly with respect to the number of siblings by religious categories. Most remarkable connections can be found in France where religious women have half a sibling more

[59] The remaining indicators are neutral.

and religious men even 0.83 siblings more than irreligious persons. In East Germany, this difference amounts to 0.65 siblings among men while religious women have – contrary to expectations – half a sibling less. It is very probable that individuals who grew up with several brothers and sisters have positive attitudes towards children and family in general. But also the opposite might be possible: a person who grew up with many siblings received too little attention and experienced a lack of money so that she or he decides to have only one child or none at all. This reaction is, however, not supported by empirical evidence.

The second characteristic that reflects the family of origin is migration background.[60] The percentage of non-Hungarians is very low because Hungary does not count among the typical destinations for immigration (see the second part of table A.8 in the appendix). Roma, including Hungarians of Roma origin, are the largest minority: 6% of the population belong to this ethnic group (they call themselves *cigány*; Hablicsek 2007 cited by Spéder/Kamarás 2008: 610–611, Hungarian Central Statistical Office 2010). Because of their high albeit slightly declining birth rate, they are on average considerably younger than the rest of the Hungarian population which is one reason why their share in the relevant (older) population in the GGS is so low (merely 2% state to have a Roma background). Individuals with a migration background are usually under-represented in population surveys especially when their national language skills are poor. Basically, poor language skills do not apply to the Roma population. Their main language is in most cases the national one. Only a small percentage of Roma still has a good command of their original mother tongue. As the questionnaire is very demanding, the larger problem concerning their under-representation is rather their low education.[61] It remains unknown if and when they migrated to Hungary and how long they have been there. As Roma seem to have a strong ethnic identification, they state they are Roma although they have been living in Hungary for many generations (Jahn 2007). They are not one homogenous group: several subgroups differing in traditions and ways of life can be distinguished (Barlai/Hartleb 2009). Their socioeconomic situation is precarious. In Hungary, 91% of them live below the poverty line which is the highest rate among Roma in Europe. Their educational level is extremely low. The same applies to their employment rate.

[60] This statement is only valid if the respondents do not belong to a first generation of migrants. In this case the family of origin naturally does not have a migration background.

[61] Education is an additional factor that strongly influences the willingness to participate in surveys.

Depending on the region, the rate of unemployment reaches 50–90%. In some villages on the border to Slovakia, where exclusively Roma dwell, the rate amounts to 100%.[62] They live unevenly distributed in the country. The majority still resides in villages, and within this category they live in the most disadvantaged rural areas (Ministry of Foreign Affairs Budapest 2004).

Before the regime change in Hungary occurred, childbearing outside of wedlock mainly took place among two groups, namely Roma and other under-educated persons (Spéder 2006: 255). Moreover, union formation patterns of non-Hungarian ethnicities in general differ substantially from those of the autochthonal population (Hoem et al. 2010: 201). Hungarians of Gypsy origin have a lower completed fertility than Gypsies (3.0 vs. 3.5) which backs up the finding that integration has an effect on fertility. Another example are Hungarians of German origin who are less fertile than respondents referring to themselves as Germans (1.8 vs. 2.2 children). The number of observations is so small however that these groups are not listed separately in the table. In general, Hungarians by naturalization have a lower fertility than the ethnic group of origin. On the whole, it is only the Roma that have a noticeably higher number of children manifesting itself in highly significant coefficients. Further group-internal variance is generated by their education. Roma with little or no education are considerably more fertile (women: 3.8; men: 3.1 children) than better educated Roma (1.5 children, both sexes taken together due to the small number of observations when it comes to higher education).[63] This permits the conclusion that more education would rapidly lower their fertility and raise their low age at first birth. All other ethnic groups – mostly people from other Eastern European countries – are summarized in the regressions. Their fertility does not significantly differ from the fertility level of the autochthonal population.[64]

According to the official French definition, immigrants are individuals who were born in another country, that means, they are "qualified" by their country of birth and not by their nationality (Institut national de la statistique et des études économiques 2010a). Inhabitants are automatically French citizens independent of

[62] Figures according to Flórián Farkas, member of parliament; taken from a text in Hungarian, cited by Barlai/Hartleb 2009: 34.

[63] In fact, the influence of education on Roma fertility is completely linear. Uneducated Roma (isced 0) have most children (4.6), followed by the next step (isced 1), etc.

[64] This does not mean that some subgroups do not have a somewhat higher or lower fertility. The single group sizes are relatively small, however.

their parents' origin if they were born in France. Therefore[65] official values cannot be meaningfully compared to the values calculated here. On the whole, the high fertility level in France has not been caused by immigrants. Immigrants from the African continent – 4% of the population originates from North Africa and a further 1.2% have another African background – form an exception and exhibit a remarkably higher completed fertility (African other: 3.2 children, Maghrebi: 2.9 children) which is reflected in highly stable and significant coefficients. These immigrants originate from countries with a lower level of modernization and an under-developed welfare state which contributes to their higher fertility. In general, the immigrants' main region of origin is Europe: more than 12% of France's inhabitants or more than one half of all migrants have a European background. A third category are *Pieds Noirs* with a share of 3.2% of the population. In the regression estimations, Europeans, *Pieds Noirs*, and "others", who have a population share of 1.1%, are pooled. Their fertility does not significantly deviate from that one of the autochthonal population.

The share of migrants in Germany among the population older than 44 years was 13.2% in 2008 (Statistisches Bundesamt 2010b: 48). Official data integrate East and West but it is known that the share in the Western part is much higher. The percentage of individuals with a migration background calculated with the GGS (15%), taking both regions together, largely corresponds to the official value, but the distribution of the immigrant groups itself is biased. Only 1% of the West German population originate from Turkey (included in category "other").[66] The share must have been higher albeit on average the population of Turkish origin is younger due to their higher fertility and specificities of the immigration history. As in France, the majority of migrants are Europeans, which cannot be itemized more precisely (7.3%). 4% of the respondents have a Russian background or lived in Russia before they migrated to Germany and 3.7% are "others". The majority of them are assumed to be *Spätaussiedler* (late repatriates). Their ancestors (mostly father or mother) or in-law family members are ethnic Germans. They immigrated to Germany between 1973 and 2004 and, according to the GGS, on average in 1991. Usually they received German citizenship at immigration.[67] The remaining migrants have been living in Germany

[65] And because the residence permit requirement for citizens of the European Union and Switzerland has been abolished (Prioux 2008: 377).

[66] This does not significantly change if it is considered that Muslims and "other" religious affiliations have been dropped from the German data set.

[67] The majority of Russian immigrants assign themselves to the ethnic group of Germans. Almost all currently have German citizenship, but only one third already had it from birth.

for almost 20 years longer, if they were born abroad.[68] The residence duration of the migrants in France is some years longer on average.

The percentage of non-ethnic East Germans is observably lower. Less than 10% of the population originate from another country. Therefore, all people with a migration background are pooled in the regressions. As in all countries considered here, the share of male migrants is higher than that of female ones. Neither female nor male migrants living in Germany have a significantly higher or lower fertility than ethnic East or West German women and men (the only exception are male migrants in West Germany). Also descriptively, the fertility of "Europeans", "Russians" or "others", each considered separately, does not diverge. In contrast, male migrants in West Germany have significantly more children than autochthonal men. European men have 1.72, Russian men have 1.81, and other migrants have 1.62 children. Taking all migrants together, as in the estimations, they have 1.72 children. It can be argued that it it not the migrants who have many children but it is the West German men who have very few (1.49).

Only 5.1% of the Norwegian respondents were not born in Norway, do not have Norwegian citizenship, or both. The main countries of origin according to GGS data are Denmark, Sweden, USA, UK, Germany, and Pakistan. Altogether, the migrants originate from 60 different countries with low numbers of individual observations. The demographic behavior of immigrants living in Norway and of Norwegians can statistically hardly be distinguished. Noticeably higher percentages of the other Christians and of non-Christians are immigrants (27%) compared with Lutherans (2.7%). This result is not surprising, because the latter are members of the Norwegian state church. While Norwegian Christians – rather "other" Christians (2.41 vs. 1.75) but also Lutherans (2.15 vs. 1.93) – have more children than immigrants, it is the other way round with respect to non-Christians (2.27 vs. 2.66 children).

It has been reported above that parental divorce (another characteristic of the family of origin) raises the later divorce risk of their children. Following the argumentation of chapter 4, the higher divorce risk should lead to lower fertility. The issue of a parental breakup could not be included into the analyses due to an accumulation of missings in the German data (84%). But descriptive results are stated.[69]

---

68 Apart from a few people, all Russians and Turkish migrants migrated on their own and were not born in Germany. The same applies to the (North) Africans and *Pieds Noirs* in France, while only half of the Europeans living in France and Germany were born abroad.

69 The question is as follows: "Did your biological parents ever break up?"

Parental breakup affects fertility behavior of Norwegian men. It is 1.8 if they experienced that decisive occurrence and 2.16 if their parents never broke up (Norwegian women: 2.01 and 2.17). In the French and Hungarian data, individuals do not differ in fertility outcome dependent on parental breakup. On the one hand, breakup is not equal to divorce and does not exclude reconciliation. On the other hand, there is no information on the age of the respondent at the time of the event. But it seems not implausible to assume that parental breakup is a more far-reaching turning point if the children are young.[70] However, in the case of Norwegian men, age makes no difference. The picture is different for French men. Those whose parents broke up and who experienced it before age 15 surprisingly have considerably more, namely 2.45, children on average. Concerning marital stability, the common finding that parental breakup boosts their children's divorce risk can be confirmed based on the French (only women), Hungarian, and Norwegian data. Persons whose parents never split up have more stable partnerships. The share of stable marriages in the group of those whose parents broke up is 10–15% lower.

Education

According to GGS data, the level of education is highest in East Germany, for both women and men, followed by West Germany (see bottom of table A.8 and the more detailed itemization in table A.11). East Germans have the lowest level of low-educated persons and the men most frequently attained a high level of education. The proportion of highly-educated individuals exceeds the expected value because access to university education was fairly restricted in the GDR (Kreyenfeld 2004: 278). The general idea was to provide the population with occupational training. While in East Germany gender-specific shares in educational attainment are by and large balanced, this is not the case in West Germany. Far more women have only a low level of education, while the percentage of men with tertiary education is significantly larger. Consequently, there is an observable difference between East and West German women. The educational level of Hungarians is lower than of East Germans. As previously mentioned, Hungary has the lowest level of modernization of all relevant countries. Gender-specific differences are noticeable[71] except for tertiary

[70] The question in the GGS has the wording: "Did you live most of your childhood up to the age of 15 with both of your own biological parents?"

[71] However, the share of women with isced 4 level education (medium) is higher than that of men.

education which is not very differently distributed. Altogether, gender equality is most pronounced in Norway and France, especially with respect to tertiary education. Referring to the countries, the level of education is lowest in France. Women however more often have completed tertiary education than in West Germany.

According to Voas 2008 material modernization[72] has not considerably influenced the level of religiosity. But for economic reasons, and as clarified in chapter 5, it should affect fertility. Education is one aspect of material modernization. If opportunity costs are measured by educational achievement rather than estimated income based on Heckman's two stage method, economist Leibenstein describes the following problem: "(...) education by itself is likely to be the significant explanatory variable (rather than its presumed indirect effect on the value of mother's time). In other words, education has significant impact on tastes rather than on the value of time" (Leibenstein 1974: 468). Basically, the possible effect of education on fertility can be threefold: education can be a proxy for wages. Education is a time investment in human capital whose returns are the wages and the investment is only effected in case it pays off, which excludes long-term employment breaks. Education may secondly bring about an ideational shift across generations as was argued for (West German) men. Education can thirdly have a delaying effect due to the longer stay in institutions which is implicitly more an economic effect because time plays an important role. The probability to bear a child is lowest during studies or training. Family formation is hence at least postponed for those years (Blossfeld/Huinink 1991).

The first result of the regressions concerning education is that the number of children of low-educated women is higher in each country compared to medium educated women, which is the reference category. Among French, Norwegian, and Hungarian women the difference is highly significant.[73] This finding is in accordance with the economic theory. As their opportunity costs are lower than those of their more educated peers, effects of long and frequent employment breaks have less severe consequences regarding the amount of wages loss, missed chances of occupational advancement, the obsolescence of knowledge and training, etc. The time these women invested in their human capital was strongly limited. This also means that they spent comparably little time in institutions which again enabled them to start family

[72] The definition can be found in section 3.2.2.

[73] This result is influenced by both lower shares of childlessness and higher shares of large families among the low-educated women. In East Germany, only large families occur more frequently: 35% have four or more children.

formation early. Interestingly, East German women with a low level of education have most children (2.61), that means their achieved fertility even exceeds low-educated women in France and Norway (2.51 and 2.32). It is not a cohort effect which is controlled for. As already mentioned, low-educated women in East Germany are merely a small group with not too much weight in total. As the whole group of East German women is small (N=545), the large numerical effect remains statistically insignificant. Thus, the reported finding that East Germany is the only country where no significant link between education and fertility exists, cannot be confirmed here.

Highly-educated women do not have significantly fewer children than medium educated women. In fact, these two categories of women cannot be distinguished in any country.[74] Thus, according to their demographic behavior women can be subdivided in two groups: low-educated and "not low" educated women. The former have a significantly higher fertility than the latter. In France, the lower educational attainment of the population seems to be only one reason for the high fertility level because even medium and highly-educated women have given birth to more children (2.0) than low-educated women in West Germany (1.88). However, it seems natural to suppose that three educational groups – which is a rough method of measuring – cannot capture the whole group-internal variability. This has been reported with a strong concentration on highly-educated women in section 5.2.[75] The coefficient for West German women is positively significant, which is a rather unexpected result, all the more with respect to the poor reconciliation situation for family and work compared to other countries. One may assume that the existing higher marital stability among West German women is responsible for this effect. However, highly-educated West German women cannot be distinguished by their marital status concerning fertility. No differences exist. Medium educated West German women have 1.62 children on average; highly-educated women have 1.64 children. The latter more often live in areas where the general fertility level is lower (cities with more than half a million inhabitants) and this fact is controlled for.[76]

[74] In East Germany highly-educated women almost strictly follow a two-child norm (53.4%).

[75] Most women at least temporarily participated in the labor force but the data do not cover the duration. Social status can only be measured if women are currently employed. Alternatively social status could be measured by partner's occupation. However, this is only possible if they are currently partnered. As a consequence, many missing values exist.

[76] In contrast to expectations, they are not more frequently unmarried.

Only low-educated men in Hungary are significantly more fertile than their medium educated peers.[77] The tendency in all other estimations for men except for East Germany is positive, but not significant. Usually and also according to GGS, low-educated men more often remain single (see section 5.2) so that their fertility should consequently be lower. The control for marital status and hence also the status "single" makes the absent negative fertility effect for low education among men explainable. This fact is of great importance for low-educated Hungarian men. This will be explained more detailed later in this section.

The fertility of highly-educated men is also higher than of medium educated men in Hungary. The effect is not significant in all estimations, however. In West Germany, the effect is persistently highly significant. One can suppose that this effect reveals the preeminence of the male breadwinner model. Highly-educated men earn higher incomes which better enable the maintenance of a whole family in a conservative surrounding. As many marriages are homogamous with respect to education, this effect may also document why highly-educated women in Germany do not have less children.[78] If the educational attainment of men who still have a partner is analyzed (which may of course be selective) it becomes obvious that highly-educated men frequently have highly-educated wives. However, West German men have most children if their wives have only a low level of education, followed by wives with a medium level of education.[79] The finding reported above, that in France no significant differences for men of different educational levels exist, can be confirmed.[80] Finally, in Norway and East Germany, signs of the effects are negative but insignificant for highly-educated men.

In the following, interactions between education and other covariates will be analyzed. In all female groups the correlations between educational attainment and birth cohort are not very pronounced (about $r = 0.25$). Correlations in the male groups are even weaker. The share of highly-educated women rises with birth cohort.

---

[77] They are frequently more often childless than medium or especially highly-educated men. But they also have many children much more often.

[78] This statement is also true for older cohorts, especially from the perspective of highly-educated women. According to the GGS only 27.6% of them are not married with an highly-educated partner.

[79] If the respondent is a woman, it is the other way round. She has most children if she has a low level of education and her partner has a high level.

[80] This changes if the isced-levels are analyzed in a more detailed form. French men with isced 5B education have 1.78 children while men with isced 5A education have 2.25 children. The number of observations is sufficiently high.

Women especially benefited from educational expansion, which is manifested in these correlations. The significant effect of a low level of education among Hungarian men is strengthened when the birth cohort is controlled for. The youngest cohort of low-educated Hungarian men is less fertile whereas, in general, cohort effects have been shown to be positive in Hungary. In that country an association between educational accomplishment and religious affiliation among men is detectable. Only 13.3% of the unaffiliated but 26.2% of the affiliated have a low level of education. The respective percentages regarding a high level of education are 24.1% and 13.7%. In socialism, religious affiliates were discriminated and marginalized also with respect to education (see further details in subsection 3.2.3). The consequence is visible in the data. However, in East Germany where low education is almost not existent, the difference is only marginal among men. Among Hungarian women, the educational gap by religious affiliation is considerable. Little more than one fifth of all unaffiliated women (21.5%) have a low level of education and 22.9% have a high level. In contrast, almost half of the affiliated women (44.5%) are low educated and only 10.9% have tertiary education. In East Germany, the gap is greater than among men, but not as large as in Hungary. For example, 26.2% of the unaffiliated have tertiary education but only 17.1% of the affiliated.

Apart from the socialist legacy, there are also associations in the remaining countries. Among men, there is no gap in France and a small gap in West Germany. In Norway, affiliated men more often have only a low or medium level of education. The most remarkable gradient can be documented for tertiary education: the share among unaffiliated individuals is almost twice as high (41.2% vs. 22%). In all three countries, affiliated women have less education than their unaffiliated peers. In France, the shares with respect to high education are 27.7% and 17.8%, which means that the difference equals the East German one. More noticeable differences can be attested for West Germany and Norway. In the former, the shares are 31.2% and 13.1%. In the latter, they are 52.2% and 22.4% which also reflect general educational levels in the respective countries.

These results lead back to an economic interpretation of the *characteristics approach*. A certain number of religiously affiliated women do not invest too much time in market-related human capital due to their (higher) fertility plans. Controlling for educational effects partly explains why religious affiliation itself is not significant in the regression analyses for women.[81] This conclusion however presupposes that the educational differences between affiliated and non-affiliated individuals are not mere cohort effects. As already ascertained, educational levels increase by birth cohort. The percentage difference between affiliated and unaffiliated persons regarding achieving a higher level of education hardly varies among women and men by birth cohort in Hungary, West Germany, and Norway which can be shown with the aid of ordered Probit regressions (not displayed here). Only among French and East German women can the difference be completely ascribed to cohort effects. A pure cohort effect can hence be excluded in most groups. However, the effect of affiliation on educational attainment slightly lowers when holding birth cohort constant. Therefore it can be said that affiliated individuals benefited even more from educational expansion.

Now, the statements made in subsection 3.2.4 should be checked. Do the Catholics have a lower level of education than the Protestants and do the Muslims have the lowest level? In France, Calvinists are much more often highly educated than all others. 39.1% are highly educated compared with 19% of the Catholics. 75% of the Muslims in France have a low level of education (in Germany it is 78.6%), which can also be interpreted as the expected finding. In Hungary, the differences between Christian affiliations are negligible except for Lutherans who more often have tertiary education and Greek Catholics whose share of those with a low level of education is considerably higher. Apart from few exceptions, hardly any Greek Catholics have tertiary education. This explains the insignificant coefficient for them in the second estimation (table 6.18). In Norway, other Christians, that means Catholics and conservative and evangelical religious groups, surprisingly more often have a high level of education than Lutherans. Differences are small however (24.4% vs. 20.9%). Non-Christians are almost as often highly educated as unaffiliated (women: 42.6% vs. 46.1%).

If the binary indicator religious affiliation is further divided into frequent attenders, affiliated rare attenders, and unaffiliated persons, the result may be surprising at first sight. Frequent attenders of religious services are better educated than rare attenders as long as the latter are affiliated. Unaffiliated individuals have the highest education apart from West German women as well as French and East German men. French and East German men who often attend are best educated, that means they also exceed the unaffiliated. Assuming that the religiosity dimension of ritual measured

[81] In principle, the human capital theory should only form the basis of the argument if all women could freely opt in favor of or against higher education. This however is doubtful.

by church attendance can – in addition to the dimension religious knowledge or more generally cognitive interest – also be interpreted as an "intellectual dimension" compared to the dimensions religious ideology, devotion, and religious experience, it more often attracts the highly educated among the affiliates. This means that the form that religiosity is expressed in depends on educational accomplishment (see also supporting details and further explanations in Sacerdote/Glaeser 2001 and Brown/Taylor 2003). The combination of church attendance and affiliation generates considerable fertility variance in most educational groups (except for East German women). In Norway, the effect exceeds that of all other countries. But it is also large among highly-educated West German men (and French men but independent of educational attainment). That means, in West Germany the combination frequent attendance of religious services and high level of education generate high fertility outcomes.

Do highly-educated women more often remain childless if they are unaffiliated? For Hungary, the question can be affirmed (unaffiliated women: 21.7%; affiliated women: 11.6%). In Norway, highly (19% vs. 13.8%) and low-educated women (17.8% vs. 8.5%) exhibit higher rates of childlessness while in France this only applies to low-educated women (15.8% vs. 7.8%). Among men affiliation also makes a difference to childlessness. Highly-educated men in East Germany (unaffiliated men: 12.7%; affiliated men: 3.9%), West Germany (26.6% vs. 17.4%), and Norway (16.8% vs. 11.3%) more frequently remain childless if they are unaffiliated. However, this phenomenon is not restricted to men with tertiary education. In West Germany and Norway, all educational groups differ in this way. In France, men with a low and medium level of education do.

The division of birth cohorts into birth cohort groups also rests on the conviction that the middle cohort group by and large has completed fertility before the transformation occurred so that the impact of the temporal collapse of fertility can be read from cohort fertility of the youngest East German cohort group, especially the better educated. This however is a fallacy because it is the middle cohort of East German men that has least children of all East German groups (1.47). Furthermore, within the middle cohort only the unaffiliated men, which is the majority, have few children (1.34). In contrast, an educational effect cannot be documented. The fact that women in the middle cohort also have fewer children, but only if they are affiliated (1.45), is striking. The result that affiliated women in East Germany contradict all assumptions – because their fertility is lower – can even be traced back to the middle cohort only. At most, slight educational effects can be attested for the middle and young cohorts, while in the older cohort highly-educated women have more children than women with a medium level of education. The assumption also does not apply to Hungarians. As already mentioned, there are even positive cohort effects and the educational effect is limited to the difference between the older and the middle cohort. Fertility of highly-educated women from the middle and young cohort basically does not differ. Among Hungarian men, fertility is strongly influenced by the interaction of educational attainment and cohort affiliation. The assumed effect can however not be found. In contrast, while middle cohort men have 1.77 children if they are highly educated, this average number rises to 2.0 in the young cohort. Among men with a low level of education, it is principally the other way round: middle cohort men have 1.96 children while young cohort men have only 1.64 children. These results also explain the strong cohort effects. In the descriptive perspective, they are suppressed by educational effects.

Marital stability

Marital status is subdivided into several subcategories. The reference category is "married for the first time" and "widowed but never divorced" (both indicating "marital stability"). If the assumptions made are confirmed, all the coefficients for alternative statuses should be negatively different from zero. The analysis effected in subsection 6.2.3 has already shown descriptively that it is not a stable marriage that leads to the highest number of children and this contradicts the presuppositions. In the following, the effects are tested again controlling for further covariates. Before doing so, it must be checked if years of exposure of the widowed were limited due to an early death of the partner. A small share of widowed women lost their partner before they reached age 44.[82] The number of men who lost their wife very early in life is negligible. Only in Norway but not in France and Hungary does the fertility of widows (and widowers) deviate downwards. The total number of respondents widowed early in Norway is very low, however, and will therefore be accepted.

The most obvious effect is treated firstly. Not too surprisingly, being single a lifelong negatively influences the fertility outcome most strongly.[83] "Lifelong single"

[82] The year of ending of the relationship in case the partner died was collected in France, Norway, and Hungary.

[83] The only exception is German women. Here, the data problems addressed are obvious.

means that the person never at least cohabited with a partner. It does not exclude living apart together relationships. Never having married (but not being lifelong single) is also a very good predictor for low fertility. If the first "step" of stability of a union is measured by a marriage itself, this part of the presupposition can be confirmed as correct. The strength of the effects is continuously stronger in the estimations for men, which leads back to the gender-difference argumentation in 5.2.1.

Women in Norway and Hungary who experienced a divorce have significantly fewer children than the reference group. The effect is somewhat stronger in Norway than in Hungary. In the remaining groups of women no negative effect can be documented. In the male groups no significant effect is visible at all. This may be associated with the higher risk of women. It is mostly they that stop work to care for the household and family. In case of divorce, their poverty risk is higher. Then they not only have the task of maintaining themselves but also of providing for the children. Before statements on the validity of the theoretical presuppositions can be made, it is important to know if fertility is not only lower due to fewer years of exposure compared to stable marriages. Among Norwegian women, age at union end and fertility are not correlated with each other. Among Hungarian women, a weak association exists. Fertility is lower if the union breaks up before the women reach age 45. However, completed fertility of women whose marriage ended after age 44 is still lower than of women whose marriage turned out to be stable. To live or have lived in a stable marriage or being divorced once does not completely exclude that the children have different biological fathers or mothers. If both statuses are limited to respondents who have children with one (ex-)partner only, those from stable marriages have more children (except for East and West German women and French men).[84]

In East and West Germany remarrying positively influences a women's number of children compared to remaining married. In East Germany hardly any remarried or more than once divorced woman is childless. 37% have three children and 19% have four or more children while merely 16.3% of the women who only married once have three or more children which is a clear picture. 12.3% of the latter remained childless. One can assume that among them are persons who anticipated divorce and therefore concentrated on gainful employment but finally remained married and also couples who stayed childless involuntarily. In West Germany the result is – in a descriptive perspective – less obvious. 11.6% of remarried women have three and 12.2% have

[84] No data for Hungarians are available to validate this information.

more than three children. Among women who married once the respective numbers are 15.4% and 5.8%. Moreover, fewer women of the former group are childless than of the latter one. Remarried Norwegian women have significantly fewer children, which again corresponds to the theoretical presuppositions. The fertility of divorced or remarried French and Hungarian women does not differ from the reference category.

Remarried men father significantly more children than men in stable marriages do. The difference between the two groups of men is only not significant in Norway. This continuous, cross-border result contradicts the theoretical presuppositions and corresponds to the findings of Klein 2003 (see section 4.4). A higher order child is rather born in a new partnership while a second child more often is born within the same partnership as the first one. This can be clearly confirmed with the aid of GGS data. A variety of preconditions have to be fulfilled to preserve the possibility to have further children in another union: it depends on early first marriage as well as its dissolution and fast re-partnering. Completely apart from the fact that empirical evidence contradicts the hypothesis, these requirements prove why the coefficients are rather significant in the male model estimations. Men are still able to produce children at a higher age. They are not as strongly limited as women are. But this is not the only reason. Most women have custody of the children after separation and divorce. They have the huge responsibility to care for their children and hence they are much more engaged in the "legacy" of the divorced marriage.

If men re-partner, the new wife could either be still childless and desires children, which leads to the man fathering further children, or she may already have children from another union. In that case, two sub-options are imaginable. On the one hand, he may opt for a stronger feeling of affiliation to his new family. He will reach it by getting his new wife pregnant. Additionally, a joint child proves commitment towards the new union (Billari 2005: 80). The second possibility is that both partners already have children so that no further child will be born. Which option the man will select also depends on the age of both partners. Here, it seems as if the first option prevails. It is obvious that remarried men much more often father children from more than one union. If men in the different statuses who have only children from one union are compared with each other, men in stable unions[85] have more children than remarried

[85] The statement can only be done for men who lived in the first marriage at the time of the interview. In no country were widowed respondents asked whether they have children with ex-partners.

men.[86] There is another possibility: all children originate from the second marriage which is anticipated as stable and hence worth investing in. But this is definitely not the case. Fewer children stem from the second marriage than from the first. This has also to do with the fact that in a considerable percentage of second marriages no further child is born. If second marriages are restricted to those with new biological children, the statement nevertheless remains true. The difference becomes smaller, however.

It has been assumed that the theoretical presuppositions always apply independent of a specific country. This is not the case. But it is surprising that of all groups they apply most to Norwegian women. In the course of this work, reasons have already been mentioned that explain why Norway should have had a lower probability to confirm the presuppositions: According to the HDI, Norway is the most modern country. Although divorce rates are high, women should be stronger willing to invest in marriage-specific capital due to their lower economic risks in case of separation and lone parenthood compared to the women in the remaining countries. The kind of welfare state and its policies are strongly supportive when it comes to female employment. Women are in the position to maintain themselves easily due to their higher level of education, the good availability of child care facilities, well-working labor markets as well as gender equality promoting measures in total. Single motherhood and female labor force participation are widely accepted. Moreover, the level of decommodification is high. Chapter 5 has reasoned these aspects in detail. But it has been shown that the presuppositions not only apply to women but – in their tendency – they also pertain to men in Norway. The 1981 Children Act established joint custody after separation and divorce as a rule and unified parental obligations – and especially the rights of fathers – independent of the question whether the child was born in or out of wedlock (Skevik/Hatland 2008: 91, Blum/Rille-Pfeiffer 2010: 32). This means that fathers usually do not risk losing contact to their children after divorce. Hence, they can invest into a marriage almost independent of the divorce probability.

Religiously affiliated people have more stable marriages and by and large also more children. It should be checked if there are interactions between religiosity, marital stability, and fertility. If the marriage is stable, the average number of children of frequent attenders exceeds the average number of rare attending affiliates. The latter's fertility in turn is higher than of the unaffiliated (except for East German

[86] For Hungary this cannot be analyzed due to the previously mentioned data restrictions.

women). The same order applies if remarried persons are regarded in isolation (except for French women and Hungarian men; Hungarian women do not differ at all). The result after having compared remarried persons with those in stable marriages at every "religiosity step" is that the first group mostly have a higher completed fertility than the latter one or at least not fewer children. There are some exceptions: Norwegian women who live in stable marriages have on each religiosity step more children than their remarried peers, e.g. frequent attending remarried women (due to the high stability of marriages composed of religious persons it is a small group) have 2.28 children while frequently attending women in stable marriages have 2.84 children. Differences between Norwegian men also exist, but are smaller.

Among West German women, the unaffiliated are more willing to invest in the marriage if the marriage is perceived as stable. Unaffiliated, remarried women have only 1.25 children while those in stable marriages have 1.58 children. French women in stable marriages have more children than remarried women as long as they are religiously affiliated (2.42 vs. 2.06). This cannot be further differentiated because there are hardly any frequent church attenders who are remarried. The will to reproduce is, especially among men, stronger than to assure that the marriage will last. If women and men in stable marriages are compared on the above mentioned religiosity steps with individuals who are once divorced, the latter are less fertile in all Norwegian groups (both genders), e.g. divorced, frequently attending women only have 1.96 children. The difference hence amounts to almost one child. Presuppositions also apply to East German and French women insofar as they are religiously affiliated. If the women are unaffiliated, the presuppositions are not true. For Hungarian women, the presuppositions apply to religiously affiliated and unaffiliated women. Both differences are rather small, however. To conclude, differences are unsystematic. Among German and Hungarian men, stability makes no difference. The only exception is unaffiliated East German men who behave like their unaffiliated, female compatriots. Apart from exceptions, hypothesis H_{2a} – that has not finally been evaluated up to now – holds with view to direct as well as indirect effects.

Size of settlement

Most people in the French sample live in an urban area, about a sixth reside in a town, and 26.7% live rurally (see table A.9). In Norway, almost two thirds of the respondents were interviewed either in Oslo or in another urban area. 19% live rurally, and one sixth lives in small towns. In Hungary, roughly one third lives in villages. Those people are evenly spread over the country and the regions. 30% of the Hungarian respondents live in towns and one fifth in cities. The rest of them resides in Budapest. Women can be found somewhat more often in urban areas and less often in rural ones. Due to extremely different population densities and categories, comparability between the countries is difficult to manage. Only in (East and West) Germany is this procedure easily possible. East Germans more often live rurally (20.2% vs. 12%). About one half of them live in towns with a maximum of 100,000 inhabitants. In West Germany, this applies to less than one third. Almost one fourth of them reside in cities with a population of more than half a million. This is far less the case in the Eastern part of the Republic.[87] The rest of the people live in agglomerations with less than half a million but more than 100,000 inhabitants.

Industrialization and urbanization were identified as important determinants of the first demographic transition that refers to the historical decline in death rates starting in the early 19th century followed by decreasing birth rates beginning around 1880 in several European populations (Lesthaeghe/Surkyn 1988, van de Kaa 1987). Today, urban areas are still "less fertile" than rural areas. According to the theoretical approach used in this work, higher divorce probabilities in cities – among other things due to a higher availability of alternative partners and lower rates of joint property ownership – can be held responsible for lower fertility. Moreover, usually the share of single people and unmarried couples is higher. In rural areas, the degree of spousal complementarity and hence mutual dependence on each other (because fewer women are in paid employment) is more pronounced, which increases the benefit of marriage and makes them invest more in their union.

Another important indicator for fertility differences by settlement size are selective movements (Kulu/Vikat/Andersson 2007, Kulu/Boyle 2009). Young and old single persons and childless couples move out of rural areas and smaller towns into the cities to work, study, have a metropolitan lifestyle, etc. These are compositional factors. Couples intending to form a family in the near future carry on residing where they have always lived. Prices and rents for housing in cities exceed those in the suburbs and rural areas so that larger apartments or houses with gardens for families are more easily affordable in the latter. The environment and infrastructure are better matched to families and the neighborhood also consists of families so that the children can play

[87] There are only two cities in total with more than half a million residents.

together. In expectation of or after the birth of their offspring, many couples move out of the cities and into suburbs or rural areas. This does not mean that all families leave the city centers, but larger families should be rather found outside of them.

The regressions show that the size of residence is significantly associated with fertility. No causal effect can be derived as long as selective movements cannot be properly excluded (this cannot be examined). The strength of the association rises with decreasing population size. This is most obvious in Hungary and among Norwegian women. Everywhere, women and men in large cities have fewest children (except for East Germany) and in non-urban areas they have most (which does not just mean "completely rural" or "village"). The fertility differences between the settlement sizes are partly considerable.

The question is whether the spatial distributional differences are responsible for varying fertility levels across countries. This question cannot be answered on the basis of the regression tables. Women and men living in Oslo or other urban areas of Norway have 2 children on average. In France, they have 1.84 children when they reside in a town. If the share of towns as a proportion of all settlement size categories were higher (it is in fact low), French fertility would fall below Norwegian fertility. In Norway the share of people who live in an "urban" area is already very high (in the GGS). At the country level, Norwegian and French fertility is equally high. In this case, it does not matter that "urban" in Norway does not really refer to a larger city. In rural areas of West Germany people have on average 1.76 children, the same applies to women in small towns (1.79). In cities with more than half a million inhabitants the value only amounts to 1.44 (women) respectively 1.34 (men). Fertility would be higher if the people lived more rurally, but even if all people did live in the country, fertility would never be as high as in Norway or France. In Budapest, women and men have 1.57 and 1.51 children while in the Hungarian villages they have 1.93 and 2.04 children on average.

Since life could be assumed to be more traditional in rural areas, people may also be more religious there. In cities the percentage of unaffiliated people is higher, while in smaller settlements the percentage of frequent attenders of religious services is higher. The exception is France, where absolutely no difference by settlement size can be measured. One reason might be that all Muslims exclusively dwell in urban areas (including towns). In Hungarian villages, almost all people are religiously affiliated while in Budapest about one fifth is unaffiliated, women somewhat less often than men.

Calvinists more often live in towns as well as villages, and Greek Catholics more often live rurally than in the capital (and than other affiliates). Greek Catholics have proven to be more fertile but this remained insignificant in the regressions. Their lower level of education and their stronger concentration in rural areas – both highly significant indicators – explain the insignificance of "being Greek Catholic". With respect to both other indicators, it is probable that people in more rural areas consider religious ceremonies at turning points in life and religious faith as child quality more important than inhabitants of urban areas and cities. The assumption holds with respect to ceremonies. The association is far from being overwhelming, but observable in many groups (French and Hungarian women and men, Norwegian women and West German men). An association between settlement size and religiosity is only observable among West German women. In rural areas 9.1% regard religious socialization as important, but only 4.5% in large cities think so (categories in-between: 7.8%).

6.3.3 Religiosity, modernization, integration, and fertility: the case of Turkish Muslims

The following subsection considers Muslims living in Germany and moved there from Turkey more closely. As they are in many respects different to the other "groups", it seems reasonable to dedicate a separate subsection to them. In this part of the work, the results of one joint model estimation integrating not only Turkish migrants but also East and West Germans will be presented. Following on, the results of the "pure" Muslim model estimations are discussed. A joint model estimation followed by group-specific estimations enables to assess whether the higher fertility among Muslims can be traced back to the lower modernization level of their country of origin – here however mainly restricted to their educational level – or to higher religiosity. The fertility behavior of migrants depends on (the modernization level of) the host country and its general fertility level, the country of origin and its culture, the duration of migrants' residence in the country of immigration (Sobotka 2008: 233, 236), their degree of integration (Spéder/Kamarás 2008: 611), as well as their socioeconomic position, i.e. educational achievement, earnings, and occupation (Algan et al. 2010). The subsection starts with a short description of the covariates.

The distributions of cohort affiliation and marital status that both strongly depend on gender have already been described jointly with all groups: Muslims are somewhat younger and more of them are still married for the first time. The composition of the

Muslims regarding educational and occupational attainment is specific. Levels are very low. One reason is that they come from a country with a much lower modernization level. The other reason is the requirement profiles at the time of their recruitment to Germany, because most of them (and/ or their spouses) are former labor migrants.[88] The government of Germany (and also France) mainly recruited semi- and unskilled workers with good physical health (see e.g. Herbert 1986, Erdoğan 2002, Wihtol de Wenden 2007). The educational situation is even more extreme with respect to the women: 85% of them have a low level of education compared to 72% of the male migrants (see tables A.8 and A.11 in the appendix). At the time of immigration, school attendance had not yet been fully enforced in many provinces of Turkey although compulsory schooling was introduced in 1924. Education was not regarded as essential, especially for girls (Unicef 2005). The result is that religious affiliation, integration aspects, and the socioeconomic status are closely associated with each other.[89]

But the (Muslim) migrants are not only lower educated, they also earn significantly less (see empirical evidence in Hubert/Althammer/Korucu-Rieger 2009: 45–51 and in Algan et al. 2010: 16–18). Moreover, only 14.2% own the apartment or house they reside in according to GGS. East Germans (43.8%) and West Germans (58.4%) own their dwelling much more often even though these are still low values in international comparison. As mentioned above, joint property can be considered marriage-specific capital stabilizing a union. In spite of the low rate of property ownership, the migrants' divorce rate is the lowest in comparison. Among them, property owners nevertheless have more stable marriages. There are only few owners whose marriages broke up. A strong connection is also true for East and West Germans.

One more reason for low property ownership rates is however that a higher share of migrants lives in large cities where prices for dwellings are much higher. 53% of the women and 45% of the men live in agglomerations with at least half a million

[88] According to the GGS, about 35% of the women have never been economically active. The variables for this measure exhibit a considerable rate of missings or unclear statements, so that the precise percentage is difficult to ascertain. The above mentioned rate refers to analyzable data only.

[89] Turkish migrants are however in no way the only migrants who have low educational and occupational attainments. This statement is indeed true for most of the former labor migrants who were recruited from abroad. Moreover, while almost all Muslims in Germany are migrants (and a large majority in France), only a small minority of all migrants are Muslims.

inhabitants (see table A.9 in the appendix).[90] Roughly one third – more male than female respondents – lives in central areas with 100,000–500,000 inhabitants or peripheral areas comprising at least 100,000 inhabitants. Finally, one sixth of the respondents reside in smaller localities (peripheral areas with 50,000–100,000 or central areas with 20,000–100,000 inhabitants). Only few Turkish migrants live in the Eastern part of the Republic. The settlement sizes just mentioned refer to the place of residence during adulthood. But according to the GGS, only 14.6% of the Turks immigrated to Germany before they were 18 years old and only few Muslims were born in Germany. Almost all of the Turks are first generation migrants. Insofar it would have been worthwhile to gather knowledge about the migrants' surroundings during childhood. Differences can be expected depending on their either stemming from rural provinces in East Anatolia or from Istanbul. The sociocultural premigration imprint should play an important role for fertility behavior. Finally, the migrants have 4.2 siblings on average. 43% have five or more siblings, a further 31% have three or four brothers and sisters. 8% are only children.

Until this point, East and West Germany have been analyzed separately from each other due to all the above mentioned differences. But now, one joint estimation is effected integrating the Muslim migrants. Table 6.28 show the results.[91] It is the only possibility to partly test whether the higher fertility among Muslims can be traced back to lower (material) modernization – here mainly restricted to educational attainment – or to higher religiosity. "Modernization" in general also comprises the modernization level of the country the migrants come from. This can however not be controlled for within the estimation. The special group composition requires the elimination of all other respondents with a migration background from the main survey.[92] Only autochthonal Germans remain in the data set.

[90] These percentages refer to the GGS data only. The real distribution deviates slightly. For data collection modalities and to avoid the danger of de-anonymization the sample was drawn in regions where sufficient migrants live.

[91] Turkish migrants quantitatively exceed East Germans. This does not reflect the real distribution of the population. Therefor, this model estimation is not unproblematic. Corrective weights are not available.

[92] The data problems force the exclusion of respondents (German and migrant data set) who have more than two children but seem to be lifelong singles or have never married. In the pure Muslim analyses the coefficient for "lifelong single" would otherwise be positive in the female case and positive for men who never married but are not lifelong single, which is impossible in reality (total number of excluded cases from all three data sets: women: N=121; men: N=45). In principle, this has no effect on the remaining coefficients.

The first finding is that under control of several covariates the fertility of Muslim migrants is significantly higher. Compared to the unaffiliated, Christians also have a higher fertility which is weakly significant among men, where the effect is induced by West German men. The latter result is a repetition of model estimation I. "Birth cohort" loses its strong negatively influence on fertility due to opposed effects in the behavior of migrants and Germans. Among migrants, the oldest cohort is least fertile while it is the other way round among Germans. Higher fertility among younger migrants counteracts the strong negative influence of Germans leading in total to no significant difference between the young and the old cohort. Only the coefficients for the middle cohort are significantly different from zero, somewhat stronger negatively for women than for men.

Compared to the reference group of a medium level of education, persons with a low and a high level of education have more children. Women are significantly more fertile if they only have a low level of education. In the descriptive perspective they have half a child more on average. Female Turkish migrants make up 50% of the respondents with a low level of education. Hence, it is they – in combination with the East German women – who cause the significant effect. The share of male migrants is almost 75% of all respondents with a low level of education and that group fathers half a child more on average. The effect is however almost captured by their being "Muslim and migrant". Being highly educated is also linked to higher fertility among both genders, but it is only significant among men. This is due to the low fertility of men with a medium level of education, also among the migrants.

Having never married remains associated with a significantly lower number of children. With respect to remarried or at least twice divorced men, the known results are again visible. They have most children. Concerning women, the effect has intensified. In the isolated model estimations the effect was only weakly significant. East Germans contribute to this result because they have an extremely high fertility (2.88). While in the isolated East German model, the effects must have been strong to become significant due to the smaller group size, this is not necessary here.

The probability for a higher number of children increases with the number of siblings. This result is highly significant among both genders but the influence is somewhat stronger among women. Settlement size loses its very strong significance for fertility levels due to the spatial distribution of the migrants. Their share is higher in areas where the fertility of Germans is traditionally lower, mainly in larger cities.

Table 6.28. Results of German models (East and West and Turkish migrants in Germany jointly)

	Women	Men
Muslim * Turkish migrant	0.233***	0.341***
Christian	0.052	0.092*
(Base category: unaffiliated		
Birth cohort 1949–1962	−0.065	−0.046
Birth cohort 1939–1952	−0.129**	−0.084*
(Base category: birth cohort 1930–1942)		
Low educ. attainment (isced 0–2)	0.133**	0.072
High educ. attainment (isced 5–6)	0.081	0.113**
(Base category: medium educational attainment (isced 3–4))		
Lifelong single	−0.603***	−1.119***
Never married but not lifelong single	−0.475***	−0.595***
Remarried/ divorced more than once	0.152**	0.256***
Divorced once	0.083	−0.092
(Base category: married for the 1st time/ widowed)		
Number of brothers and sisters	0.045***	0.032***
Up to 19,999 inhabitants	0.129*	0.170**
Peripheral area from 50–100,000/ central area from 20–100,000 inh.	0.095*	0.100*
Peripheral area from 100,000/ central area from 100–500,000 inh.	0.119**	0.055
(Base category: more than 500,000 inhabitants)		
East Germany	0.112*	0.105*
(Base category: West Germany)		
Constant	0.312***	0.219***
Numbers of observations	2409	2349
Wald chi^2	360.35	361.08
Pr $> \chi^2$	0.0000	0.0000
McFadden's pseudo R^2	0.040	0.055

Estimations are based on Poisson regression. Significance levels: * $p < 0.05$, ** $p < 0.01$, *** $p < 0.001$.

The second reason is the lack of fertility variance by settlement size among East German women. Among men, the linearity of effect strengths remains preserved. It is still men in rural areas who are most fertile (holding all other variables constant).

In direct comparison, East Germans have – controlling for religious affiliation – significantly more children than West Germans and this statements applies to both genders. To conclude, the higher fertility of Muslim migrants cannot be explained by the covariates. A robust significant effect supporting hypotheses H_{2a} and the second part of H_{2b} can again be documented. But currently it cannot yet be determined whether it is a mere modernization or a religiosity effect that is responsible.

Within the migrant group, religiosity hardly causes any variance with respect to fertility, neither among women nor among men (see table 6.29).[93] This means that (also) migrants who rarely or never participate in collective prayer, who regard religious ceremonies at turning points in life not as important or who do not define religious faith as an important child quality have more children than Germans. Among women, this statement even applies if non-religious Turkish migrants are compared with religious Germans. If two religiosity indicators are considered jointly, female Turkish migrants who frequently take part in religious services and moreover regard religious faith as an important child quality indeed have a higher fertility (2.57) than all other three combinations of female migrants. Frequent attending men who moreover consider religious faith as important have as many children as those both does not apply to. In this perspective, men who regularly join collective prayer but do not regard religious faith as important have most children (2.33), followed by the other way round (2.22).

Male Muslims who belong to the young birth cohort have significantly more children than the older cohort. This effect is very significant. Men in the middle cohort also have more children compared to the base category, but the effect is only significant in the second model estimation. In the model estimations for women, no coefficient differs significantly from zero. Fertility variance is smaller and the base category is much more fertile than the respective category of men.

Remarried men have proven to be more fertile than men who live in stable unions. This finding also applies to Turkish migrants. In contrast and hence in accordance with expectations, divorced men have a significantly lower fertility. These results accord with exceptions. However, both groups are very small due to great homogeneity of the Turkish migrants when it comes to their marital status. Apart from those who never married, the fertility of Turkish women cannot be discriminated by their marital status. The current settlement size does not play a major role for fertility behavior.

93 Religiosity only makes a difference in the group of women with more than a low level of education. In the group of women with a low level of education, fertility is equally high. In the young and middle cohorts, fertility differences by religiosity are hardly measurable. Only in the small group of women belonging to the oldest cohort is the attendance frequency of great importance. Both however do not explain why the coefficients have a negative sign.

This has already been reasoned in advance. The socialization period which mostly still occurred in Turkey (apart from a few exceptions all of the respondents were born there) has apparently left a stronger imprint on values and attitudes. Beyond this reason, selective movements – which among other things are assumed to be an important factor for the strong influence of the settlement size on fertility – may have played a minor role. However, among women the tendency is towards the expected because their fertility is somewhat lower in large cities than in areas with fewer inhabitants.

One childhood trait is available: the number of siblings. It can (again) be assumed that the number of siblings is higher when a person grew up rurally. The influence on fertility is strong and highly significant. The value of a bivariate correlation coefficient is $r = 0.31$ for women but only $r = 0.11$ for men. Among women, frequent participants of religious services have half a sibling more than rare attenders (4.67 vs. 4.15). The people with the lowest level of education also have most siblings. The number of brothers and sisters does not differ by participation frequency among men.

Migrants with a low level of education have more children but it is only (weakly) significant among women. In contrast, the educational effect among men does not exist in the young cohort (which in turn is very significant). It is restricted to the other two cohorts. Due to the very low educational level of the migrants, the category "low education" should be further differentiated into "primary level", which corresponds to isced 1, and "lower secondary level", which is isced 2. Quantitatively, migrants with primary level education are the largest group, especially among women. If the models are re-estimated with stronger particularized (low) education categories (not tabulated here), it becomes obvious that the significant effect mainly rests upon the very low educational level of women (primary level), whose significance rises, while the coefficient indicating women with a lower secondary level does not significantly deviate from zero. In a descriptive perspective, women with a very low educational level have 2.5 children (primary level), women with a low educational level have 2.08 (lower secondary level) and the remaining women have 1.93 children on average. In an additional model estimation for men, both coefficients remain insignificant (numbers of children: 2.15, 2.32, 1.81). Women who attended school only briefly (or even not at all) also began family formation earlier. And those who attended for a longer time, began later. Women with a very low educational level exhibit the lowest rate of ever having been economically active. From the perspective of the human

Table 6.29. Results of the models of Turkish migrants

	Women	Men	Women	Men	Women	Men
Frequent attendance of religious services	−0.065	0.054				
Religious ceremonies important			−0.013	0.003		
Religious faith important					0.103	−0.004
Birth cohort 1949–1962	0.079	0.349**	0.086	0.372**	0.129	0.325**
Birth cohort 1939–1952	−0.034	0.208	−0.032	0.236*	0.007	0.201
(Base category: birth cohort 1930–1942)						
Low educ. attainment (isced 0–2)	0.244*	0.117	0.239*	0.107	0.238*	0.127
(Base category: medium or high educational attainment (isced 3–6))						
Lifelong single	−0.396**	−1.409***	−0.376*	−1.351***	−0.372*	−1.418***
Never married but not lifelong single	−1.166***	−0.991*	−1.145**	−1.005*	−1.206***	−1.022*
Remarried/ divorced more than once	0.000	0.299*	0.027	0.298*	0.028	0.294*
Divorced once	−0.027	−0.739*	−0.057	−0.746*	0.008	−0.756*
(Base category: married for the 1st time/ widowed)						
Number of brothers and sisters	0.054***	0.039***	0.057***	0.041***	0.055***	0.041***
Peripheral area from 50–100,000/ central area from 20–100,000 inhabitants	0.126	0.101	0.148	0.103	0.150	0.087
Peripheral area from 100,000/ central area from 100–500,000 inhabitants	0.067	−0.026	0.072	−0.024	0.066	−0.015
(Base category: more than 500,000 inhabitants)						
Constant	0.349	0.238	0.424	0.211	0.229	0.273
Numbers of observations	432	478	416	461	426	471
Wald chi^2	61.222	69.915	57.711	68.130	61.089	70.239
Pr > χ^2	0.0000	0.0001	0.0000	0.0001	0.0000	0.0001
McFadden's pseudo R^2	0.045	0.040	0.039	0.041	0.040	0.041

Estimations are based on negative binomial models. Significance levels: * $p < 0.05$, ** $p < 0.01$, *** $p < 0.001$

capital theory, this behavior is comprehensible. It should not be forgotten however that the earnings capacities of the spouse who often has also only little education is restricted, making a second income indispensable. With respect to fertility however, women who were never economically active do not differ from women who were workers or are still employed as workers.[94]

The absence of category isced 0 (preprimary education) can be compensated by additional information on writing and speaking skills (see table 6.30). They measure literacy but also one dimension of integration (linguistic integration) and the results again makes the gender gap obvious. Women have less skills due to less education. As expected, almost all speak Turkish fluently. Only one in ten has outstanding speaking skills in the German language. 38% speak German at least "good". A relative majority has medium language skills and almost one fourth speaks German "rather bad" or even "not at all". One tenth is not able to write Turkish, and one fourth has no skills in writing German. Less than one fifth evaluate their skills as good or even better. If writing skills of both languages are crossed, it becomes apparent that 9% of the women are illiterate (men: 0.6%). If percentages of "rather bad" and "not at all" are summed up, the share amounts to 17% (men: 2.6%).[95] This procedure helps to further differentiate the isced 1 group and also provides further information regarding demographic behavior. Illiterate women have 2.84 children on average. This means that the significant effect has by and large been finally generated by these women. This is not the case for men. The effect is only measurable if men are restricted to those who cannot write German at all. That minority has 3.11 children. The remaining male groups have less than 2 children and men with very good skills have least children (1.7).

Speaking practice can be interpreted as an integration indicator.[96] Women who mainly communicate in Turkish at home have 2.4 children, women who mainly

[94] The spouses of the migrants resemble them with respect to citizenship, country of birth, and native language. 54% have the same level of education. In most of the other cases, the male spouse is better educated. Fertility in the partner perspective (dependent on the condition that there is a partner of course) among women is highest if both partners have only primary level education (2.94). Such a clear statement cannot be made for men.

[95] Principally, all ascribed themselves to category "isced 1".

[96] It is plausible to assume that the degree of integration influences fertility. However, in principle this cannot be measured correctly because as speaking and writing skills are a continuous developmental process while fertility has been concluded. On the one hand, the following analyses must be interpreted with care. On the other hand, this process does not occur in people who are not inclined or able to learn the language of the host country, also in written form.

speak German have only 1.9 children. Finally, women who mix both languages are in between ("partly ... partly": 2.24 children). Men exhibit absolutely no difference concerning language practice.

Table 6.30. Speaking and writing skills of Turkish migrants

	Speaking				Writing			
	Turkish		German		Turkish		German	
	Women	Men	Women	Men	Women	Men	Women	Men
Very good	69.3	65.6	8.5	11.3	44.0	48.7	4.3	5.5
Good	28.9	30.0	24.2	31.6	28.3	37.2	9.9	16.8
Medium	1.3	3.9	36.9	40.0	10.8	10.8	23.0	28.1
Rather bad	0.5	0.4	28.2	16.1	7.8	2.6	29.6	33.7
Not at all	0.0	0.2	2.4	1.0	9.2	0.8	33.2	15.9
Nobs	462	501	462	500	462	501	462	500

Age group 45–74, birth cohorts 1930–1962. In %; weighted data.

To summarize, Muslims have more children than the unaffiliated and Christians but this mainly does not seem to be an effect of religiosity. Rather, it is a "modernization (and integration) effect".[97] First, the migrants originate from Turkey which – compared to Germany – has a noticeably lower HDI rank (83 vs. 10 in 2010; United Nations Development Programme (UNDP) 2010). Secondly, there is a pronounced fertility effect for education among women. In many cases this is equal to the lack of any education or means that merely elementary school has been completed. Thirdly, family structures and gender roles are still traditional (Just 2011: 191). However, these statements are only valid if religiosity has been measured reliably. Findings from other studies show that their values on other religiosity indicators are higher (Bertelsmann Stiftung 2008, Haug/Müssig/Stichs 2009: 137–166, Just 2011: 193–201). This is of special importance as it is well known that women practice religiosity more privately. The relevance for fertility must remain untested. The controlled indicators available here have already documented a generally higher religiosity level. The result can moreover be interpreted as accuracy of the socialization hypothesis postulating that migration does not influence fertility (Schmid/Kohls 2011: 34). Rather, the values and norms women and men grew up with during childhood in the country of origin are

[97] Basically, modernization can be interpreted as a third variable that has an impact on both religiosity and fertility.

more decisive. A hint is given by the absence of a notable correlation between age at immigration (restricted to persons below the age of 41) and the number of children.

7 Conclusion

These final paragraphs summarize the dissertation. It has investigated the impact of religiosity of both genders born between 1930 and 1962 on the completed number of (biological and adopted) children in comparative perspective. The goal was to provide evidence that religiosity has a positive effect on the realized number of children. The study has been based on a design of several European countries with differing demographic and denominational patterns, institutional and legal contexts, social norms, degrees of religious vitality, and state-church relations. These countries are France, Hungary, Norway, as well as East and West Germany. The selection of countries rested upon the expectation that religiosity influences fertility decisions independent of all these differences. The countries have been systematically compared with each other resulting in a cross-country study. It has not only taken account of women but also men to observe gender-specific behavior as well as effects. A relatively broad time period (roughly 1950–2010) has been considered during which fertility has experienced the second demographic transition whose consequence was a remarkable decline in the number of children born (per woman). Due to the assumption that religiosity is not only able to affect fertility at the individual level, the macrolevel has been explicitly integrated as well. As fertility decisions are usually made by a couple, preferences of both partners have been regarded. One specific characteristic of this work has consequently been the consideration of several dimensions.

The theoretical approach was embedded in the economic theory of the family and adopted its assumptions. It has combined economic factors with religiosity and argued that religiosity promotes fertility both directly and indirectly. The direct effect referred to denomination-specific norms and rules with respect to family behavior as well as religious socialization, identification with one's own religious tradition and other affiliates, the religious network, and organizational characteristics (theological strictness, hierarchy of the structure, communicability of teachings). The indirect effect was derived from the religious composition of a couple that either stabilizes a marriage or endangers its stability. A pronounced stability was supposed to promote a higher number of children. Confidence in marital stability has for several reasons been assumed to be especially elevated if both spouses are either religious Catholics or Muslims. Couples with a heterogamous religious affiliation and religiosity or in which both partners are unaffiliated may be confronted with insecurity and decisions enforcing compromises. The anticipation of instability or a high divorce risk discourages the partners from investing in children and further marriage-specific capital. Instead, both concentrate on their commitment in the labor market. A so-called marital stability effect and a bargaining effect have been assumed to result. Since not only religiosity has an impact on marital stability, one part of the work has dealt with characteristics that promote or threaten the stability of a union. Among these are e.g. parental divorce, (female) full-time employment, the age at marriage, the size of settlement, and joint property. Some of them are associated with religiosity on their own.

One part of the study has dealt with the definition of religion and religiosity. While the religiosity definition is of a psychological nature, the multi-dimensional measurement concept of religiosity originates from sociology. The aggregated influence of religiosity on fertility depends on the population share of religious individuals. The national level of religious vitality itself is affected by three historical-cultural patterns that interact with each other: the degree of modernization, state-church relations, and the dominating denominational cultural tradition. Modernization processes or a high degree of modernization and church-hostile politics (e.g. in socialist states) lower religious vitality. Concerning the last pattern, predominantly Catholic countries show a higher religious vitality than countries with a Protestant imprint. Several reasons have been discussed. For example, a higher degree of internal rationalization can be ascribed to Protestantism and it has a stronger anchorage in contemporary societies. Moreover, it is more individualistic. In contrast, Catholicism is more conservative in its theological perspective and the church is the mediator between God and the affiliates which raises the frequency of attendance. Church traditions have normative orientation power. France is an exception: although most people are affiliated to the Catholic Church, religiosity is at a very low level.

Empirically, the hypotheses have been tested by estimating Poisson and negative binomial regression models on the basis of the *Generations and Gender Study* (GGS, wave I). It could be demonstrated that religious affiliation and religiosity are linked to a higher fertility supporting the direct effects proposed for religiosity. Religiously affiliated individuals have on average more children than unaffiliated people. Among the affiliated, Muslims have more children than all other affiliates. Moreover, Muslims in France have noticeably more children than Muslims in Germany though they are less religious. Due to the non-negligible share of Alevis among the Turkish Muslims in Germany, their total religiosity level could have been assumed as lower. Catholics are – against expectations – not more fertile than Protestants. Only the religious minority of Greek Catholics in Hungary gave birth to or fathered more children than Protestants (in a national perspective). Frequent attenders of religious services have on average more children than people who rarely or never attend and persons who approve of religious ceremonies at turning points in life complete fertility on average at higher levels. The same affirmative finding cannot be repeated for individuals who think that religious faith is an important child quality. While frequency of participation in religious services is an indicator for the dimension of ritual, the last two indicators cannot be assigned to one of the religiosity dimensions of the elaborate concept introduced in this study but have been included for explorative reasons. Not all reported effects of religiosity are statistically significant after having controlled for further important determinants of fertility – mainly birth cohort, educational attainment, marital status, size of settlement, and migration background. The interpretation has been that not all effects are directly observable. Religiosity is correlated with many of these determinants, what has been attested.

Religiosity, marital stability, and fertility interact. A stable marriage has been used as an ex-post indicator to measure a divorce risk that was perceived ex-ante as low by both spouses and led to the non-restriction of their marital investments. The effects of religious affiliation and religiosity on marital stability have been shown to be noticeable. Contrary to expectations however, marital stability – among men – is not associated with the highest number of children. Rather, they are most fertile when they are remarried. The positive fertility effects of remarriage are (apart from Norwegian men) stable and statistically significant. When it comes to women, results are more mixed. The proposed effects of instability hold in some cases (Norwegian and Hungarian women have significantly fewer children). Men's completely absent negative effect may also be explained with their lower risks in case of a divorce compared to women. It is mainly women who bear the consequences of divorce: in case of employment breaks due to family tasks they have to accept lower wages and find more unfavorable conditions after their re-entry into the labor market and they are confronted with lone parenthood. Remarriage is often linked to having children from more than one union. When different marital status groups are limited to people who have children from one union only and then compared with each other, it could be shown that stable marriages (mostly) produce more children. Apart from marital stability, persons who have married at least once have more children than persons who never married (excluding lifelong singles). As the fragility of unmarried unions is higher than of married ones, a marriage itself can be interpreted as an indicator for relationship stability increasing the willingness to invest in the relationship.

One model estimation varied religiosity by birth cohort because in older birth cohorts both fertility and religiosity levels were higher. This procedure prevented the confounding of religiosity and cohort effects. For Spain, Alicia Adsera found that in younger birth cohorts religious practice is necessary to discriminate people's demographic behavior, while in older birth cohorts affiliation itself was a sufficiently informative indicator. This result could be by and large reproduced in this work, which is due to the fact that fertility among religious people has decreased least. It had been assumed that behavioral changes (falling numbers of children) not only occurred among the growing group of unaffiliated people, but also among the affiliated, while only highly religious individuals were excluded. They tend to marry homogamously which keeps their divorce risk low. Moreover, people who plan large families (according to the argumentation here: people who have a functionally autonomous religious motivational system) are not affected too much by environmental – institutional, political, and societal – circumstances and changing general conditions such as the increasing cost of time.

As part of the German GGS, a supplemental survey of migrants originating from Turkey and living in Germany for many years was conducted so that the opportunity to involve Muslims into the analysis could be used. Usually, both migrants and Muslims are under-represented in surveys. The goal was to assess whether their significantly higher fertility (compared to Christians and unaffiliated individuals) is a religiosity effect or rather a consequence of the lower (material, institutional, and ideological) modernization level of their country of origin. Moreover, most of the migrants are former guest workers with very low levels of educational and occupational attainment. First, the Muslims' degree of religiosity is much higher (compared to Christians and others). Second, religiosity hardly causes variance with respect to fertility, neither among women nor among men. Illiterate women who are neither able to write Turkish nor German have the highest number of children. This is however not the case for men. The effect is only measurable if men are restricted to the small minority of those men who cannot write German at all. This however rather reminds of an integration effect. Results are subject to the correct measurement of religiosity; it could however not be fully measured.

In addition to religiosity, the significance of further, already well-researched determinants of fertility could be confirmed. The family of origin, if measured by the number of siblings, exerts a consistently highly positive and significant impact on family size. According to the argumentation of the theoretical approach, individuals with many siblings were raised by religious parents and probably experienced a religious socialization. The second indicator representing the family of origin was the migration background or ethnic group. Roma in Hungary and (North) Africans in France have significantly more children compared to the respective autochthonal population. Their high fertility does not rest upon high religiosity. Women with a low level of education gave birth to significantly more children than women with a medium or high educational level while the latter two groups could not be distinguished on the basis of their birth behavior. Results for men were not so clear: only Hungarians are significantly more fertile if they have a low level of education and only in West Germany do highly-educated men have significantly more children. Concerning the time dimension, it could be shown that fertility has not decreased linearly. The oldest cohort (people born between 1930 and 1942) who had their fertile period in the 1950s and 1960s gave birth to most children. The remaining cohorts did not differ very much from each other. Concerning the size of settlement, the common finding of other studies that people in larger cities have (in all countries) smaller families than people in rural or peripheral areas has also been supported here.

A literature-based analysis was carried out to demonstrate an intermediate influence of religious institutions on fertility (macrolevel). The differentiation of levels has revealed that contradictory effects on fertility are possible: while individual religiosity in general positively affects fertility, church influences on policy-making and arrangements as well as on social norms (e.g. towards maternal employment) can have negative effects. It could be shown that (in some countries) a strong Catholic Church promoting traditional family life has probably contributed to decreasing fertility, lower female labor supply, and less gender equality. West Germany, where state-church relations are in general cooperative and the principles of Catholic social teachings build one foundation of policy-making, serves as a good example. In contrast, the Protestant (state) church with its individualistic principles has been supporting gender equality (e.g. in Norway) which has lead to policies promoting female labor force participation and the availability of public child care. These results have made the divergence between the societal and individual level obvious. While individual secularization has proceeded far (rather in Norway than in West Germany), the churches keep power over policy-making and public opinion. In Hungary, East Germany, and France, laicism as the result of struggles between church and state prevented church influences on policy-making and outcomes. Especially in France, but also in Hungary, this has led to a relatively high fertility because the arrangement of family policies was strongly motivated by pro-natalism. While the fertility outcome and the degree of state support are similarly high in Norway and France, the kinds of support, the ideological background, motives, and justification for state interventions differ quite considerably. Hence, state-church relations do not only influence the level of religious vitality at the individual level but also the degree of secularization at the macrolevel.

This work has tried to uncover all paths and mechanisms through which religious institutions and religiosity can affect fertility. The total (multifold) effect of religiosity, religious institutions, and religious traditions on demographic behavior can however not be evaluated. Nevertheless, religiosity should definitely not be underestimated when it comes to fertility (and still less in the case of marital stability). Norwegians in general have confirmed the presuppositions and hypotheses best: religiosity has strong direct and indirect effects on completed fertility. Marital stability leads to more children among Norwegian women but this is independent of their level of religiosity. All the religiosity indicators used have led to significant results and the effects have been largest compared to the other countries. This is a rather surprising result because Norway is a country where economic security and the level of decommodification are high and the rights of fathers after separation are far-reaching. Therefore, investing in marriage-specific capital is connected to a lower risk even if the partners anticipate a certain divorce probability. This statement is especially valid in the comparative perspective. The share of religious people related to the population is small, however, so that the total fertility effect generated by individual religiosity is not very pronounced. Referring to the macrolevel, the influence of the Protestant state church on policy-making and attitudes presumably also contributed to a high general fertility level among Norwegians who cannot be characterized as religious at the microlevel. Results with respect to other countries are more mixed. Some assumptions hold while others do not. Direct religiosity effects have been shown to be stronger among men while indirect effects only applied to women. The effects of religiosity on fertility are mainly restricted to countries without a socialist past (i.e. Hungary and East Germany).

In this work, the emphasis was on the comparison between countries. One reason for this must be seen in data limitations. The GGS does not have a multi-actor design and hence does not offer much information on the current partner and no information on former partners. A proper examination of the theoretical approach would have required taking account of characteristics of both partners and not only of the interviewed person. So, future research should concentrate on the dimension of the couple.

References

AASSVE, ARNSTEIN, BILLARI, FRANCESCO C., SPÉDER, ZSOLT (2006): Societal transition, policy changes and family formation: evidence from Hungary. In: *European Journal of Population*, 22 No. 2, pp. 127–152

ADSERA, ALICIA (2004): Marital fertility and religion: recent changes in Spain. In: *IZA Discussion Paper* No. 1399

ADSERA, ALICIA (2005): Where are the babies? Labor market conditions and fertility in Europe. In: *IZA Discussion Paper* No. 1576

ADSERA, ALICIA (2006): Marital fertility and religion in Spain, 1985 and 1999. In: *Population Studies*, 60 No. 2, pp. 205–221

ADSERA, ALICIA (2007): Reply to the note by Neuman: is fertility indeed related to relgiosity? In: *Population Studies*, 61 No. 2, pp. 225–230

ADSERA, ALICIA (2008): Fertility in developed countries. In: *Durlauf, Steven N./Blume, Lawrence E., editors:* The new Palgrave dictionary of economics. Basingstoke and Hampshire: Palgrave Macmillan, pp. 287–290

AHN, NAMKEE, MIRA, PEDRO (2002): A note on the changing relationship between fertility and female employment rates in developed countries. In: *Journal of Population Economics*, 15 No. 13, pp. 667–682

ALESINA, ALBERTO, GIULIANO, PAOLA (2006): Divorce, fertility and the shot gun marriage. In: *NBER Working Paper* No. 12375

ALESINA, ALBERTO, GIULIANO, PAOLA (2007): The power of the family. In: *IZA Discussion Paper* No. 2750

ALGAN, YANN ET AL. (2010): The economic situation of first- and second-generation immigrants in France, Germany, and the UK. In: *Economic Journal*, 120 No. 542, pp. F4–F30

ALLPORT, GORDON W. (1950): The individual and his religion: a psychological interpretation. New York: MacMillan

ALLPORT, GORDON W. (1961): Pattern and growth in personality. New York: Holt Rinehart & Winston

ALLPORT, GORDON W., ROSS, J. MICHAEL (1967): Personal religious orientation and prejudice. In: *Journal of Personality and Social Psychology*, 5 No. 4, pp. 432–443

ALTHAMMER, JÖRG (2000): Ökonomische Theorie der Familienpolitik: Theoretische und empirische Befunde zu ausgewählten Problemen staatlicher Familienpolitik. Heidelberg: Physica

AMATO, PAUL R. (1996): Explaining the intergenerational transmission of divorce. In: *Journal of Marriage and Family*, 58 No. 3, pp. 628–640

ANDERSSON, GUNNAR (2003): Dissolution of unions in Europe: a comparative overview. In: *MPIDR Working Paper* No. 004

ANDERSSON, GUNNAR (2004): Childbearing developments in Denmark, Norway, and Sweden from the 1970s to the 1990s: a comparison. In: *Demographic Research*, 3 No. 7, pp. 155–176

ANDERSSON, GUNNAR ET AL. (2009): Cohort fertility patterns in the Nordic countries. In: *Demographic Research*, 20 No. 14, pp. 313–352

APPS, PATRICIA, REES, RAY (2004): Fertility, taxation, and family policy. In: *Scandinavian Journal of Economics*, 106 No. 4, pp. 745–763

AUFFARTH, CHRISTOPH, MOHR, HUBERT (2006a): Introduction: the academic study of religion - historical and contemporary issues. In: *Stuckrad, Kocku von, editor:* The Brill dictionary of religion. Leiden: Brill, pp. xi–xxxvi

AUFFARTH, CHRISTOPH, MOHR, HUBERT (2006b): Religion. In: *Stuckrad, Kocku von, editor:* The Brill dictionary of religion. Leiden: Brill, pp. 1607–1619

AZZI, CORRY, EHRENBERG, RONALD G. (1975): Household allocation of time and church attendance. In: *Journal of Political Economy*, 83 No. 1, pp. 27–56

BACLET, ALEXANDRE ET AL. (2005): Verteilungseffekte der staatlichen Familienförderung – Ein empirischer Vergleich zwischen Deutschland und Frankreich: Kurzexpertise. Forschungsprojekt im Auftrag der Hans-Böckler-Stiftung. Forschungsschwerpunkt "Zukunft des Sozialstaats". In: *DIW Berlin: Politikberatung kompakt* No. 9

BAHLE, THOMAS (1995): Familienpolitik in Westeuropa: Ursprünge und Wandel im internationalen Vergleich. Frankfurt am Main and New York: Campus

Banchoff, Thomas F., editor (2007): Democracy and the new religious pluralism. Oxford and New York: Oxford University Press

BARGAIN, OLIVIER ET AL. (2012): Female labor supply and divorce: new evidence from Ireland. In: *European Economic Review*, 56 No. 8, pp. 1675–1691

BARLAI, MELANI, HARTLEB, FLORIAN (2007): Ungarn – vom Musterknaben zum Sorgenkind der Europäischen Union. In: *Politische Studien*, 58 No. 411, p. 95

BARLAI, MELANI, HARTLEB, FLORIAN (2009): Die Roma in Ungarn. In: *Aus Politik und Zeitgeschichte (APuZ)*, No. 29-30, pp. 33–39

BEAUFTRAGTE DER BUNDESREGIERUNG FÜR MIGRATION, FLÜCHTLINGE UND INTEGRATION (2007): 7. Bericht der Beauftragten der Bundesregierung für Migration, Flüchtlinge und Integration über die Lage der Ausländerinnen und Ausländer in Deutschland. Berlin

BEBLO, MIRIAM (2001): Bargaining over time allocation: economic modeling and econometric investigation of time use within families. Heidelberg: Physica

BECKER, GARY S. (1960): An economic analysis of fertility. In: *Becker, Gary S., editor:* Demographic and economic change in developed countries. Princeton: University Press, pp. 209–231

BECKER, GARY S. (1965): A theory of the allocation of time. In: *Economic Journal*, 75 No. 299, pp. 493–517

BECKER, GARY S. (1973): A theory of marriage: part I. In: *Journal of Political Economy*, 81 No. 4, pp. 813–846

BECKER, GARY S. (1981): A treatise on the family. Cambridge and London: Harvard University Press

BECKER, GARY S., LANDES, ELISABETH M., MICHAEL, ROBERT T. (1977): An economic analysis of marital instability. In: *Journal of Political Economy*, 85 No. 6, pp. 1141–1187

BECKER, GARY S., LEWIS, H. GREGG (1973): On the interaction between the quantity and quality of children. In: *Journal of Political Economy*, 81 No. 2 (Part 2: New Economic Approaches to Fertility), pp. S279–S288

BECKER, GARY S., TOMES, NIGEL (1976): Child endowments and the quantity and quality of children. In: *Journal of Political Economy*, 84 No. 4, pp. S143–62

BECKER, SASCHA O., WOESSMANN, LUDGER (2008): Luther and the girls: Religious denomination and the female education gap in 19th century Prussia. In: *CESIFO Working Paper* No. 2414

BECKER, SASCHA O., WOESSMANN, LUDGER (2009): Was Weber wrong? A human capital theory of Protestant economic history. In: *Quarterly Journal of Economics*, 124 No. 2, pp. 531–596

BERGER, PETER L. (1963): A market model for the analysis of ecumenicity. In: *Social Research*, 30 No. 1, pp. 77–93

BERGER, PETER L. (1969): The sacred canopy: Elements of a sociological theory of religion. New York: Doubleday

Berger, Peter L. ET AL., *editors* (2005): The desecularization of the world: Resurgent religion and world politics. Washington D.C.: Ethics and Public Policy Center

BERGGREN, NICLAS (1997): Rhetoric or reality? An economic analysis of the effects of religion in Sweden. In: *Journal of Socio-Economics*, 26 No. 6, pp. 571–596

BERINDE, DIANA (1999): Pathways to a third child in Sweden. In: *European Journal of Population*, 15 No. 4, pp. 349–378

Bertelsmann Stiftung, editor (2008): Religion monitor. Muslim religiousness in Germany. Overview of religious attitudes and practices. Gütersloh: Bertelsmann Stiftung

BESEMERES, JOHN F. (1980): Socialist population politics: The political implications of demographic trends in the USSR and Eastern Europe. White Plains: M.E. Sharpe

BILLARI, FRANCESCO C. (2005): Partnership, childbearing and parenting: Trends of the 1990s. In: *Macura, Miroslav/Macdonald, Alphonse L./Haug, Werner, editors:* The new demographic regime: Population challenges and policy responses. New York: United Nations, pp. 63–94

BISCHOF STENGER, MARC (2009): Laicité und ihre Bedeutung für die Verfassung Europas. In: *Kranemann, Benedikt/Wijlens, Myriam, editors:* Religion und Laicité in Frankreich: Entwicklungen, Herausforderungen und Perspektiven. Würzburg: Echter, pp. 69–78

BISIN, ALBERTO, VERDIER, THIERRY A. (2000): "Beyond the melting pot": Cultural transmission, marriage, and the evolution of ethnic and religious traits. In: *Quarterly Journal of Economics*, 115 No. 3, pp. 955–988

BISIN, ALBERTO, VERDIER, THIERRY A. (2010): The economics of cultural transmission and socialization. In: *NBER Working Paper* No. 16512

BJÖRKLUND, ANDERS (2006): Does family policy affect fertility? In: *Journal of Population Economics*, 19 No. 1, pp. 3–24

BLASCHKE, OLAF (2006): Catholicism. In: *Stuckrad, Kocku von, editor:* The Brill dictionary of religion. Leiden: Brill, pp. 265–270

BLASI, ANTHONY J. (1998): Definition of religion. In: *Swatos Jr., William H., editor:* Encyclopedia of religion and society. Walnut Creek: AltaMira Press, pp. 129–132

BLAU, FRANCINE D., FERBER, MARIANNE A., WINKLER, ANNE E. (2002): The economics of women, men, and work. Upper Saddle River: Prentice Hall

BLAU, FRANCINE D., KAHN, LAWRENCE M. (2000): Gender differences in pay. In: *Journal of Economic Perspectives*, 14 No. 4, pp. 75–99

BLOOM, DAVID E. ET AL. (2007): Fertility, female labor force participation, and the demographic dividend. In: *NBER Working Paper* No. 13583

BLOSSFELD, HANS-PETER, HUININK, JOHANNES (1991): Human capital investments or norms of role transition? How women's schooling and career affect the process of family formation. In: *American Journal of Sociology*, 97 No. 1, pp. 143–168

BLUM, SONJA, RILLE-PFEIFFER, CHRISTIANE (2010): Existential Field 3: Major trends of state family policies in Europe. In: *FAMILYPLATFORM Working Report*

BLUME, CARSTEN, RAMSEL, CARSTEN, GRAUPNER, SVEN (2006): Religiosity as a demographic factor – an underestimated connection? In: *Marburg Journal of Religion*, 11 No. 1, pp. 1–22

BODENMANN, GUY ET AL. (2006): Attractors and barriers to divorce: A retrospective study in three European countries. In: *Journal of Divorce & Remarriage*, 45 No. 3/4, pp. 1–23

BOELE-WOELKI, KATHARINA ET AL. (2004): Principles of European family law regarding divorce and maintenance between former spouses. Anwerp: Intersentia

BOEREE, C. GEORGE (2006): Personality theories. George Kelly. ⟨URL: `http://webspace.ship.edu/cgboer/kelly.html`⟩ – visited on 05 Mar 2012

BOROOAH, VANI K. (2004): The politics of demography: A study of inter-community fertility differences in India. In: *European Journal of Political Economy*, 20 No. 3, pp. 551–578

BÖTTCHER, KARIN (2006): Scheidung in Ost-und Westdeutschland. Der Einfluss der Frauenerwerbstätigkeit auf die Ehestabilität. In: *MPIDR Working Paper* No. 016

BRAÑAS-GARZA, PABLO, NEUMAN, SHOSHANA (2006): Is fertility related to religiosity? – Evidence from Spain. In: *IZA Discussion Paper* No. 2192

BRAÑAS-GARZA, PABLO, NEUMAN, SHOSHANA (2007): Parental religiosity and daughters' fertility: The case of Catholics in southern Europe. In: *Review of Economics of the Household*, 5 No. 3, pp. 305–327

BREUER, RITA (2008): Familienleben im Islam: Traditionen, Konflikte, Vorurteile. Freiburg: Herder

BREWSTER, KARIN L., RINDFUSS, RONALD R. (2000): Fertility and women's employment in industrialized countres. In: *Annual Review of Sociology*, 26, pp. 271–296

BRIEN, MICHAEL J., LILLARD, LEE A., STERN, STEVEN (2006): Cohabitation, marriage, and divorce in a model of match quality. In: *International Economic Review*, 47 No. 2, pp. 451–494

BROWN, SARAH, TAYLOR, KARL (2003): Religion and education: evidence from the National Child Development Study. In: *Discussion Papers in Economics* No. 16

BRUCE, STEVE (2002): God is dead: Secularization in the West. Oxford: Blackwell

BRÜDERL, JOSEF, KALTER, FRANK (2001): The dissolution of marriages: The role of information and marital-specific capital. In: *Journal of Mathematical Sociology*, 25 No. 4, pp. 403–421

BUJARD, MARTIN ET AL. (2012): (Keine) Lust auf Kinder? Geburtenentwicklung in Deutschland. Wiesbaden: Bundesinstitut für Bevölkerungsforschung

BUMPASS, LARRY L., SWEET, JAMES A. (1972): Differentials in marital instability: 1970. In: *American Sociological Review*, 37 No. 6, pp. 754–766

BUNDESMINISTERIUM DES INNERN (2008): Migration und Integration: Aufenthaltsrecht, Migrations- und Integrationspolitik in Deutschland. Berlin

BUNDESMINISTERIUM FÜR FAMILIE, SENIOREN, FRAUEN UND JUGEND (2006): Familie zwischen Flexibilität und Verlässlichkeit. Perspektiven für eine lebenslaufbezogene Familienpolitik. Siebter Familienbericht: Stellungnahme der Bundesregierung zum Bericht der Sachverständigenkommission. Bericht der Sachverständigenkommission. Berlin

CALL, VAUGHN R. A., HEATON, TIM B. (1997): Religious influence on marital stability. In: *Journal for the Scientific Study of Religion*, 36 No. 3, pp. 382–392

CASANOVA, JOSÉ (1994): Public religions in the modern world. Chicago: University of Chicago Press

CASANOVA, JOSÉ (2003): Beyond European and American exceptionalisms: Towards a global perspective. In: *Davie, Grace/Heelas, Paul/Woodhead, Linda, editors:* Predicting religion: Christian, secular and alternative futures. Aldershot: Ashgate, pp. 17–29

CASANOVA, JOSÉ (2007): Die religiöse Lage in Europa. In: *Joas, Hans/Wiegandt, Klaus, editors:* Säkularisierung und die Weltreligionen. Frankfurt am Main: Fischer Taschenbuch Verlag, pp. 322–357

CHÉLINI-PONT, BLANDINE (2007): French Catholics, secularization, and politics. In: *Hargreaves, Alec G., editor:* Politics and religion in France and the United States. Lanham: Lexington Books, pp. 79–93

CHRISTOFIDES, LOUIS N., POLYCARPOU, ALEXANDROS, VRACHIMIS, KONSTANTINOS (2010): The gender wage gaps, 'sticky floors' and 'glass ceilings' of the European Union. In: *IZA Discussion Paper* No. 5044

Clarke, Peter B., editor (2009): The Oxford handbook of the sociology of religion. Oxford and New York: Oxford University Press

COPPOLA, LUCIA, DI CESARE, MARIACHIARA (2008): How fertility and union stability interact in shaping new family patterns in Italy and Spain. In: *Demographic Research*, 18 No. 4, pp. 117–144

COUNCIL OF EUROPE (2003): Hungary. ⟨URL: `http://www.coe.int/t/e/social_cohesion/population/demographic_year_book/2003_edition/04%20country%20data/Member%20States/Hungary/Hungary%20General%20Page.asp`⟩ – visited on 01 Nov 2012

CROMM, JÜRGEN (1998): Familienbildung in Deutschland: Soziodemographische Prozesse, Theorie, Recht und Politik unter besonderer Berücksichtigung der DDR. Opladen: Westdeutscher Verlag

D'ADDIO, ANNA C., D'ERCOLE, MARCO M. (2005): Trends and determinants of fertility rates: The role of policies. In: *OECD Social Employment and Migration Working Papers* No. 27

DALY, MARY (2005): Changing family life in Europe: Significance for state and society. In: *European Societies*, 7 No. 3, pp. 379–398

DAVIE, GRACE (2002): Europe: The exceptional case: Parameters of faith in the modern world. London: Darton Longman & Todd

DAVIE, GRACE (2008): The sociology of religion. Los Angeles: Sage

DEL BOCA, DANIELA (2002): The effect of child care and part time opportunities on participation and fertility decisions in Italy. In: *Journal of Population Economics*, 15 No. 3, pp. 549–573

DEL BOCA, DANIELA, LOCATELLI, MARILENA (2006): The determinants of motherhood and work status: a survey. In: *IZA Discussion Paper* No. 2414

DEL BOCA, DANIELA, PASQUA, SILVIA, PRONZATO, CHIARA (2008): Market work and motherhood decisions in contexts. In: *IZA Discussion Paper* No. 3303

DENZ, HERMANN (2000): Postmodernisierung von Religion in Deutschland – Ost-West-Vergleich im Europäischen Kontext. In: *Pollack, Detlef/Pickel, Gert, editors:* Religiöser und kirchlicher Wandel in Ostdeutschland 1989–1999. Opladen: Leske + Budrich, pp. 70–86

DIEKMANN, ANDREAS, ENGELHARDT, HENRIETTE (1995): Die soziale Vererbung des Scheidungsrisikos. Eine empirische Untersuchung der Transmissionshypothese mit dem deutschen Familiensurvey. In: *Zeitschrift für Soziologie*, 24 No. 3, pp. 215–228

DOBBELAERE, KAREL (2004): Secularization: An analysis at three levels. Bruxelles: PIE Lang

DORBRITZ, JÜRGEN (2008): Germany: Family diversity with low actual and desired fertility. In: *Demographic Research*, 19 No. 17, pp. 557–598

DORBRITZ, JÜRGEN, LENGERER, ANDREA, RUCKDESCHEL, KERSTIN (2005): Einstellungen zu demographischen Trends und zu bevölkerungsrelevanten Politiken: Ergebnisse der Population Policy Acceptance Study in Deutschland. Wiesbaden: Bundesinstitut für Bevölkerungsforschung

DURKHEIM, ÉMILE (1965 [1915]): The elementary forms of the religious life (translated from the French by Joseph W. Swain). New York: Free Press

DUSCHEK, KLAUS-JÜRGEN, WIRTH, HEIKE (2005): Kinderlosigkeit von Frauen im Spiegel des Mikrozensus. Eine Kohortenanalyse der Mikrozensen 1987–2003. In: *Wirtschaft und Statistik*, No. 8, pp. 800–820

ECCLESIA CATHOLICA (1994): Catechism of the Catholic Church. London: Chapman

EHRENBERG, RONALD G., SMITH, ROBERT S. (2009): Modern labor economics: Theory and public policy. 10th edition. Boston: Pearson/ Addison Wesley

ERDOĞAN, MEHMET SARPER (2002): Berufskrankheiten türkischer Arbeitnehmer in Deutschland. Sankt Augustin: HVBG

ERMISCH, JOHN F. (1989): Purchased child care, optimal family size and mother's employment. Theory and econometric analysis. In: *Journal of Population Economics*, 2 No. 2, pp. 79–102

ESPING-ANDERSEN, GØSTA (1990): The three worlds of welfare capitalism. Princeton/ New York: Polity Press

ESPING-ANDERSEN, GØSTA (2002): Why we need a new welfare state. New York: Oxford University Press

ETTE, ANDREAS ET AL. (2007): Generations and Gender Survey Dokumentation der Befragung von türkischen Migranten in Deutschland. In: *Materialien zur Bevölkerungswissenschaft* No. 121b

EUROPEAN COMMISSION (2007): EU research on social sciences and humanities. Population Policy Acceptance Study – the viewpoint of citizens and policy actors regarding the management of population related change. Final report. ⟨URL: `http://cordis.europa.eu/documents/documentlibrary/100124311EN6.pdf`⟩ – visited on 21 Dec 2010

EUROPEAN UNION (2010): Europe in figures. Eurostat yearbook 2010. Luxembourg: Publications Office of the European Union

EUROSTAT (2010a): Life expectancy at birth, by gender. ⟨URL: `http://epp.eurostat.ec.europa.eu/tgm/table.do?tab=table&init=1&language=en&pcode=tps00025&plugin=1`⟩ – visited on 13 Dec 2010

EUROSTAT (2010b): Live births outside marriage. ⟨URL: `http://epp.eurostat.ec.europa.eu/tgm/table.do?tab=table&init=1&language=en&pcode=tps00018&plugin=1`⟩ – visited on 06 Dec 2010

EUROSTAT (2010c): Mean age at childbirth. ⟨URL: `http://epp.eurostat.ec.europa.eu/tgm/table.do?tab=table&init=1&language=en&pcode=tps00017&plugin=1`⟩ – visited on 07 Dec 2010

EUROSTAT (2010d): Total fertility rate. ⟨URL: http://epp.eurostat.ec.europa.eu/tgm/table.do?tab=table&init=1&language=en&pcode=tsdde220&plugin=1⟩ – visited on 30 Nov 2010

EUROSTAT (2012a): Crude divorce rate. ⟨URL: http://appsso.eurostat.ec.europa.eu/nui/show.do?dataset=demo_ndivind&lang=en⟩ – visited on 15 Sep 2012

EUROSTAT (2012b): Crude marriage rate. ⟨URL: http://appsso.eurostat.ec.europa.eu/nui/show.do?dataset=demo_nind&lang=en⟩ – visited on 15 Sep 2012

EUROSTAT (2012c): Employment rate, by sex. ⟨URL: http://epp.eurostat.ec.europa.eu/tgm/table.do?tab=table&init=1&language=en&pcode=tsdec420&plugin=1⟩ – visited on 01 Oct 2012

EUROSTAT (2012d): Fertility indicators (total fertility rate, proportion of live births outside marriage, mean age of women at childbirth). ⟨URL: http://appsso.eurostat.ec.europa.eu/nui/show.do?dataset=demo_find&lang=en⟩ – visited on 15 Sep 2012

EUROSTAT (2012e): Gender pay gap in unadjusted form. ⟨URL: http://epp.eurostat.ec.europa.eu/tgm/table.do?tab=table&init=1&language=en&pcode=tsdsc340&plugin=1⟩ – visited on 01 Oct 2012

EVANGELISCHE KIRCHE IN DEUTSCHLAND (2004): Rolle der Frau in der EKD. Anhörung vor dem Gleichstellungsausschuss des Europarats "Frauen und Religion". ⟨URL: http://www.ekd.de/bevollmaechtigter/stellungnahmen/52400.html⟩ – visited on 22 Feb 2012

EVANGELISCHE KIRCHE IN DEUTSCHLAND (2008): EKD-Statistik. Christen in Deutschland 2007. ⟨URL: http://www.ekd.de/statistik/mitglieder.html⟩ – visited on 31 Jan 2010

FAGNANI, JEANNE (2002): Why do French women have more children than German women? Family policies and attitudes towards child care outside home. In: *Community, Work, and Family*, 5 No. 1, pp. 103–120

FATH, SÉBASTIEN (2007): Putting God into the city: Protestants in France. In: *Hargreaves, Alec G., editor:* Politics and religion in France and the United States. Lanham: Lexington Books, pp. 49–61

FEDERAL INSTITUTE FOR POPULATION RESEARCH (2012a): Durchschnittliches Heiratsalter nach dem bisherigen Familienstand der Ehepartner in Deutschland, 1971 bis 2010. ⟨URL: http://www.bib-demografie.de/DE/DatenundBefunde/04/Abbildungen/a_04_14_durchschnittl_heiratsalter_familienstand_d_1971_2010.html?nn=3073946⟩ – visited on 01 Nov 2012

FEDERAL INSTITUTE FOR POPULATION RESEARCH (2012b): Eheschließungen und rohe Eheschließungsziffer in Ostdeutschland, 1950 bis 2010. ⟨URL: http://www.bib-demografie.de/DE/DatenundBefunde/04/Abbildungen/a_04_02b_eheschl_o_1950_2010.html?nn=3073946⟩ – visited on 01 Nov 2012

FEDERAL INSTITUTE FOR POPULATION RESEARCH (2012c): Eheschließungen und rohe Eheschließungsziffer in Westdeutschland, 1950 bis 2010. ⟨URL: http://www.bib-demografie.de/DE/DatenundBefunde/04/Abbildungen/a_04_02a_eheschl_w_1950_2010.html?nn=3073946⟩ – visited on 01 Nov 2012

FEDERAL INSTITUTE FOR POPULATION RESEARCH (2012d): Rohe Ehescheidungsziffer für West- und Ostdeutschland, 1950 bis 2010. ⟨URL: http://www.bib-demografie.de/DE/DatenundBefunde/05/Abbildungen/a_05_03_rohe_ehescheidungsziffer_w_o_1950_2010.html?nn=3073800⟩ – visited on 01 Nov 2012

FEDERAL INSTITUTE FOR POPULATION RESEARCH (2012e): Scheidungsziffern der Ehen in Deutschland, West- und Ostdeutschland, 1960 bis 2010. ⟨URL: http://www.bib-demografie.de/EN/Facts_Figures/Divorces/Figures/a_05_04_ehescheidungsziffern_d_w_o_1960_2010.html?nn=3214408⟩ – visited on 01 Nov 2012

FEDERAL INSTITUTE FOR POPULATION RESEARCH (2012f): Zusammengefasste Ehescheidungsziffern in Deutschland, West- und Ostdeutschland, 1970 bis 2010. ⟨URL: http://www.bib-demografie.de/EN/Facts_Figures/Divorces/Figures/a_05_06_zusgef_ehescheidungsziffer_d_w_o_1950_2010.html?nn=3214408⟩ – visited on 01 Nov 2012

FELLA, GIULIO, MANZINI, PAOLA, MARIOTTI, MARCO (2002): Does divorce law matter? In: *IZA Discussion Paper* No. 439

FETZER, JOEL S., SOPER, J. CHRISTOPHER (2006): Muslims and the state in Britain, France, and Germany. Cambridge: University Press

FIX, BIRGIT (2001): Religion und Familienpolitik. Wiesbaden: Westdeutscher Verlag

FÖLDHÁZI, ERZSÉBET (2010): Divorce. In: *HCSO Demographic Research Institute, editor:* Demographic Portrait of Hungary 2009: Report on the conditions of the Hungarian population. Budapest: HCSO, pp. 19–27

FRASER, SEAN (2012): Norway abolishes state-sponsored Church of Norway. ⟨URL: http://digitaljournal.com/article/324906#ixzz2Sp71C1zn⟩ – visited on 15 May 2012

FREJKA, TOMAS (2008a): Birth regulation in Europe: completing the contraceptive revolution. In: *Demographic Research*, 19 No. 5, pp. 73–84

FREJKA, TOMAS (2008b): Determinants of family formation and childbearing during the societal transition in Central and Eastern Europe. In: *Demographic Research*, 19 No. 7, pp. 139–170

FREJKA, TOMAS, CALOT, GÉRARD (2001): Cohort reproductive patterns in the Nordic countries. In: *Demographic Research*, 5 No. 5, pp. 125–186

FREJKA, TOMAS, SARDON, JEAN-PAUL (2007): Cohort birth order, parity progression ratio and parity distribution trends in developed countries. In: *Demographic Research*, 16 No. 11, pp. 315–374

FREJKA, TOMAS, WESTOFF, CHARLES F. (2006): Religion, religiousness, and fertility in the U.S. and in Europe. In: *MPIDR Working Paper* No. 013

FRERICH, JOHANNES, FREY, MARTIN (1996): Sozialpolitik in der Deutschen Demokratischen Republik. München: Oldenbourg

FRIEDBERG, LEORA (1998): Did unilateral divorce raise divorce rates? Evidence from panel data. In: *NBER Working Paper* No. 6398

FUCHS, JOHANN, WEBER, BRIGITTE (2004): Frauen in Ostdeutschland. Erwerbsbeteiligung weiter hoch. In: *IAB-Kurzbericht* No. 4

GÁBOS, ANDRÁS, GÁL, RÓBERT I., KÉZDI, GÁBOR (2009): The effects of child-related benefits and pensions on fertility by birth order: a test on Hungarian data. In: *Population Studies*, 63 No. 3, pp. 215–231

Gabriel, Karl, editor (1996): Religiöse Individualisierung oder Säkularisierung: Biographie und Gruppe als Bezugspunkte moderner Religiösität. Gütersloh: Chr. Kaiser Gütersloher Verlagshaus

GABRIEL, KARL (2003): (Post-)Moderne Religiosität zwischen Säkularisierung, Individualisierung und Deprivatisierung. In: *Waldenfels, Hans, editor:* Religion: Entstehung – Funktion – Wesen. Freiburg: Alber, pp. 109–131

GABRIEL, KARL, KAUFMANN, FRANZ-XAVER (1988): Der Katholizismus in den deutschsprachigen Ländern. In: *Kaufmann, Franz-Xaver, editor:* Religion, Kirchen und Gesellschaft in Deutschland. Opladen: Leske + Budrich, pp. 31–57

GALOR, ODED, WEIL, DAVID N. (1996): The gender gap, fertility, and growth. In: *American Economic Review*, 86 No. 3, pp. 374–387

GAUTHIER, ANNE H. (2002): Family policies in industrialized countries: Is there convergence? In: *Population Research and Policy Review*, 57 No. 3, pp. 447–474

GERLACH, IRENE (2010): Familienpolitik. 2nd edition. Wiesbaden: VS Verlag für Sozialwissenschaften

GERTH, HANS, MILLS, C. WRIGHT (1958): From Max Weber: essays in sociology. New York: Oxford University Press

GLASENAPP, HELMUTH VON (2005): Die fünf Weltreligionen: Hinduismus, Buddhismus, chinesischer Universismus, Christentum, Islam. Kreuzlingen: Hugendubel

GLOCK, CHARLES Y. (1962): On the study of religious commitment. In: *Religious Education*, 57 No. 4 (supplement), pp. 98–110

Glock, Charles Y./Stark, Rodney, editors (1965): Religion and society in tension. Chicago: Rand McNally & Co

GOLDBERG, ANDREAS, HALM, DIRK, ŞEN, FARUK (2004): Die deutschen Türken. Münster: Lit

GOLDSCHEIDER, CALVIN (1971): Population, modernization, and social structure. Boston: Little, Brown and Company

GONZÁLEZ, LIBERTAD, VIITANEN, TARJA K. (2009): The effect of divorce laws on divorce rates in Europe. In: *European Economic Review*, 53 No. 2, pp. 127–138

GOODY, JACK (1961): Religion and ritual: the definitional problem. In: *British Journal of Sociology*, 12 No. 2, pp. 142–164

GOTTSCHALL, KARIN, HAGEMANN, KAREN (2002): Die Halbtagsschule in Deutschland: Ein Sonderfall in Europa? In: *Aus Politik und Zeitgeschichte (APuZ)*, No. 41, pp. 12–22

GOUJON, ANNE ET AL. (2007): New times, old beliefs: projecting the future size of religions in Austria. In: *Lutz, Wolfgang, editor:* Vienna yearbook of population research. Wien: Verlag der österreichischen Akademie der Wissenschaften, pp. 237–270

GRAF, FRIEDRICH WILHELM (2007): Der Protestantismus. In: *Joas, Hans/Wiegandt, Klaus, editors:* Säkularisierung und die Weltreligionen. Frankfurt am Main: Fischer Taschenbuch Verlag, pp. 78–124

GREENE, WILLIAM H. (2012): Econometric analysis. 7th edition. Upper Saddle River: Pearson Prentice Hall

GROSSER, ALFRED (2009): Katholische Kirche in Frankreich. In: *Kranemann, Benedikt/Wijlens, Myriam, editors:* Religion und Laicité in Frankreich: Entwicklungen, Herausforderungen und Perspektiven. Würzburg: Echter, pp. 57–66

GRUESCU, SANDRA, RÜRUP, BERT (2005): Nachhaltige Familienpolitik. In: *Aus Politik und Zeitgeschichte (APuZ)*, No. 23-24, pp. 3–5

GRÜNHEID, EVELYN (2011): Wandel des Heiratsverhaltens in Deutschland. In: *BiB Working Paper* No. 2

HAAN, PETER, WROHLICH, KATHARINA (2009): Can child care policy encourage employment and fertility? Evidence from a structural model. In: *IZA Discussion Paper* No. 4503

HAAS, BARBARA ET AL. (2006): Household employment patterns in an enlarged European Union. In: *Work, Employment & Society*, 20 No. 4, pp. 751–771

HADAWAY, C. KIRK, MARLER, PENNY L., CHAVES, MARK (1998): Overreporting church attendance in America: Evidence that demands the same verdict. In: *American Sociological Review*, 63 No. 1, pp. 122–130

HALL, ANJA (1997): "Drum prüfe, wer sich ewig bindet". Eine empirische Untersuchung zum Einfluss vorehelichen Zusammenlebens auf das Scheidungsrisiko. In: *Zeitschrift für Soziologie*, 26 No. 4, pp. 275–295

HANK, KARSTEN, KREYENFELD, MICHAELA (2002): A multilevel analysis of child care and the transition to motherhood in western Germany. In: *DIW Discussion Papers* No. 290

HANK, KARSTEN, KREYENFELD, MICHAELA, SPIESS, C. KATHARINA (2003): Kinderbetreuung und Fertilität in Deutschland. In: *DIW Diskussionspapiere* No. 002

HAUG, SONJA, MÜSSIG, STEPHANIE, STICHS, ANJA (2009): Muslimisches Leben in Deutschland. Nürnberg: Bundesamt für Migration und Flüchtlinge

HEINECK, GUIDO (2001): The determinants of church attendance and religious human capital in Germany. Evidence from panel data. In: *DIW Discussion Papers* No. 263

HEINECK, GUIDO (2006): The relationship between religion and fertility: evidence for Austria. In: *Papers on Economics of Religion* No. 06/01

HERBERT, ULRICH (1986): Geschichte der Ausländerbeschäftigung in Deutschland 1880 bis 1980: Saisonarbeiter, Zwangsarbeiter, Gastarbeiter. Berlin [etc.]: Dietz

HERVIEU-LÉGER, DANIÈLE (1998): Secularization and religious modernity in Western Europe. In: *Shupe, Anson D./Misztal, Bronislaw, editors:* Religion, mobilization, and social action. Religion in the age of transformation. Westport: Praeger, pp. 15–31

HERVIEU-LÉGER, DANIÈLE (2007): Islam and the Republic: the French case. In: *Banchoff, Thomas F., editor:* Democracy and the new religious pluralism. Oxford and New York: Oxford University Press, pp. 203–221

HINRICHS, ERNST, HAUPT, HEINZ-GERHARD (2008): Kleine Geschichte Frankreichs. Stuttgart: Reclam

HOBCRAFT, JOHN N., KIERNAN, KATHLEEN (1995): Becoming a parent in Europe: Plenary paper for European Population Conference. In: *EAPS/IUSSP Proceedings of European Population Conference Milan,*, pp. 27–65

HOEM, JAN M. (2008): The impact of public policies on European fertility. In: *Demographic Research*, 19 No. 10, pp. 249–260

HOEM, JAN M. ET AL. (2010): Levels of recent union formation: six European countries compared. In: *Demographic Research*, 22 No. 9, pp. 199–210

HOEM, JAN M., NEYER, GERDA, ANDERSSON, GUNNAR (2006a): Education and childlessness. The relationship between educational field, educational level, and childlessness among Swedish women born in 1955-59. In: *Demographic Research*, 14 No. 15, pp. 331–380

HOEM, JAN M., NEYER, GERDA, ANDERSSON, GUNNAR (2006b): Educational attainment and ultimate fertility among Swedish women born in 1955-59. In: *Demographic Research*, 14 No. 16, pp. 381–404

HOFSTEDE, GEERT H. (1980): Culture's consequences: international differences in work-related values. Beverly Hills: Sage

HÖHN, CHARLOTTE, ETTE, ANDREAS, RUCKDESCHEL, KERSTIN (2006): Kinderwünsche in Deutschland. Konsequenzen für eine nachhaltige Familienpolitik. Stuttgart: Robert-Bosch-Stiftung

HÖLLINGER, FRANZ (1996): Volkskirche und Herrschaftsreligion. Die Wurzeln des religiösen Verhaltens in westlichen Gesellschaften. Opladen: Leske + Budrich

HOLST, ELKE, SCHIMETA, JULIA (2011): 29 von 906: Weiterhin kaum Frauen in Top-Gremien großer Unternehmen. In: *DIW Wochenbericht*, No. 3, pp. 2–10

HUBER, STEFAN (2003): Zentralität und Inhalt: Ein neues multidimensionales Messmodell der Religiosität. Opladen: Leske + Budrich

HUBER, STEFAN (2009): Religion Monitor 2008: structuring principles. In: *Bertelsmann Stiftung, editor:* What the world believes: analyses and commentary on the religion monitor 2008. Gütersloh: Bertelsmann Stiftung, pp. 17–33

HUBERT, SANDRA (2011): Die Effekte von Religion auf die Kinderzahl. In: *Brüderl, Josef/ Castiglioni, Laura/Schumann, Nina, editors:* Partnerschaft, Fertilität und intergenerationale Beziehungen: Ergebnisse der ersten Welle des Beziehungs- und Familienpanels. Würzburg: Ergon, pp. 203–226

HUBERT, SANDRA, ALTHAMMER, JÖRG, KORUCU-RIEGER, CANAN (2009): Soziodemographische Merkmale und psychopysisches Befinden älterer türkischer Migrantinnen und Migranten in Deutschland: Eine Untersuchung auf Basis der Haupt- und Zusatzbefragung des Generations and Gender Survey der ersten Welle. Berlin: Pro Business

HUININK, JOHANNES, KREYENFELD, MICHAELA (2004): Family formation in times of social and economic change: an analysis of the 1971 east German cohort. In: *MPIDR Working Paper* No. 013

HUNGARIAN CENTRAL STATISTICAL OFFICE (2010): Foreign citizens residing in Hungary by continents, countrys, sex, 1 January (1995-). ⟨URL: `http://portal.ksh.hu/pls/ksh/docs/eng/xstadat/xstadat_annual/i_wnvn001b.html`⟩ – visited on 18 Jan 2011

HUNT, STEPHEN J. (2011): Book review: The promise of salvation: A theory of religion by Martin Riesebrodt, translated by Steven Rendall. In: *Contemporary Sociology: A Journal of Reviews*, 40 No. 1, pp. 75–76

IANNACCONE, LAURENCE R. (1994): Why strict churches are strong. In: *American Journal of Sociology*, 99 No. 5, pp. 1180–1211

INSTITUT NATIONAL DE LA STATISTIQUE ET DES ÉTUDES ÉCONOMIQUES (2009): Marriages, nuptialité, divorces, pactes civils de solidarité: Évolution du divorce. Séries depuis 1960 pour la France. ⟨URL: `http://www.insee.fr/fr/themes/detail.asp?ref_id=ir-sd2008&page=irweb/sd2008/dd/sd2008_nuptialite.htm#SD2008_DIVORCE_TAB`⟩ – visited on 04 Dec 2010

INSTITUT NATIONAL DE LA STATISTIQUE ET DES ÉTUDES ÉCONOMIQUES (2010a): Immigrant. ⟨URL: `http://www.insee.fr/en/methodes/default.asp?page=definitions/immigre.htm`⟩ – visited on 18 Jan 2011

INSTITUT NATIONAL DE LA STATISTIQUE ET DES ÉTUDES ÉCONOMIQUES (2010b): Population totale par sexe et âge au 1er janvier 2010, France métropolitaine. ⟨URL: `http://www.insee.fr/fr/themes/detail.asp?reg_id=0&ref_id=bilan-demo&page=donnees-detaillees/bilan-demo/pop_age2.htm`⟩ – visited on 01 Dec 2010

INSTITUT NATIONAL DE LA STATISTIQUE ET DES ÉTUDES ÉCONOMIQUES (2012): Nuptialité: Pourcentage de femmes déja mariées a divers ages par génération. Séries depuis 1928. ⟨URL: http://http://www.insee.fr/fr/themes/detail.asp?ref_id=ir-sd2008&page=irweb/sd2008/dd/sd2008_nuptialite.htm#SD2008_MARIAGES⟩ – visited on 01 Nov 2012

INSTITUT NATIONAL D'ÉTUDES DÉMOGRAPHIQUES (2009a): Total divorce rate. ⟨URL: http://www.ined.fr/en/lexicon/bdd/mot/Divorce/motid/149/⟩ – visited on 03 Dec 2010

INSTITUT NATIONAL D'ÉTUDES DÉMOGRAPHIQUES (2009b): Total marriage rate. ⟨URL: http://www.ined.fr/en/lexicon/bdd/mot/Total+marriage+rate/motid/152/⟩ – visited on 03 Dec 2010

INSTITUT NATIONAL D'ÉTUDES DÉMOGRAPHIQUES (2010a): Civil solidarity pact. ⟨URL: http://www.ined.fr/en/lexicon/bdd/mot/Civil+solidarity+pact/motid/150/⟩ – visited on 03 Dec 2010

INSTITUT NATIONAL D'ÉTUDES DÉMOGRAPHIQUES (2010b): Civil Unions (Pacs). ⟨URL: http://www.ined.fr/en/pop_figures/france/marriages_divorces_pacs/pacs/⟩ – visited on 03 Dec 2010

INSTITUT NATIONAL D'ÉTUDES DÉMOGRAPHIQUES (2010c): Est-il vrai qu'en France, un enfant sur deux naît de parents non mariés? ⟨URL: http://www.ined.fr/en/everything_about_population/faq/naissances_natalite/bdd/q_text/is_it_true_that_half_of_all_babies_in_france_are_born_to_unmarried_parents_/question/226/⟩ – visited on 06 Dec 2010

INSTITUT NATIONAL D'ÉTUDES DÉMOGRAPHIQUES (2012): Cohort nuptiality. ⟨URL: http://http://www.ined.fr/en/pop_figures/france/marriages_divorces_pacs/nuptiality_generations/⟩ – visited on 01 Nov 2012

INSTITUTE FOR JEWISH COMMUNITY RESEARCH (2006): The American Jewish yearbook. Estimates of world Jewish populations. ⟨URL: bechollashon.org/img/charts/World_Pop_01.pdf⟩ – visited on 04 May 2012

JAGODZINSKI, WOLFGANG (2000): Religiöse Stagnation in den neuen Bundesländern: Fehlt das Angebot oder fehlt die Nachfrage? In: *Pollack, Detlef/Pickel, Gert, editors:* Religiöser und kirchlicher Wandel in Ostdeutschland 1989–1999. Opladen: Leske + Budrich, pp. 48–69

JAHN, EGBERT (2007): Ethnische, religiöse und nationale Minderheiten. Begriffe und Statusoptionen. In: *Osteuropa*, 57 No. 11, pp. 7–25

JALOVAARA, MARIKA (2003): The joint effects of marriage partners' socioeconomic positions on the risk of divorce. In: *Demography*, 40 No. 1, pp. 67–81

JAMES, WILLIAM (1925): The varieties of religious experience: A study in human nature. London: Longmans, Green, and Company

JUST, WOLF-DIETER (2011): Religionsausübung. In: *Fischer, Veronika/Springer, Monika, editors:* Handbuch Migration und Familie. Grundlagen für die Soziale Arbeit mit Familien Schwalbach Wochenschau. Schwalbach: Wochenschau, pp. 189–207

KAA, DIRK VAN DE (1987): Europe's second demographic transition. In: *Population Bulletin*, 42 No. 1, pp. 2–57

KALMIJN, MATTHIJS (2007): Explaining cross-national differences in marriage, cohabitation, and divorce in Europe, 1990-2000. In: *Population Studies*, 61 No. 3, pp. 243–263

KALMIJN, MATTHIJS, LOEVE, ANNEKE, MANTING, DORIEN (2007): Income dynamics in couples and the dissolution of marriage and cohabitation. In: *Demography*, 44 No. 1, pp. 159–179

KAUFMANN, FRANZ-XAVER (1989): Religion und Modernität: Sozialwissenschaftliche Perspektiven. Tübingen: Mohr

KAUFMANN, FRANZ-XAVER (2002): Politics and policies towards the family in Europe: a framework and an inquiry into their differences and convergences. In: *Kaufmann, Franz-Xaver* ET AL., *editors:* Family life and family policies in Europe: Problems and issues in comparative perspective. Oxford: University Press, pp. 419–490

KAUFMANN, FRANZ-XAVER (2004): Verkirchlichung des Christentums und das Diffus-Werden der Religion: Franz-Xaver Kaufmanns Analyse der Religionsentwicklung in der Moderne. In: *Gabriel, Karl/Reuter, Hans-Richard, editors:* Religion und Gesellschaft: Texte zur Religionssoziologie. Paderborn: Schöningh, pp. 213–232

KECSKES, ROBERT, WOLF, CHRISTOF (1993): Christliche Religiosität: Konzepte, Indikatoren, Messinstrumente. In: *Kölner Zeitschrift für Soziologie und Sozialpsychologie*, 45 No. 2, pp. 270–287

KELLER, BERNDT, SCHULZ, SUSANNE, SEIFERT, HARTMUT (2012): Entwicklung und Strukturmerkmale der atypisch Beschäftigten in Deutschland bis 2010. In: *WSI-Diskussionspapier* No. 182

KELLY, A. GEORGE (1955): The psychology of personal constructs: Theory and personality. New York: Norton

KIPPENBERG, HANS G. (2009): Max Weber: Religion and modernization. In: *Clarke, Peter B., editor:* The Oxford handbook of the sociology of religion. Oxford and New York: Oxford University Press, pp. 63–78

KLEIN, THOMAS (2003): Die Geburt von Kindern in paarbezogener Perspektive. In: *Zeitschrift für Soziologie*, 32 No. 6, pp. 506–527

KNAUFT, WOLFGANG (1980): Katholische Kirche in der DDR. Gemeinden in der Bewährung 1945–1980. Mainz: Grünewald

KNEIP, THORSTEN, BAUER, GERRIT (2007): Effects of different divorce probabilities on female labor force participation and fertility. In: *MZES Working Paper* No. 102

KNEIP, THORSTEN, BAUER, GERRIT (2009): Did unilateral divorce laws raise divorce rates in western Europe? In: *Journal of Marriage and Family*, 71 No. 3, pp. 592–607

KNEIP, THORSTEN, BAUER, GERRIT, REINHOLD, STEFFEN (2011): Direct and indirect effects of unilateral divorce law on marital stability. In: *Munich Center for the Economics of Aging Discussion Paper* No. 248

KNOBLAUCH, HUBERT (1999): Religionssoziologie. Berlin: de Gruyter

KNOESTER, CHRIS, BOOTH, ALAN (2000): Barriers to divorce: When are they effective? When are they not? In: *Journal of Family Issues*, 21 No. 1, pp. 78–99

KÖGEL, THOMAS (2004): Did the association between fertility and female employment within OECD countries really change its sign? In: *Journal of Population Economics*, 17 No. 1, pp. 45–65

KÖPPEN, KATJA (2004): The compatibility between work and family life – an empirical study of second birth risks in West Germany and France. In: *MPIDR Working Paper* No. 015

KÖPPEN, KATJA (2006): Second births in Western Germany and France. In: *Demographic Research*, 14 No. 14, pp. 295–330

KÖPPEN, KATJA, MAZUY, MAGALI, TOULEMON, LAURENT (2007): Kinderlosigkeit in Frankreich. In: *Konietzka, Dirk/Kreyenfeld, Michaela, editors:* Ein Leben ohne Kinder.

Kinderlosigkeit in Deutschland. Wiesbaden: VS Verlag für Sozialwissenschaften, pp. 83–104

KRAFT, KORNELIUS, NEIMANN, STEFANIE (2009): Impact of educational and religious homogamy on marital stability. In: *IZA Discussion Paper* No. 4491

Kranemann, Benedikt/Wijlens, Myriam, editors (2009): Religion und Laicité in Frankreich: Entwicklungen, Herausforderungen und Perspektiven. Würzburg: Echter

KRAVDAL, ØYSTEIN (2001): The high fertility of college educated women in Norway: an artefact of the separate modelling of each parity transition. In: *Demographic Research*, 5 No. 6, pp. 187–216

KREYENFELD, MICHAELA (2004): Fertility decisions in the FRG and GDR: An analysis with data from the German Fertility and Family Survey. In: *Demographic Research*, 3 No. 11, pp. 273–318

KREYENFELD, MICHAELA (2006): Der Einfluss der 'Wende' auf bildungsspezifische Fertilitätsunterschiede in Ostdeutschland. In: *MPIDR Working Paper* No. 025

KREYENFELD, MICHAELA, HORNUNG, ANNE, KUBISCH, KAROLIN (2010): Fertility and union histories from German GGS data: Some critical reflections. In: *MPIDR Working Paper* No. 023

KREYENFELD, MICHAELA, KONIETZKA, DIRK (2004): Angleichung oder Verfestigung von Differenzen? Geburtenentwicklung und Familienformen in Ost- und Westdeutschland. In: *MPIDR Working Paper* No. 025

KREYENFELD, MICHAELA ET AL. (2007): Gibt es eine zunehmende bildungsspezifische Polarisierung der Erwerbsmuster von Frauen? Analysen auf Basis der Mikrozensen 1976-2004. In: *MPIDR Working Paper* No. 013

KULU, HILL, BOYLE, PAUL J. (2009): High fertility in city suburbs: compositional or contextual effects? In: *European Journal of Population*, 25 No. 2, pp. 157–174

KULU, HILL, BOYLE, PAUL J., ANDERSSON, GUNNAR (2009): High suburban fertility: evidence from four Northern European countries. In: *Demographic Research*, 21 No. 31, pp. 915–944

KULU, HILL, VIKAT, ANDRES, ANDERSSON, GUNNAR (2007): Settlement size and fertility in the Nordic countries. In: *Population Studies*, 61 No. 3, pp. 265–285

LAMPERT, HEINZ, ALTHAMMER, JÖRG (2007): Lehrbuch der Sozialpolitik. Berlin: Springer

LAPPEGÅRD, TRUDE (2000): New fertility trends in Norway. In: *Demographic Research* 2 No. 3

LEHRER, EVELYN L. (1995): The effects of religion on the labor supply of married women. In: *Social Science Research*, 24 No. 3, pp. 281–301

LEHRER, EVELYN L. (1996): Religion as a determinant of marital fertility. In: *Journal of Population Economics*, 9 No. 2, pp. 173–196

LEHRER, EVELYN L. (1998): Religious intermarriage in the United States: determinants and trends. In: *Social Science Research*, 27 No. 3, pp. 245–263

LEHRER, EVELYN L. (2004): Religion as a determinant of economic and demographic behavior in the United States. In: *Population and Development Review*, 30 No. 4, pp. 707–726

LEHRER, EVELYN L. (2008): Age at marriage and marital instability: revisiting the Becker-Landes-Michael-hypothesis. In: *Journal of Population Economics*, 21 No. 2, pp. 463–484

LEHRER, EVELYN L., CHISWICK, CARMEL U. (1993): Religion as a determinant of marital stability. In: *Demography*, 30 No. 3, pp. 385–404

LEIBENSTEIN, HARVEY (1974): An interpretation of the economic theory of fertility: promising path oder blind alley? In: *Journal of Economic Literature*, 12 No. 2, pp. 457–479

LESTHAEGHE, RON, SURKYN, JOHAN (1988): Cultural dynamics and economic theories of fertility change. In: *Population and Development Review*, 14 No. 1, pp. 1–45

LETABLIER, MARIE-THÉRÈSE (2002): Kinderbetreuungspolitik in Frankreich und ihre Rechtfertigung. In: *WSI Mitteilungen*, No. 3, pp. 169–175

LETABLIER, MARIE-THÉRÈSE (2003): Fertility and family policies in France. In: *Journal of Population and Social Security (Population), Supplement to Volume 1*, No. 6, pp. 245–261

LEWIS, H. GREGG (1972): Income and substitution effects in labor force participation and hours of work. In: *Center for Econmic Research Discussion Paper* No. 18

LIBRERIA EDITRICE VATICANA (1983): Code of Canon law. ⟨URL: `http://www.vatican.va/archive/ENG1104/_INDEX.HTM`⟩ – visited on 20 Dec 2012

LILLARD, LEE A., WAITE, LINDA J. (1993): A joint model of marital childbearing and marital disruption. In: *Demography*, 30 No. 4, pp. 653–681

LIVANOS, ILIAS, POULIAKAS, KONSTANTINOS (2009): The gender wage gap as a function of educational degree choices in an occupationally segregated EU country. In: *IZA Discussion Paper* No. 4636

LUCKMANN, THOMAS (1970): The invisible religion: the problem of religion in modern society. New York: MacMillan

LUHMANN, NIKLAS (1977): Funktion der Religion. Frankfurt am Main: Suhrkamp

LUHMANN, NIKLAS (2002): Die Religion der Gesellschaft. Frankfurt am Main: Suhrkamp

LUHMANN, NIKLAS (2005): Einführung in die Theorie der Gesellschaft. Heidelberg: Auer

LYNGSTAD, TORKILD HOVDE, JALOVAARA, MARIKA (2010): A review of the antecentdents of union dissolution. In: *Demographic Research*, 23 No. 10, pp. 257–292

MARTIN, DAVID (1978): A general theory of secularization. Oxford: Blackwell

MATYSIAK, ANNA, VIGNOLI, DANIELE (2008): Fertility and women's employment: A meta-analysis. In: *European Journal of Population*, 24 No. 4, pp. 363–384

MAX PLANCK INSTITUTE FOR DEMOGRAPHIC RESEARCH, VIENNA INSTITUTE OF DEMOGRAPHY (2012): Human Fertility Database. ⟨URL: `www.humanfertility.org`⟩ – visited on 01 Oct 2012

MCCLEARY, RACHEL M., BARRO, ROBERT J. (2006): Religion and political economy in an international panel. In: *Journal for the Scientific Study of Religion*, 45 No. 2, pp. 149–175

MCGUE, MATT, LYKKEN, DAVID T. (1992): Genetic influences on risk of divorce. In: *Psychological Science*, 3 No. 6, pp. 368–373

MCQUILLAN, KEVIN (2004): When does religion influence fertility? In: *Population and Development Review*, 30 No. 1, pp. 25–56

MEGGIOLARO, SILVIA, ONGARO, FAUSTA (2010): The implications of marital instability for a woman's fertility: Empirical evidence from Italy. In: *Demographic Research*, 23 No. 34, pp. 963–996

MINCER, JACOB (1963): Market prices, opportunity costs and income effects. In: *Christ, Carl F., editor:* Measurement in economics: Studies in mathematical economics and econometrics in memory of Yehuda Grunfeld. Stanford: University Press, pp. 67–82

MINCER, JACOB (1974): Schooling, experience, and earnings. New York: Columbia University Press, National Bureau of Economic Research

MINCER, JACOB, POLACHEK, SOLOMON (1974): Family investments in human capital: earnings of women. In: *Journal of Population Economics*, 82 No. 2, pp. S76–S108

MINISTERIUM FÜR GENERATIONEN, FAMILIE, FRAUEN UND INTEGRATION DES LANDES NORDRHEIN-WESTFALEN (2006): Familienpolitik und Familie in Europa. Literaturbericht. Düsseldorf

MINISTRY OF FOREIGN AFFAIRS BUDAPEST (2004): Fact sheets on Hungary. Gypsies/ Roma in Hungary. ⟨URL: http://www.mfa.gov.hu/NR/rdonlyres/05DF7A51-99A5-4BFE-B8A5-210344C02B1A/0/Roma_en.pdf⟩ – visited on 31 Jan 2011

MOLNÁR, ATTILA K. (2006): Civil or ethnic religion: the case of Hungary. In: *Borowik, Irena, editor:* Religions, churches and religiosity in post-communist Europe. Kraków: Nomos, pp. 279–290

MORGAN, S. PHILIP ET AL. (2002): Muslim and non-Muslim differences in female autonomy and fertility: evidence from four Asian countries. In: *Population and Development Review*, 28 No. 3, pp. 515–537

MÜLLER, OLAF (2008): Religion in Central and Eastern Europe: Was there a re-awakening after the breakdown of communism? In: *Pollack, Detlef/Olson, Daniel V. A., editors:* The role of religion in modern societies. New York: Routledge, pp. 63–92

MÜLLER, OLAF (2009): Religiosity in Central and Eastern Europe: results from the PCE 2000 survey in comparison. In: *Pickel, Gert/Müller, Olaf, editors:* Church and religion in contemporary Europe: results from empirical and comparative research. Wiesbaden: VS Verlag für Sozialwissenschaften, pp. 65–88

NADERI, ROBERT, DORBRITZ, ROBERT, RUCKDESCHEL, KERSTIN (2009): Einleitung – Der Generations and Gender Survey in Deutschland: Zielsetzung, Verortung, Einschränkungen und Potenziale. In: *Zeitschrift für Bevölkerungswissenschaft*, 34 No. 1-2, pp. 5–30

NAUCK, BERNHARD (1993): Ausländerinnen in Westdeutschland. In: *Helwig, Gisela/Nickel, Hildegard Maria, editors:* Frauen in Deutschland, 1945-1992. Berlin: Akademie, pp. 364–395

NETHERLANDS INTERDISCIPLINARY DEMOGRAPHIC INSTITUTE (NIDI), UNITED NATIONS ECONOMIC COMMISSION FOR EUROPE (UNECE) (2011): Generations and Gender Programme (GGP). ⟨URL: http://www.ggp-i.org/, http://www.unece.org/pau/pub/ggp_concepts_guidelines.html⟩ – visited on 14 Dec, 2011

NEYER, GERDA (2003): Family policies and low fertility in western Europe. In: *MPIDR Working Paper* No. 021

NEYER, GERDA, ANDERSSON, GUNNAR (2007): Consequences of family policies on childbearing behavior: Effects or artifacts? In: *MPIDR Working Paper* No. 021

NIENTIEDT, KLAUS (2009): Kirche und postkirchliche Gesellschaft in Frankreich. In: *Kranemann, Benedikt/Wijlens, Myriam, editors:* Religion und Laicité in Frankreich: Entwicklungen, Herausforderungen und Perspektiven. Würzburg: Echter, pp. 125–139

NORRIS, PIPPA, INGLEHART, RONALD (2006): Sacred and secular: religion and politics worldwide. Cambridge: University Press

NORRIS, PIPPA, INGLEHART, RONALD (2007): Uneven secularization in the United States and Western Europe. In: *Banchoff, Thomas F., editor:* Democracy and the new religious pluralism. Oxford and New York: Oxford University Press, pp. 31–57

OBERTREIS, GESINE (1986): Familienpolitik in der DDR, 1945-1980. Opladen: Leske + Budrich

OECD (2007): Babies and bosses - reconciling work and family life: A synthesis of findings for OECD countries. Paris: OECD

OECD (2008): Growing unequal — Income distribution and poverty in OECD countries. Paris ⟨URL: `http://www.oecd.org/els/socialpoliciesanddata/growingunequalincomedistributionandpovertyinoecdcountries.htm`⟩ – visited on 14 Dec 2010

OECD (2010): PISA 2009 Results: Overcoming social background – Equity in learning opportunities and outcomes (Volume II). Paris: OECD

OECD FAMILY DATABASE (2011): Mean age of mothers at first childbirth. ⟨URL: `http://www.oecd.org/els/socialpoliciesanddata/41919586.pdf`⟩ – visited on 01 Oct 2012

OLÁH, LIVIA SZ, FRATCZAK, EWA (2004): Becoming a mother in Hungary and Poland during state socialism. In: *Demographic Research*, 3 No. 9, pp. 213–244

OLSON, DANIEL V. A., PERL, PAUL M. (2001): Variations in strictness and religious commitment within and among five denominations. In: *Journal for the Scientific Study of Religion*, 40 No. 4, pp. 757–764

OTT, NOTBURGA (2001): Der Erklärungsansatz der Familienökonomik. In: *Huinink, Johannes/Strohmeier, Klaus Peter/Wagner, Michael, editors:* Solidarität in Partnerschaft und Familie: Zum Stand familiensoziologischer Theoriebildung. Würzburg: Ergon, pp. 129–143

PERELLI-HARRIS, BRIENNA ET AL. (2012): Changes in union status during the transition to parenthood in eleven European countries, 1970s to early 2000s. In: *Population Studies*, 66 No. 2, pp. 167–182

PERELLI-HARRIS, BRIENNA ET AL. (2009): Examining nonmarital childbearing in Europe: How does union context differ across countries? In: *MPIDR Working Paper* No. 021

PEUCKERT, RÜDIGER (2008): Familienformen im sozialen Wandel. Wiesbaden: VS Verlag für Sozialwissenschaften

PHILIPOV, DIMITER, BERGHAMMER, CAROLINE (2007): Religion and fertility ideals, intentions and behaviour: A comparative study of European countries. In: *Lutz, Wolfgang, editor:* Vienna yearbook of population research. Wien: Verlag der österreichischen Akademie der Wissenschaften, pp. 271–305

PICKEL, GERT (2003): Areligiosität, Antireligiosität, Religiosität: Ostdeutschland als Sonderfall niedriger Religiosität im osteuropäischen Rahmen? In: *Gärtner, Christel/Pollack, Detlef/Wohlrab-Sahr, Monika, editors:* Atheismus und religiöse Indifferenz. Opladen: Leske + Budrich, pp. 247–269

PICKEL, GERT (2009): Secularization as a European fate? – Results from the church and religion in an enlarged Europe project 2006. In: *Pickel, Gert/Müller, Olaf, editors:* Church and religion in contemporary Europe: results from empirical and comparative research. Wiesbaden: VS Verlag für Sozialwissenschaften, pp. 89–122

PICKEL, GERT (2011): Ostdeutschland im europäischen Vergleich. Immer noch ein Sonderfall oder ein Sonderweg. In: *Pickel, Gert/Sammet, Kornelia, editors:* Religion und Religiosität im vereinigten Deutschland: Zwanzig Jahre nach dem Umbruch. Wiesbaden: VS Verlag für Sozialwissenschaften, pp. 165–190

POLLACK, DETLEF (1996): Individualisierung statt Säkularisierung? Zur Diskussion eines neueren Paradigmas in der Religionssoziologie. In: *Gabriel, Karl, editor:* Religiöse Individualisierung oder Säkularisierung: Biographie und Gruppe als Bezugspunkte moderner Religiösität. Gütersloh: Chr. Kaiser Gütersloher Verlagshaus, pp. 57–85

POLLACK, DETLEF (2000): Der Wandel der religiös-kirchlichen Lage in Ostdeutschland nach 1989: Ein Überblick. In: *Pollack, Detlef/Pickel, Gert, editors:* Religiöser und kirchlicher Wandel in Ostdeutschland 1989–1999. Opladen: Leske + Budrich, pp. 18–47

POLLACK, DETLEF (2003): Säkularisierung – ein moderner Mythos? Studien zum religiösen Wandel in Deutschland. Tübingen: Mohr Siebeck

POLLACK, DETLEF, PICKEL, GERT (2009): Church-state relations and the vitality of religion in European comparison. In: *Pickel, Gert/Müller, Olaf, editors:* Church and religion in contemporary Europe: results from empirical and comparative research. Wiesbaden: VS Verlag für Sozialwissenschaften, pp. 145–166

POPULATION REFERENCE BUREAU (2007): World population data sheet. ⟨URL: `www.prb.org/pdf07/07WPDS_Eng.pdf`⟩ – visited on 25 Mar 2010

POPULATION REFERENCE BUREAU (2008): Fertility rates for low birth-rate countries, 1995 to most recent year. ⟨URL: `http://www.prb.org/pdf08/TFRTable.pdf`⟩ – visited on 20 Dec 2010

PRIOUX, FRANCE (2005): Recent demographic developments in France. In: *Population-E*, 60 No. 4, pp. 371–414

PRIOUX, FRANCE (2006): Recent demographic developments in France. In: *Population-E*, 61 No. 4, pp. 323–364

PRIOUX, FRANCE (2008): Recent demographic developments in France. In: *Population-E*, 63 No. 3, pp. 375–414

RENDALL, MICHAEL S. ET AL. (1999): Incomplete reporting of mens' fertility in the United States and Britain: A research note. In: *Demography*, 36 No. 1, pp. 135–144

REUTER, ASTRID (2009): Religionsmigration. Der Islam in Frankreich und Deutschland. In: *Kranemann, Benedikt/Wijlens, Myriam, editors:* Religion und Laicité in Frankreich: Entwicklungen, Herausforderungen und Perspektiven. Würzburg: Echter, pp. 35–56

RIESEBRODT, MARTIN (2010): The promise of salvation: A theory of religion. Chicago: University of Chicago Press

ROBERT, PETER, BLOSSFELD, HANS-PETER (1995): Hungary. In: *Blossfeld, Hans-Peter, editor:* The new role of women: Family formation in modern societies. Boulder: Westview Press, pp. 211–226

ROBERT-BOBÉE, ISABELLE, MAZUY, MAGALI (2005): Calendriers de constitution des familles et âge de fin des études. In: *Lefevre, Cécile/Filhon, Alexandra, editors:* Histoires de familles, histoires familiales, les Cahiers de l'INED. Paris, pp. 175–200

RØNSEN, MARIT (2004a): Fertility and family policy in Norway – A reflection on trends and possible connections. In: *Demographic Research*, 10 No. 10, pp. 265–286

RØNSEN, MARIT (2004b): Fertility and public policies – Evidence from Norway and Finland. In: *Demographic Research*, 10 No. 6, pp. 143–170

RØNSEN, MARIT, SKREDE, KARI (2010): Can public policies sustain fertility in the Nordic countries? Lessons from the past and questions for the future. In: *Demographic Research*, 22 No. 13, pp. 321–346

RUTHVEN, MALISE (2001): Der Islam: Eine kurze Einführung. Stuttgart: Reclam

SACERDOTE, BRUCE, GLAESER, EDWARD L. (2001): Education and religion. In: *NBER Working Paper* No. 8080

SALLES, ANNE, ROSSIER, CLÉMENTINE, BRACHET, SARA (2010): Understanding the long term effects of family policies on fertility: The diffusion of different family models in France and Germany. In: *Demographic Research*, 22 No. 34, pp. 1057–1096

SCHMEISSER, CLAUDIA ET AL. (2012): Atypische Beschäftigung in Europa 1996 – 2009. In: *WZB Discussion Paper* No. 001

SCHMID, SUSANNE, KOHLS, MARTIN (2011): Generatives Verhalten und Migration. Eine Bestandsaufnahme des generativen Verhaltens von Migrantinnen in Deutschland. Nürnberg: Bundesamt für Migration und Flüchtlinge

SCHMITT, CHRISTIAN, WINKELMANN, ULRIKE (2005): Wer bleibt kinderlos? Sozialstrukturelle Daten zur Kinderlosigkeit von Frauen und Männern. In: *DIW Discussion Papers* No. 473

SCHRAGE, ANDREA (2007): Low fertility of highly educated women: the impact of child care infrastructure. In: *University of Regensburg Working Papers in Business, Economics and Management Information Systems* No. 421

SCHRATZENSTALLER, MARGIT (2002): Familienpolitik – wozu und für wen? Die aktuelle familienpolitische Debatte. In: *WSI-Mitteilungen* No. 03

SCHRÖDER, JETTE, BRÜDERL, JOSEF (2008): Der Effekt der Erwerbstätigkeit von Frauen auf die Fertilität: Kausalität oder Selbstselektion? In: *Zeitschrift für Soziologie*, 37 No. 2, pp. 117–136

SCHULTZ, PAUL (2008): Fertility in developing countries. In: *Durlauf, Steven N./Blume, Lawrence E., editors:* The new Palgrave dictionary of economics. Basingstoke and Hampshire: Palgrave Macmillan, pp. 291–295

SCHWARTZ, MICHAEL (2005): Emanzipation zur sozialen Nützlichkeit: Bedingungen und Grenzen von Frauenpolitik in der DDR. In: *Hoffmann, Dierk/Schwartz, Michael, editors:* Sozialstaatlichkeit in der DDR: Sozialpolitische Entwicklungen im Spannungsfeld von Diktatur und Gesellschaft 1945/49-1989. München: Oldenbourg, pp. 47–88

SCHWARTZ, RÉMY (2007): Historical and constitutional relations between churches and the state in France. In: *Hargreaves, Alec G., editor:* Politics and religion in France and the United States. Lanham: Lexington Books, pp. 15–25

Sengers, Erik/Sunier, Thijl, editors (2010): Religious newcomers and the nation state: Political culture and organized religion in France and the Netherlands. Delft: Eburon

SKEVIK, ANNE, HATLAND, AKSEL (2008): Family policies in Norway. In: *Ostner, Ilona/Schmitt, Christoph, editors:* Family policies in the context of family change. Wiesbaden: VS Verlag für Sozialwissenschaften, pp. 89–107

SKIRBEKK, VEGARD (2008): Fertility trends by social status. In: *Demographic Research*, 18 No. 5, pp. 145–180

SLEEBOS, JOËLLE (2003): Low fertility rates in OECD countries: Facts and policy responses. In: *OECD Labour Market and Social Policy Occasional Papers* No. 15

SMITH, IAN (2002): European divorce laws, divorce rates, and their consequences. In: *Dnes, Antony W./Rowthorn, Robert, editors:* The law and economics of marriage and divorce. Cambridge: University Press, pp. 212–229

SOBOTKA, TOMÁŠ (2008): The rising importance of migrants for childbearing in Europe. In: *Demographic Research*, 19 No. 9, pp. 225–248

SOBOTKA, TOMÁŠ, TOULEMON, LAURENT (2008): Changing family and partnership behaviour: Common trends and persistent diversity across Europe. In: *Demographic Research*, 19 No. 6, pp. 85–138

SÖKEFELD, MARTIN (2008): Alevis in Germany. In: *Bertelsmann Stiftung, editor:* Religion monitor. Muslim religiousness in Germany. Overview of religious attitudes and practices. Gütersloh: Bertelsmann Stiftung, pp. 32–37

SONTHEIMER, KURT, BLEEK, WILHELM (2005): Grundzüge des politischen Systems Deutschlands. München: Piper

SOUTH, SCOTT J., BOSE, SUNITA, TRENT, KATHERINE (2004): Anticipating divorce: Spousal agreement, predictive accuracy, and effects on labor supply and fertiliy. In: *Journal of Divorce & Remarriage*, 40 No. 3/4, pp. 1–22

SPÉDER, ZSOLT (2006): Rudiments of recent fertility decline in Hungary: Postponement, educational differences, and outcomes of changing partnership forms. In: *Demographic Research*, 15 No. 8, pp. 253–288

SPÉDER, ZSOLT, KAMARÁS, FERENC (2008): Hungary: Secular fertility decline with distinct period fluctuations. In: *Demographic Research*, 19 No. 18, pp. 599–664

SPIRO, MELFORD E. (1966): Religion: problems of definition and explanation. In: *Banton, Michael, editor:* Anthropological approaches to the study of religion. London: Routledge, pp. 85–126

STARK, RODNEY, BAINBRIDGE, WILLIAM SIMS (1985): The future of religion: Secularization, revival, and cult formation. Berkeley: University of California Press

STARK, RODNEY, GLOCK, CHARLES Y. (1968): American piety: The nature of religious commitment. Berkeley: University of California Press

STATISTICS NORWAY (2005): Part-time employment practices. One in four works part-time. ⟨URL: http://www.ssb.no/english/magazine/art-2005-02-01-01-en.html⟩ – visited on 03 Nov 2012

STATISTICS NORWAY (2012a): Adoptions, 2011. ⟨URL: http://www.ssb.no/en/adopsjon/⟩ – visited on 01 Dec 2012

STATISTICS NORWAY (2012b): Average age at marriage. Marriages between persons of opposite sex. Males and females. 1961–2011. ⟨URL: http://www.ssb.no/english/subjects/02/02/30/ekteskap_en/tab-2012-08-23-06-en.html⟩ – visited on 01 Nov 2012

STATISTICS NORWAY (2012c): Continued high population increase. ⟨URL: http://www.ssb.no/english/subjects/02/02/folkendrkv_en/⟩ – visited on 01 Oct 2012

STATISTICS NORWAY (2012d): Fewer births and older first-time parents. ⟨URL: http://www.ssb.no/english/subjects/02/02/10/fodte_en/⟩ – visited on 01 Oct 2012

STATISTICS NORWAY (2012e): Marriages between persons of opposite sex , by previous marital status of the spouses. 1961–2011. ⟨URL: http://www.ssb.no/english/subjects/02/02/30/ekteskap_en/tab-2012-08-23-05-en.html⟩ – visited on 01 Nov 2012

STATISTICS NORWAY (2012f): Marriages dissolved. Separations. 1961–2011. ⟨URL: http://www.ssb.no/english/subjects/02/02/30/ekteskap_en/tab-2012-08-23-08-en.html⟩ – visited on 01 Nov 2012

STATISTICS NORWAY (2012g): Number of children distributed, by age and cohort. ⟨URL: http://www.ssb.no/english/subjects/02/02/10/fodte_en/tab-2012-04-11-09-en.html⟩ – visited on 01 Oct 2012

STATISTICS NORWAY (2012h): Religious communities and life stance communities. ⟨URL: http://www.ssb.no/en/trosamf/⟩ – visited on 12 Jan 2013

STATISTICS NORWAY (2012i): Total fertility rate. ⟨URL: http://www.ssb.no/english/subjects/02/02/10/fodte_en/⟩ – visited on 01 Oct 2012

STATISTISCHES BUNDESAMT (2007): Geburten in Deutschland. Wiesbaden: Statistisches Bundesamt

STATISTISCHES BUNDESAMT (2008): Datenreport 2008: Ein Sozialbericht für die Bundesrepublik Deutschland. Bonn: Bundeszentrale für Politische Bildung

STATISTISCHES BUNDESAMT (2009a): Anteile der geschiedenen Ehen bei den Eheschließungsjahrgängen 1964 bis 2003 in Deutschland. ⟨URL: http://www.bib-demografie.de/cln_099/nn_1881292/DE/DatenundBefunde/05/Abbildungen/a__05__12__anteil__gesch__ehen__eheschl__jahrgaenge__d__1964__2003.html⟩ – visited on 08 Dec 2010

STATISTISCHES BUNDESAMT (2009b): Mikrozensus 2008. Neue Daten zur Kinderlosigkeit. Wiesbaden: Statistisches Bundesamt

STATISTISCHES BUNDESAMT (2010a): Pressemitteilung Nr. 079 vom 05.03.2010. Gender pay gap 2008: Deutschland weiterhin eines der Schlusslichter in der EU. ⟨URL: http://www.destatis.de/jetspeed/portal/cms/Sites/destatis/Internet/DE/Presse/pm/2010/03/PD10__079__621,templateId=renderPrint.psml⟩ – visited on 26 Jan 2011

STATISTISCHES BUNDESAMT (2010b): Statistical Yearbook 2010 for the Federal Republic of Germany. Wiesbaden: Statistisches Bundesamt

STATISTISCHES BUNDESAMT (2012a): Eheschließungen, Ehescheidungen und durchschnittliches Heiratsalter Lediger. ⟨URL: https://www.destatis.de/DE/ZahlenFakten/GesellschaftStaat/Bevoelkerung/Eheschliessungen/Tabellen/EheschliessungenScheidungen.html⟩ – visited on 01 Nov 2012

STATISTISCHES BUNDESAMT (2012b): Population movement. First marriage and remarriage. ⟨URL: https://www.destatis.de/EN/FactsFigures/SocietyState/Population/Marriages/Tables/FirstMarriageRemarriage.html⟩ – visited on 01 Nov 2012

STLOUKAL, LIBOR (1999): Understanding the "abortion culture" in Central and Eastern Europe. In: *David, Henry P./Skilogianis, Joanna/Posadskaya-Vanderbeck, Anastasia, editors:* From abortion to contraception: a resource to public policies and reproductive behavior in Central and Eastern Europe from 1917 to the present. Westport: Greenwood Press, pp. 23–47

STORCH, KERSTEN (2003): Konfessionslosigkeit in Ostdeutschland. In: *Gärtner, Christel/ Pollack, Detlef/Wohlrab-Sahr, Monika, editors:* Atheismus und religiöse Indifferenz. Opladen: Leske + Budrich, pp. 231–245

STROHMEIER, KLAUS PETER (2002): Family policy – how does it work? In: *Kaufmann, Franz-Xaver* ET AL., *editors:* Family life and family policies in Europe: Problems and issues in comparative perspective. Oxford: University Press, pp. 321–362

SURKYN, JOHAN, LESTHAEGHE, RON (2004): Values orientations and the second demographic transition (SDT) in northern, western and southern Europe: An update. In: *Demographic Research*, 3 No. 3, pp. 47–86

TAN, DURSUM (1999): Aleviten in Deutschland. Zwischen Selbstethnizierung und Emanzipation. In: *Jonker, Gerdien, editor:* Kern und Rand. Religiöse Minderheiten aus der Türkei in Deutschland. Berlin: Das Arabische Buch, pp. 65–89

TEACHMAN, JAY D. (2002): Stability across cohorts in divorce risk factors. In: *Demography*, 39 No. 2, pp. 331–351

TESTA, MARIA RITA, GRILLI, LEONARDO (2006): The influence of childbearing regional contexts on ideal family size in Europe. In: *Population-E*, 61 No. 1-2, pp. 109–137

THE WORLD BANK (2011): GNI per capita, Atlas method (current US-Dollar). ⟨URL: http://data.worldbank.org/indicator/NY.GNP.PCAP.CD⟩ – visited on 23 Jun 2011

THOMSON, ELIZABETH ET AL. (2012): Union instability as an engine of fertility? A microsimulation model for France. In: *Demography*, 49 No. 1, pp. 175–195

TÖLKE, ANGELIKA (2004): Die Bedeutung von Herkunftsfamilie, Berufsbiografie und Partnerschaften für den Übergang zur Ehe und Vaterschaft. In: *MPIDR Working Paper*, No. 007, pp. 1–33

TOMKA, MIKLÓS (1999): Religion und Kirche in Ungarn nach dem Ende des Kommunismus. In: *Tomka, Miklós/Maslauskaitçe, Ausra/Zulehner, Paul M., editors:* Religion und Kirchen in Ost(Mittel)-Europa: Ungarn, Litauen, Slowenien. Ostfildern: Schwabenverlag, pp. 21–133

TOMKA, MIKLÓS (2006): Catholics and Protestants in post-communist Europe. In: *Borowik, Irena, editor:* Religions, churches and religiosity in post-communist Europe. Kraków: Nomos, pp. 37–51

TOMKA, MIKLÓS, ZULEHNER, PAUL M. (1999): Religion in den Reformländern Ost(Mittel)Europas. Ostfildern: Schwabenverlag

TOULEMON, LAURENT, MAZUY, MAGALI (2001): Les naissances sont retardées mais la fécondité est stable. In: *Population*, 56 No. 4, pp. 611–644

TOULEMON, LAURENT, PAILHÉ, ARIANE, ROSSIER, CLÉMENTINE (2008): France: high and stable fertility. In: *Demographic Research*, 19 No. 16, pp. 503–556

UNECE POPULATION ACTIVITIES UNIT (2006): Generations and Gender Programme. Summary Description. ⟨URL: http://www.unece.org/pau/_docs/ggp/GGP_2006_SumDescr.pdf⟩ – visited on 14 Dec, 2011

UNICEF (2005): "Auf in die Schule, Mädchen!". ⟨URL: www.unicef.de/presse/pm/2005/auf-in-die-schule-maedchen⟩ – visited on 17 Aug 2012

United Nations Development Programme (UNDP), editor (2009): Overcoming barriers: Human mobility and development. Houndmills: Palgrave Macmillan

UNITED NATIONS DEVELOPMENT PROGRAMME (UNDP) (2010): Human Development Report 2010. The real wealth of nations: pathways to human development. ⟨URL: http://hdr.undp.org/en/media/HDR_2010_EN_Complete_reprint.pdf⟩ – visited on 14 Dec 2010

UNITED NATIONS EDUCATIONAL, SCIENTIFIC AND CULTURAL ORGANIZATION (UNESCO) (2006): International Standard Classification of Education I S C E D 1997. ⟨URL: http://www.uis.unesco.org/Library/Documents/isced97-en.pdf⟩ – visited on 03 Apr 2011

VEIL, MECHTHILD (2002): Ganztagsschule mit Tradition: Frankreich. In: *Aus Politik und Zeitgeschichte (APuZ)*, No. 41, pp. 29–37

VEIL, MECHTHILD (2005): Der Einfluss des republikanischen Modells auf die Geschlechterkulturen in Frankreich. In: *gender ... politik ... online*,, pp. 1–8

VEIL, MECHTHILD (2007): Geteilte Verantwortung. Neuere Entwicklungen in der französischen Familienpolitik. In: *Dokumente*, No. 1, pp. 31–37

VELLENGA, SIPCO (2003): Wie "Gott" in den Niederlanden verblasst: Ein kultureller Trend in einem säkularen Staat. In: *Gärtner, Christel/Pollack, Detlef/Wohlrab-Sahr, Monika, editors:* Atheismus und religiöse Indifferenz. Opladen: Leske + Budrich, pp. 197–214

VIKAT, ANDRES ET AL. (2007): Generations and Gender Survey (GGS): towards a better understanding of relationships and processes in the life course. In: *Demographic Research*, 17 No. 14, pp. 389–440

VOAS, DAVID (2008): The continuing secular transition. In: *Pollack, Detlef/Olson, Daniel V. A., editors:* The role of religion in modern societies. New York: Routledge, pp. 25–48

VOAS, DAVID, CROCKETT, ALASDAIR (2005): Religion in Britain: Neither believing nor belonging. In: *Sociology*, 39 No. 1, pp. 11–28

WAGNER, MICHAEL (1993): Soziale Bedingungen des Ehescheidungsrisikos aus der Perspektive des Lebensverlaufs. In: *Diekmann, Andreas/Weick, Stefan, editors:* Der Familienzyklus als sozialer Prozess. Bevölkerungssoziologische Untersuchungen mit den Methoden der Ereignisanalyse. Berlin: Duncker & Humblot, pp. 372–393

WAGNER, MICHAEL, WEISS, BERND (2003): Bilanz der deutschen Scheidungsforschung. Versuch einer Meta-Analyse. In: *Zeitschrift für Soziologie*, 32 No. 1, pp. 29–49

WAGNER, MICHAEL, WEISS, BERND (2006): On the variation of divorce risks in Europe: Findings from a meta-analysis of European longitudinal studies. In: *European Sociological Review*, 22 No. 5, pp. 483–500

WAITE, LINDA J., LILLARD, LEE A. (1991): Children and marital disruption. In: *American Journal of Sociology*, 96 No. 4, pp. 930–953

WEBER, MAX (1919): Wissenschaft als Beruf. München: Duncker & Humblot

WEBER, MAX (1922): Gesammelte Aufsätze zur Religionssoziologie. Tübingen: Mohr

WEBER, MAX (1930 [1904]): The Protestant ethic and the spirit of capitalism. Translated by Talcott Parson. New York: Scribner

WEICHSELBAUMER, DORIS, WINTER-EBMER, RUDOLF (2005): A meta-analysis of the international gender wage gap. In: *Journal of Economic Surveys*, 19 No. 3, pp. 479–511

WENDEN, CATHERINE WIHTOL DE (2007): From migrants to citizens: Muslims in France. In: *Hargreaves, Alec G., editor:* Politics and religion in France and the United States. Lanham: Lexington Books, pp. 139–153

WHITE, LYNN K. (1990): Determinants of divorce: A review of research in the eighties. In: *Journal of Marriage and Family*, 52 No. 4, pp. 904–912

WHITE, ROBERT G., BERNARDI, LAURA (2008): Close kin influences on fertility behavior. In: *MPIDR Working Paper* No. 024

WICK, VOLKER (2007): Die Trennung von Staat und Kirche: Jüngere Entwicklungen in Frankreich im Vergleich zum deutschen Kooperationsmodell. Tübingen: Mohr Siebeck

WILLMS-HERGET, ANGELIKA (1985): Frauenarbeit: Zur Integration der Frauen in den Arbeitsmarkt. Frankfurt am Main and New York: Campus

WINKELMANN, RAINER (1994): Count data models. Econometric theory and an application to labor mobility. Berlin [etc.]: Springer

WIRTH, HEIKE (2007): Kinderlosigkeit von hoch qualifizierten Frauen und Männern im Paarkontext – Eine Folge von Bildungshomogamie? In: *Konietzka, Dirk/Kreyenfeld, Michaela, editors:* Ein Leben ohne Kinder. Kinderlosigkeit in Deutschland. Wiesbaden: VS Verlag für Sozialwissenschaften, pp. 167–199

WOLFERS, JUSTIN (2006): Did unilateral divorce laws raise divorce rates? A reconciliation and new results. In: *American Economic Review*, 96 No. 5, pp. 1802–1820

WROHLICH, KATHARINA, DELL, FABIEN, BACLET, ALEXANDRE (2005): Steuerliche Familienförderung in Frankreich und Deutschland. In: *DIW Wochenbericht*, 72 No. 33, pp. 479–486

WULFF, DAVID M. (1991): Psychology of religion: Classic and contemporary views. New York: Wiley

WUNN, INA (2008): Religiousness of Muslim women in Germany. In: *Bertelsmann Stiftung, editor:* Religion monitor. Muslim religiousness in Germany. Overview of religious attitudes and practices. Gütersloh: Bertelsmann Stiftung, pp. 60–67

ZENTRALARCHIV FÜR EMPIRISCHE SOZIALFORSCHUNG (2001): ISSP 1998. Coodbook. ZA Study 3190. Religion II. ⟨URL: `info1.gesis.org/dbksearch/file.asp?file=ZA3190_cdb.pdf`⟩ – visited on 20 Mar 2010

Appendix

Table A.1. Attitudes towards religious ceremonies at turning points of life structured by country and gender

	FRANCE		HUNGARY		NORWAY		GERMANY					
							East		West		Tr. migs	
	Women	Men	Women	Men	Women	Men	Women	Men	Women	Men	Women	Men
I am going to read out some statements about religious ceremonies and I would like you to tell me to what extent do you agree or disagree with each one.												
Baptism: It is important for an infant to be registered in the appropriate religious ceremony.												
Strongly agree	51.6	45.5	60.1	50.6	32.8	25.5	5.4	5.5	33.3	29.6	31.9	31.1
Agree	14.5	17.0	10.1	11.5	17.9	18.8	21.2	19.5	44.1	41.4	22.1	23.6
Neither agree nor disagree	12.3	14.1	16.4	19.1	13.9	13.7	16.6	21.0	11.4	13.2	11.4	14.6
Disagree	4.2	4.3	3.1	4.4	6.1	6.0	22.9	19.8	6.6	8.9	11.5	12.8
Strongly disagree	16.7	17.9	9.5	13.0	8.8	9.8	32.4	31.8	4.1	5.9	16.5	9.2
No response/ refusal	0.7	1.2	0.8	1.4	20.6	26.3	1.5	2.5	0.6	1.1	6.6	8.7
Wedding: It is important for people who marry in registry offices to have a religious wedding too.												
Strongly agree	36.9	32.3	49.1	42.4	27.2	23.0	5.2	5.1	24.8	20.4	45.9	44.8
Agree	15.1	16.4	9.7	11.1	18.3	19.7	16.6	12.2	31.7	33.1	32.8	32.0
Neither agree nor disagree	19.5	21.2	20.0	22.6	19.2	16.6	19.2	27.0	20.6	20.9	7.0	8.7
Disagree	6.2	6.7	5.6	6.0	6.7	5.9	26.6	24.8	15.2	16.4	3.8	6.1
Strongly disagree	21.7	22.4	14.6	16.8	7.9	8.5	31.4	29.0	7.3	8.4	7.5	4.9
No response/ refusal	0.6	1.0	0.9	1.0	20.8	26.3	1.1	2.0	0.4	0.8	3.2	3.5
Funeral: It is important for a funeral to include a religious ceremony.												
Strongly agree	52.8	47.4	63.4	55.1	42.8	35.6	8.4	7.4	34.9	28.0	52.1	53.0
Agree	15.9	17.8	7.7	10.8	17.8	19.8	16.0	15.8	39.0	38.4	31.9	34.3
Neither agree nor disagree	11.3	13.6	14.0	16.0	10.4	9.5	17.4	25.5	12.2	14.7	6.9	5.9
Disagree	4.2	4.4	3.3	4.3	2.8	3.4	25.7	24.2	8.5	11.1	3.1	3.5
Strongly disagree	15.2	15.9	10.6	12.5	5.6	5.5	31.5	25.8	4.9	7.2	3.6	1.2
No response/ refusal	0.6	0.9	1.0	1.3	20.7	26.3	1.0	1.3	0.5	0.7	2.4	2.0
Numbers of observations	2,640	2,122	3,837	2,821	3,542	3,484	463	444	1,856	1,790	482	501

Age group 45–74; birth cohorts 1930–1962. In %; weighted data. Tr. migs: Turkish migrants.

Table A.2. Correlation matrix of attitudes towards religious ceremonies at turning points of life structured by country and gender

	FRANCE		HUNGARY		NORWAY		GERMANY					
							East		West		Tr. migs	
	Women	Men	Women	Men	Women	Men	Women	Men	Women	Men	Women	Men
Baptism – wedding												
Spearman's ρ	0.68	0.71	0.74	0.78	0.81	0.80	0.84	0.85	0.66	0.71	0.95	0.96
Wedding – funeral												
Spearman's ρ	0.69	0.69	0.70	0.74	0.74	0.77	0.86	0.85	0.71	0.75	0.73	0.69
Funeral – baptism												
Spearman's ρ	0.66	0.66	0.70	0.74	0.77	0.76	0.80	0.81	0.71	0.71	0.88	0.84

Age group 45–74; birth cohorts 1930–1962. In %; weighted data. Tr. migs: Turkish migrants. Values of Turkish migrants for "baptism" already replaced by the mean of the sum of both other values.

Table A.3. Attitudes towards religious ceremonies at turning points of life (*rites de passage*) by country, gender, and religious affiliation

	FRANCE		HUNGARY		NORWAY		GERMANY			
							East		West	
	Women	Men	Women	Men	Women	Men	Women	Men	Women	Men
With religious affiliation										
Values 0–3	14.6	15.7	8.5	10.4	9.3	10.3	13.3	4.7	5.5	5.9
Values 4–7	19.1	20.2	16.3	19.8	19.8	21.5	33.1	33.2	21.1	24.1
Values 8–10	25.1	27.8	22.6	22.4	32.3	33.5	38.3	44.0	44.4	43.8
Values 11–12	41.2	36.1	52.4	47.4	38.7	34.7	15.3	18.3	29.0	26.3
Nobs	2,478	1,950	3,455	2,420	2,661	2,399	173	121	1,649	1,453
Without religious affiliation										
Values 0–3	68.6	67.9	45.8	49.4	50.8	53.8	69.4	63.2	40.2	49.1
Values 4–7	13.6	16.7	24.9	27.9	29.4	22.6	25.2	32.1	51.0	37.6
Values 8–10	10.8	10.2	14.4	12.2	13.3	14.5	5.1	4.7	7.1	11.9
Values 11–12	7.0	5.3	14.9	10.6	6.5	9.2	0.4	0.0	1.8	1.5
Nobs	129	142	320	342	193	206	365	308	189	305

Age group 45–74; birth cohorts 1930–1962. In %; weighted data.

Table A.4. Attitudes towards religious ceremonies at turning points of life (*rites de passage*) by country, gender, and religious affiliation

	FRANCE						HUNGARY								NORWAY					
	Roman Catholic		Protestant		Muslim		Roman Catholic		Greek Catholic		Reformed (Calvinist)		Lutheran		Church of Norway		Christianity outside the Church of Norway		Other	
	W	M	W	M	W	M	W	M	W	M	W	M	W	M	W	M	W	M	W	M
Values 0–3	15.0	16.1	6.0	19.7	8.9	7.4	7.3	10.1	6.7	5.4	12.1	12.9	11.1	8.4	6.6	7.7	2.7	6.7	56.3	60.1
Values 4–7	18.6	18.3	36.1	14.6	10.5	31.4	15.3	18.6	8.1	20.0	19.5	22.5	20.9	23.5	20.0	22.0	16.6	17.3	18.7	15.1
Values 8–10	25.8	28.8	19.8	24.7		15.7	22.7	22.2	18.2	17.1	23.2	23.7	23.7	23.1	33.4	34.6	29.1	26.7	17.4	18.0
Values 11–12	40.6	36.8	38.1	41.0	80.5	45.4	54.8	49.1	66.9	57.5	45.3	40.9	44.3	44.9	39.9	35.7	51.5	49.4	7.6	6.8
Nobs	2,177	1,684	49	38	43	65	2,366	1,695	112	86	821	524	156	115	2,368	2,188	127	91	166	120

Age group 45–74; birth cohorts 1930–1962. In %; weighted data. W: Women, M: Men.

Table A.5. Frequency of attending religious services and attitudes towards religious ceremonies at turning points of life (*rites de passage*) by country, gender, and birth cohort

	FRANCE		HUNGARY		NORWAY		GERMANY					
							East		West		Tr. migs	
Birth cohort	Women	Men	Women	Men	Women	Men	Women	Men	Women	Men	Women	Men
Frequency of attending religious services (in %)												
1949–1962												
Intense attendance	11.3	5.5	87.5	83.6	7.1	4.1	6.2	7.7	22.4	17.1	43.0	59.7
Rare attendance (* affiliated)	82.0	86.6			85.1	85.4	17.4	16.6	66.1	65.5	57.0	40.3
Unaffiliated	6.8	7.9	12.5	16.4	7.8	10.4	76.4	75.7	11.5	17.5		
1939–1952												
Intense attendance	16.3	10.0	91.4	88.1	8.3	6.5	11.2	6.7	30.6	18.0	52.1	66.0
Rare attendance (* affiliated)	79.5	84.5			86.8	87.9	21.0	27.7	60.2	63.8	47.9	34.0
Unaffiliated	4.1	5.5	8.6	11.9	4.9	5.6	67.8	65.7	9.3	18.2		
1930–1942												
Intense attendance	25.7	13.9	95.2	92.7	10.8	10.1	13.6	6.0	43.7	31.8	62.5	72.0
Rare attendance (* affiliated)	71.8	80.8			85.7	85.7	30.7	22.1	51.9	58.4	37.5	28.0
Unaffiliated	2.5	5.3	4.9	7.3	3.5	4.2	55.7	71.9	4.4	9.9		
Attitudes towards religious ceremonies at turning points of life (*rites de passage*) (mean)												
1949–1962	7.2	7.1	8.0	7.7	7.8	7.5	3.5	3.8	7.7	7.3	9.5	9.2
1939–1952	8.3	7.9	8.9	8.4	9.0	8.5	4.1	4.8	8.2	7.8	9.4	9.6
1930–1942	9.4	8.6	10.1	9.3	9.5	9.4	5.2	4.7	9.3	8.8	10.4	10.3

Weighted data. Tr. migs: Turkish migrants. For numbers of observation, see tables 6.6 and 6.7.

Table A.6. Completed fertility by country, gender, and cohort*religiosity

	FRANCE		HUNGARY		NORWAY		GERMANY					
							East		West		Tr. migs	
Birth cohort	Women	Men	Women	Men	Women	Men	Women	Men	Women	Men	Women	Men
1949–1962												
Intense attendance	2.61	3.04	1.93	1.72	2.53	2.47			1.76	1.80	2.45	2.11
Rare attendance (* affiliated)	2.05	1.88			2.08	1.91	1.61	(1.85)	1.63	1.44	2.40	2.38
Unaffiliated	1.97	1.89	1.74	1.79	1.72	1.73	1.78	1.73	1.38	0.95		
1939–1952												
Intense attendance	2.24	2.70	1.86	1.81	2.53	2.79	1.62	2.14	1.63	1.57	2.17	2.29
Rare attendance (* affiliated)	2.12	2.16			2.08	2.09	1.57	1.64	1.60	1.44	2.17	2.01
Unaffiliated	1.93	1.70	1.68	2.0	1.88	1.88	1.89	1.34	1.52	1.49		
1930–1942												
Intense attendance	2.75	2.73	1.77	1.78	2.65	3.14			1.85	1.91	2.51	2.06
Rare attendance (* affiliated)	2.55	2.31			2.41	2.27	2.16	1.90	1.87	1.64		(1.14)
Unaffiliated	(2.37)	2.12	1.43	1.67	(1.88)	2.02	1.97	1.87	1.39	1.54		

Weighted data. Tr. migs: Turkish migrants. For numbers of observation, see table 6.6. Empty cells indicate low numbers of observation (<19). Observations between N=19 and N=29 are in brackets.

Table A.7. Parity distribution by country, gender, and religiosity

	FRANCE		HUNGARY		NORWAY		GERMANY					
							East		West		Tr. migs	
	W	M	W	M	W	M	W	M	W	M	W	M
Intense attendance												
0	11.3	12.6			12.2	6.7	18.6	0.8	21.2	20.9	18.9	21.7
1	14.7	7.2			7.4	8.1	17.8	25.7	21.0	19.4	13.9	17.1
2	24.6	26.3			26.8	26.6	54.6	46.9	30.4	35.2	22.4	23.2
3	26.9	24.0			34.0	30.2	5.1	13.8	19.7	14.9	22.2	20.6
4	12.5	14.7			15.0	18.7	1.5	10.2	5.1	5.7	11.5	7.2
5+	9.9	15.2			4.6	9.8	2.4	2.5	2.6	3.9	11.1	10.2
Nobs	417	194			317	220	50	29	550	389	216	325
Rare attendance (* affiliated)												
0	9.8	12.4	9.0	13.1	10.5	13.7	15.4	12.1	17.0	23.9	12.8	19.9
1	19.9	19.2	25.7	22.9	13.2	11.3	27.4	22.9	27.9	28.1	17.9	19.8
2	37.2	36.3	46.0	46.0	40.2	39.8	34.6	47.2	36.4	30.6	26.9	25.7
3	20.0	19.1	13.7	13.3	26.8	25.3	14	14.2	11.7	11.9	27.0	24.1
4	6.6	8.2	3.2	3.1	7.2	7.1	2.3	0.3	3.9	3.3	9.4	3.4
5+	6.3	4.8	2.3	1.6	2.1	2.8	6.3	3.3	3.0	2.1	6.0	7.1
Nobs	2,077	1,776	3,505	2,465	2,995	2,987	126	96	1,119	1,093	247	176
Unaffiliated												
0	13.5	17.2	13.6	8.8	15.0	20.3	13.1	14.9	19.9	30.4		
1	22.2	25.8	27.2	23.2	25.2	16.0	26.6	31.3	33.9	28.0		
2	32.5	24.6	44.2	49.0	33.3	37.3	38.5	36.8	33.9	28.7		
3	20.6	21.4	10.5	14.8	20.3	17.5	11.5	11.6	9.4	10.4		
4	7.5	8.8	3.2	2.8	5.7	7.6	5.9	3.9	1.4	2.4		
5+	3.7	2.1	1.4	1.5	0.4	1.3	4.4	1.5	1.6	0.2		
Nobs	130	141	332	356	230	277	376	319	187	308		

Weighted data. W: Women, M: Men, Tr. mig: Turkish migrants. The values of Hungarians in the middle of the table refer to all affiliated (including frequent attenders) because those people cannot be kept apart.

Table A.8. Distribution of covariates: cohorts, migration background and ethnic group, number of siblings, and educational attainment by country and gender

	FRANCE		HUNGARY		NORWAY		GERMANY					
							East		West		Tr. migs	
	Women	Men	Women	Men	Women	Men	Women	Men	Women	Men	Women	Men
45–54 (birth cohorts 1949–1962)	41.5	36.1	38.9	43.5	40.9	41.3	37.4	40.2	37.1	39.1	36.7	29.1
55–64 (birth cohorts 1939–1952)	32.6	39.9	33.3	33.8	35.4	36.2	31.9	32.6	33.0	33.5	45.9	42.2
65–74 (birth cohorts 1930–1942)	25.9	23.9	27.8	22.7	23.6	22.6	30.8	27.2	29.9	27.4	17.4	28.6
Autochthonal population	80.7	75.3	96.9	96.0	94.6	94.1	92.9	90.0	86.0	84.1	0.0	0.0
Immigrant population	19.3	24.7	3.1	4.0	5.4	5.9	7.1	10.0	14.0	15.9	100.0	100.0
European (EU and non EU)	11.4	13.7					3.8	6.6	7.3	7.4		
Maghrebi/ African other	4.0	6.4										
Pieds Noirs	3.2	3.2										
Russian									3.3	4.6		
Gypsy/ Hungarian of Gypsy origin			1.7	2.0								
East European/ German/ Hungarian of German origin			1.4	2.0								
Other	0.8	1.5					3.2	3.4	3.5	3.9		
No siblings	8.0		10.2		11.2		20.0		19.3		8.0	
1 brother or sister	18.2		28.2		22.3		31.3		26.0		6.6	
2 siblings	21.2		21.3		25.3		23.7		23.0		11.4	
3 siblings	16.7		13.9		17.6		11.3		13.6		15.8	
4 siblings	10.6		8.6		10.2		6.1		7.7		15.3	
5 and more siblings	25.3		17.9		13.4		7.6		10.4		43.0	
Mean number of siblings	3.4		2.7		2.5		1.8		2.1		4.2	
Low educational attainment (isced 0–2, other)	48.8	40.2	42.5	24.6	31.2	25.0	10.2	4.2	26.0	9.5	85.1	72.2
Medium educational attainment (isced 3–4)	33.0	40.3	45.6	60.4	44.6	51.5	66.6	63.7	59.3	60.2	13.2	23.8
High educational attainment (isced 5–6)	18.2	19.6	11.9	15.0	24.3	23.5	23.2	32.1	14.7	30.3	1.7	4.0
Nobs	2,640	2,122	3,837	2,821	3,542	3,484	552	444	1,856	1,790	463	501
Nobs (siblings: women and men aggregated)	4,762		6,640		7,026		996		3,646		964	

Age group 45–74, birth cohorts 1930–1962. In %; weighted data. Tr. migs: Turkish migrants. Migration background and ethnic group: categories are country-specific. Notations according to original. Original distribution of ISCED in table A.11.

Table A.9. Distribution of covariates: living region

	FRANCE		NORWAY		HUNGARY		GERMANY					
							East		West		Tr. migs	
	Women	Men	Women	Men	Women	Men	Women	Men	Women	Men	Women	Men
FRA: rural	26.0	27.4										
FRA: urban	57.4	57.5										
FRA: town	16.6	15.1										
NOR: centrality level 0: completely rural			11.9	14.9								
NOR: centrality level 1			5.9	5.3								
NOR: centrality level 2			16.1	16.8								
NOR: centrality level 3: urban/ capital			66.1	63.1								
HUN: capital					16.5	13.7						
HUN: city					20.7	19.8						
HUN: town					30.2	30.6						
HUN: village					32.7	35.9						
GER: > 500,000 inhabitants							13.4	14.1	24.7	23.5	52.9	44.9
GER: peripheral area from 100,000/ central area from 100–500,000 inhabitants							33.1	32.8	43.3	44.6	31.3	38.7
GER: peripheral area from 50–100,000/ central area from 20–100,000 inhabitants							32.9	33.4	19.8	20.2	15.9	16.4
GER: up to 19,999 inhabitants							20.6	19.7	12.2	11.7	–	–
Numbers of observations	2,640	2,122	3,541	3,484	552	444	1,856	1,790	463	501		

Age group 45–74, birth cohorts 1930–1962. In %; weighted data. Tr. migs: Turkish migrants. Migration background and ethnic group: categories are country-specific.

Table A.10. Marital status by country and gender

	FRANCE		HUNGARY		NORWAY		GERMANY					
							East		West		Tr. mig	
	Women	Men	Women	Men	Women	Men	Women	Men	Women	Men	Women	Men
Never married	**12.1**	**12.0**	**4.7**	**7.8**	**8.8**	**12.5**	**16.8**	**12.5**	**17.1**	**13.4**	**16.5**	**7.5**
Single (never had partnership)	6.0	4.8	3.1	4.9	3.0	4.2	12.3	8.0	12.5	8.0	12.9	6.0
Married (1st time)	**58.3**	**67.3**	**48.6**	**65.0**	**52.5**	**61.0**	**57.2**	**67.4**	**58.3**	**68.6**	**65.4**	**84.1**
Widowed (never divorced)	**10.7**	**2.8**	**21.8**	**4.2**	**9.1**	**2.8**	**8.7**	**3.8**	**7.3**	**2.1**	**7.0**	**0.2**
Separated (never divorced)	**1.0**	**0.7**	**1.3**	**1.1**	**0.5**	**0.3**	**0.8**	**0.5**	**1.1**	**1.2**	**0.8**	**0.9**
Divorced	**11.7**	**9.0**	**17.0**	**12.4**	**20.9**	**9.7**	**10.3**	**10.1**	**8.7**	**7.0**	**8.1**	**3.3**
once	10.9	8.5	14.4	10.6	15.3	9.5	9.7	8.4	7.1	6.0	7.9	2.6
more than once	0.9	0.5	2.6	1.8	5.6	0.2	0.6	1.6	1.5	1.1	0.2	0.7
Remarried	**6.2**	**8.2**	**6.7**	**9.6**	**7.9**	**10.1**	**5.0**	**5.2**	**4.6**	**5.6**	**1.5**	**2.9**
(at least one) previous marriage divorced	5.3	7.4	5.6	8.2	7.2	9.0	4.7	4.7	4.1	4.9	1.1	2.0
Inconsistent data/ incomplete information	**0.0**	**0.0**	**0.0**	**0.0**	**0.2**	**0.2**	**1.3**	**0.6**	**3.0**	**2.1**	**0.7**	**1.2**
Nobs	2,640	2,122	3,837	2,821	3,534	3,478	545	443	1,807	1,753	460	494
Married (1st time)	**66.4**	**76.5**	**51.0**	**70.5**	**57.6**	**69.6**	**68.7**	**77.1**	**70.3**	**79.2**	**78.3**	**90.9**
Widowed (never divorced)	**12.2**	**3.2**	**22.9**	**4.5**	**10.0**	**3.2**	**10.4**	**4.3**	**8.8**	**2.4**	**8.4**	**0.3**
Separated (never divorced)	**1.1**	**0.7**	**1.4**	**1.2**	**0.6**	**0.4**	**1.0**	**0.5**	**1.2**	**1.3**	**0.9**	**0.9**
Divorced	**13.4**	**10.3**	**17.8**	**13.4**	**22.9**	**15.1**	**12.4**	**11.4**	**10.4**	**8.2**	**9.7**	**3.6**
once	12.4	9.7	15.1	11.5	16.8	10.9	11.7	9.6	8.6	6.9	9.5	2.8
more than once	1.0	0.6	2.7	1.9	6.1	4.2	0.7	1.8	1.8	1.3	0.2	0.8
Remarried	**7.0**	**9.3**	**7.0**	**10.4**	**8.7**	**11.5**	**6.0**	**6.0**	**5.6**	**6.5**	**1.8**	**3.1**
(at least one) previous marriage divorced	6.1	8.4	5.9	8.9	7.9	10.4	5.7	5.4	5.1	5.8	1.3	2.2
Inconsistent data/ incomplete information	**0.0**	**0.0**	**0.0**	**0.0**	**0.2**	**0.2**	**1.5**	**0.7**	**3.7**	**2.5**	**0.9**	**1.3**
Nobs (without respondents who never married)	2,228	1,804	3,697	2,655	3,224	3,064	447	386	1,500	1,525	393	461

Age group 45–74; birth cohorts 1930–1962. In %; weighted data. W: Women, M: Men, Tr. migs: Turkish migrants. Sum of boldly marked proportions amounts to 100%. In regression analysis "remarried" and "divorced more than once" build one joint category.

Table A.11. Educational attainment structured by country and gender (ISCED 1997) – original distribution of values

	FRANCE		HUNGARY		NORWAY		GERMANY East		GERMANY West		GERMANY Tr. migs	
	Women	Men	Women	Men	Women	Men	Women	Men	Women	Men	Women	Men
0: preprimary education	1.2	2.2	0.6	0.3	0.1	0.2						
1: primary level			8.5	5.1	0.3	0.1	0.7	0.2	0.9	0.4	46.9	29.7
1 – 2	47.5	38.0										
2: lower secondary level			33.3	19.2	30.8	24.8	9.2	3.8	23.4	7.5	30.9	32.5
3A	8.7	5.7										
3B	0.4	0.6										
3C	24.0	33.9										
3: upper secondary level			17.8	39.8	42.2	47.0	66.0	62.9	57.3	58.3	12.7	23.3
4: post secondary non-tertiary education			27.8	20.7	2.4	4.5	0.6	0.8	2.1	1.9	0.6	0.4
5A – 6	11.2	14.8										
5: first stage of tertiary education			11.9	15.0	23.9	22.8	22.2	29.8	13.6	27.9	1.7	4.0
5B	7.0	4.7										
6: second stage of tertiary education					0.4	0.7	1.0	2.4	1.1	2.5		
Other education							0.3	0.2	1.7	1.6	7.3	10.1
Nobs	2,640	2,122	3,837	2,821	3,530	3,467	552	444	1,856	1,790	461	498

Age group 45–74; birth cohorts 1930–1962. In %; weighted data. Tr. migs: Turkish migrants. Categories according to country-specific list.

MIX
Papier aus verantwortungsvollen Quellen
Paper from responsible sources
FSC® C105338

If you have any concerns about our products, you can contact us on
ProductSafety@springernature.com

In case Publisher is established outside the EU, the EU authorized representative is:
Springer Nature Customer Service Center GmbH
Europaplatz 3, 69115 Heidelberg, Germany

Printed by Libri Plureos GmbH
in Hamburg, Germany